ALPHA-FETOPROTEIN AND HEPATOMA

Japanese Cancer Association
GANN Monographs on Cancer Research

GANN Monographs on Cancer Research are intended for the publication of the proceedings of international conferences and symposia dealing with cancer or closely related research fields, and series of papers on specific subjects of importance to cancer research. Publication of each individual monograph is to be decided by the Editorial Board of the Japanese Cancer Association with the final approval of the Board of Directors of the said Association. It is hoped that series of GANN Monographs on Cancer Research will serve as an important source of international information in cancer research.

Tomizo Yoshida, M.D.

JAPANESE CANCER ASSOCIATION

GANN Monograph on Cancer Research No. 14

ALPHA-FETOPROTEIN AND HEPATOMA

Edited by HIDEMATSU HIRAI
TORU MIYAJI

UNIVERSITY PARK PRESS
Baltimore · London · Tokyo

UNIVERSITY PARK PRESS
Baltimore · London · Tokyo

Library of Congress Cataloging in Publication Data

Japanese Cancer Association Symposium on Alpha-Fetoprotein and Hepatoma, 11th, Tokyo, 1971.
Alpha-fetoprotein and hepatoma.

(GANN monograph on cancer research no. 14)
1. Cancer—Diagnosis—Congresses. 2. Alpha fetoproteins—Congresses. I. Hirai, Hidematsu, ed. II. Miyaji, Toru, 1912– ed. III. Nippon Gan Gakkai. IV. Title. V. Series: Gann monograph on cancer research no. 14. [DNLM: 1. Antigens, Neoplasm—Congresses. 2. Fetal globulins—Congresses. 3. Hepatoma—Diagnosis—Congresses. 4. Liver neoplasms—Diagnosis—Congresses. W3 Ca163 v. 14 1973/

Library of Congress Cataloging in Publication Data

WI735 J35a 1971]
RC270. J36 1971 616.9'94'36 73-7966
ISBN 0-8391-0712-9

UTP 3047-67882-5149
Printed in Japan.

Originally published by
UNIVERSITY OF TOKYO PRESS

PREFACE

Of the methods developed for the diagnosis of cancer using body fluids, the diagnosis of primary liver cancer based on the detection of α-fetoprotein (AFP) by precipitin reaction in gel has been considered the most reliable one. When this protein is detected in the blood, diagnosis of primary liver cancer can, with rare exceptions, be made with reasonable certainty.

In Japan it has been only three years since the study of this protein began, nevertheless the procedure mentioned has been widely employed, and more than several hundred cases of primary liver cancer have already been examined.

The fact that liver cells undergoing cancerous change can resynthesize protein of the embroyonic stage provides an important lead in understanding the true nature of cancer. Considerable advances have been made in experimental studies conducted along this line.

In light of this background it was opportune that the Japanese Cancer Association held a symposium on "Alpha-Fetoprotein and Hepatoma" focussing on the following points:

1. Evaluation of the procedure using AFP for the diagnosis of primary liver cancer;
2. Pathohistological differences between AFP-producing hepatoma and AFP-non-producing hepatoma;
3. Appearance of AFP in diseases other than primary liver cancer;
4. Determination and significance of low levels of AFP under limit of sensitivity of precipitin reaction in gel;
5. Analyses of the mechanism of AFP appearance in animal experiments.

The results of this symposium are given in this monograph. We look forward to a further delineation of the relation of hepatitis to liver cancer through microdetermination of AFP by radio-immunoassay and more sensitive detection of Australia antigen together with the support of pathological findings. Determination of the association among hepatitis, liver cirrhosis, and liver cancer must wait for future studies; in Japan, with a high incidence of these three diseases, it is a matter requiring early resolution.

At this symposium the diagnostic value of AFP based on the studies made to date was established and the direction in which future studies will be pursued was determined.

This volume is a compilation of the presentations made at the 11th Japanese Cancer Association Symposium on "Alpha-Fetoprotein and Hepatoma" held in Tokyo in December 1971 and arranged by us. We wish to express our appreciation to Drs. L. R. Purves, R. F. Masseyeff, J. Uriel, and D. Buffe for contributing, at our invitation, papers on their valuable studies.

June 1972

Hidematsu Hirai
Toru Miyaji

CONTENTS

PATHOLOGY OF HUMAN HEPATOMAS AND AFP

EXPERIMENTS IN HEPATOMA AND AFP

GENERAL

GANN Monograph on Cancer Research 14, 1973

FACTORS INFLUENCING α-FETOPROTEIN BIOSYNTHESIS IN PATIENTS WITH PRIMARY LIVER CANCER AND OTHER DISEASES

René F. MASSEYEFF

*École de Médecine et Centre de Lutte contre le Cancer**

Factors influencing α-fetoprotein (AFP) production in primary liver cancer patients are reviewed. Considering the frequency of positive blood samples amongst patients and the level of this protein whenever present, age, sex, and size of the tumor definitely influence positivity rates, while geographic or ethnic influences remain to be proven in the author's view. Investigation by fluorescent antibody technique has shown that only a small proportion of cancer cells do produce AFP. α-Fetoprotein levels tend to increase with time in those patients, sometimes with temporary peaks.

Preliminary findings on low rate production of AFP in normal and pathological people as estimated by radioimmunoassay are indicated. Finally hypotheses on the mechanisms of AFP production by cancerous liver cells are reviewed.

Since the demonstration by Abelev (*1*) that experimental liver tumors of mice produce an α-globulin identical with a protein present in fetal blood, and the demonstration by Tatarinov (*62*) that a similar situation occurs in human primary liver tumors, the detection of α-fetoprotein (AFP) has become a valuable aid in the diagnosis of human primary liver cancer (PLC).

A number of studies (*2, 12, 40, 45, 65*), have shown that a positive test with the conventional Ouchterlony method for the demonstration of AFP is found only in PLC and in a rarer cancer, teratoblastoma of the gonads (TRB) (*5*). Our personal experience in Africa coincides completely with this common conclusion. Only 3 false positive cases were found, out of more than 70,000 tests covering a wide range of normal and pathological individuals. Indeed, these 3 false positives were not documented sufficiently to completely rule out the occurrence of a small, hidden primary liver tumor.

Thus, to a first approximation, this Ouchterlony test for AFP appears to be highly satisfactory from a diagnostic point of view. Few biological tests, indeed, show such a high specificity. However, this specificity is not absolute and a number of facts show that the process of AFP biosynthesis is quite complex.

Some specific points deserve special comments and studies.

1) A percentage of patients with PLC (ranging from 20 to 60%) do not have

* Chemin de Vallombrose-06100, Nice, France .

a detectable level of AFP. Moreover, in the same patient some cells produce AFP and some others do not.
2) The level of AFP is not constant during the evolution of the disease. The dynamics of AFP production raise some interesting questions.
3) An increasing number of "false positive cases" have occurred, *i.e.*, cases where neither PLC nor TRB can be demonstrated in patients with a positive serum AFP test.

α-Fetoprotein Levels in Patients with PLC

We have investigated 304 patients suffering from PLC in Senegal, Africa (*37*, *40*). The diagnosis was made in 177 cases only by clinical examination.

TABLE I. Frequency of Occurrence of Serum AFP in Patients with PLC

	First author	No. of cases	% Pos.	Ref.
Africa				
Congo Kinshasa	O'Conor[a]	22	77	(*45*)
Ghana	Foli[a]	35	72	(*20*)
Kenya	O'Conor[a]	14	71	(*45*)
Mozambique	Portugal	37	68	(*48*)
Nigeria	O'Conor[a]	14	71	(*45*)
Senegal	Masseyeff	304	72	(*40*)
South Africa	Purves[a]	130	78	(*50*)
Uganda	Alpert	40	50	(*10*)
	Alpert[b]	28	86	(*8*)
America				
U.S.A.	Hull Caucasian	32	31	(*27–29*)
	Negro	7	71	(*27–29*)
	Alpert[b] Caucasian	41	51	(*8*)
	Non-Caucasian	21	76	(*8*)
Asia				
Hong Kong	Smith	60	65	(*57–60*)
Indonesia	Kresno[a]	100	87	(*31, 32*)
Japan	Endo[a]	24	67	(*18*)
Malaya	O'Conor[a]	29	72	(*45*)
Taiwan	Alpert[b]	15	93	(*8*)
	Lin	26	65	(*34*)
Europe				
France	Economopoulos	30	60	(*17*)
	Hirsch-marie	84	59	(*26*)
	Sauger	27	59	(*55, 56*)
	Uriel	22	55	(*65*)
Great Britain	Foli[a]	35	40	(*20*)
Greece	Economopoulos	35	51	(*17*)
Spain	Teres[a]	17	42	(*63*)
U.S.S.R.	Abelev[a]	28	60	(*4*)

[a] All cases confirmed histologically.
[b] Results obtained by immunoelectrodiffusion.

In 127 cases it was confirmed by microscopic examination of the liver. Using a conventional micro-Ouchterlony method, AFP was present in 72% of these patients, the percentage being nearly identical in both groups. Table I compares this figure with some data collected from the literature. The homogeneity of the results obtained in Africa and Asia is striking.

The prevalence rates calculated from the results obtained in Europe or America are smaller: This point will be discussed later. It was found that 28% of the sera remained negative in our series. Does this mean that they contain AFP, but at a concentration beyond the sensitivity threshold of our method, or are they actually devoid of AFP? The answer to this question can be obtained by using more sensitive methods. Abelev *et al.* (*3*, *6*) have tested 48 negative sera from our collection using a radioimmunodiffusion method which is said to be 16 to 32 times more sensitive than the conventional Ouchterlony method. The presence of AFP was demonstrated in about half of these sera. Thus, with this extremely sensitive method, about 15% of the cases remained negative. From more recent studies using radioimmunoassay methods (*38*) it may be concluded that even in these negative cases AFP can be found in the serum, but at trace levels not differing significantly from those found in other hepatic diseases. Thus it appears to be established that some PLC's are not secreting AFP.

The extent of AFP production varies in a wide range in PLC patients. AFP concentration was assayed in the sera of 156 patients using a radial immunodiffusion method (*36*). Figure 1 shows the distribution of these levels. Average AFP concentration reaches 0.4 mg/ml (or 0.6 mg/ml if the negative patients are excluded). From the shape of this distribution curve, one may guess that most of the negative cases are, in fact, cases beyond the sensitivity threshold of the

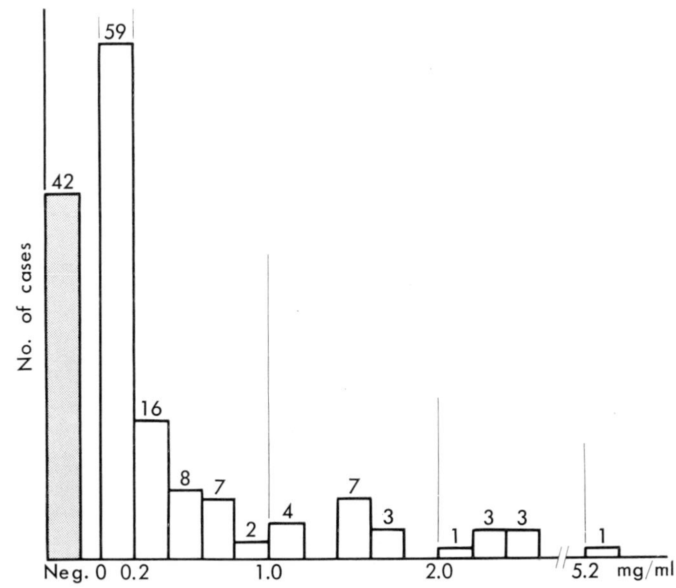

FIG. 1. Distribution of AFP levels in 156 patients with PLC

assay technique. We hoped that analysis of the clinical or biological features of these patients would show some correlation when related to these scattered AFP levels. This analysis was disappointing, since not one characteristic could be related to the AFP level (*40*). However, different conclusions were reached by two other groups. Purves *et al.* (*50*) found that AFP level seems to be related at borderline significance to the levels of cholesterol, hemoglobin, and serum protein, which increase with AFP, while mucoprotein and α_2-globulin decrease. The same group also obtained some evidence that nodular tumors achieved the highest degree of production when compared to massive and diffuse tumors. The microscopic features also seem to influence AFP production, the average serum level being 0.16 mg/ml in the anaplastic forms, 0.32 mg/ml in the poorly differentiated, and 0.25 mg/ml in the well-differentiated tumors. Alpert *et al.* (*8*) also found that the AFP level is influenced by the size of the tumor, being higher in large tumors.

None of these conclusions can be derived from our survey. However, very significant trends can be observed if one considers not the level of AFP but the positivity rate (Ouchterlony method) in different patients.

The influence of age is clearly shown in Fig. 2. Very young patients are most often positive. AFP prevalence is slightly less in adults and decreases distinctly over 40 (*40*). Other groups (*8*, *41*) have confirmed this finding.

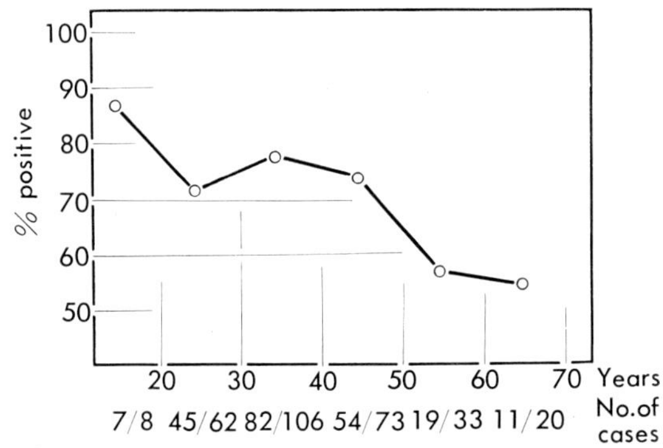

FIG. 2. Frequency of serum AFP-positivity in relation to age in patients suffering from PLC

The influence of sex is clearly apparent from Table II, showing that the positivity rate is 20% higher in males than in females. This fact has been noted by O'Conor *et al.* (*45*) and Alpert *et al.* (*8*). The reason for this sex disparity

TABLE II. Incidence of AFP in the Serum of Patients with PLC in Relation to Sex

	Males	Females	Total
AFP-positive	182 (75.9%)	38 (56.3%)	220 (72.4%)
AFP-negative	58 (24.1%)	26 (43.7%)	84 (27.6%)
Total	240	64	304

From Masseyeff *et al.* (*40*).

is unknown. There is no evidence of a direct role of male hormone. The recent discovery of Nunez *et al.* (*44*) that AFP possesses strong binding activity for oestrone and oestradiol, but not for other steroid hormones, should be mentioned at this point, since it is possibly related to this fact.

Turning now to pathological features, one striking fact is apparent from our series: Patients with large tumors are more often positive than those with smaller ones (Table III). All tumors heavier than 5 kg induced serum positivity. However, as already stated, there was no correlation between tumor weight and AFP level.

TABLE III. Incidence of AFP in the Serum of Patients with PLC in Relation to the Weight of the Tumoral Liver

	Tumoral liver weight					
	Less than 2 (kg)	2–3 (kg)	3–4 (kg)	4–5 (kg)	More than 5 (kg)	Total
AFP-positive	3	12	11	8	8	42
AFP-negative	3	6	3	1	0	13
Percent positive	50	67	79	89	100	76

From Masseyeff *et al.* (*40*) (postmortem examination).

Results collected in Table I indicate that AFP prevalence in PLC varies significantly in different countries. While the average frequency is 63%, in Europe it is only 53%, and in the group Africa/Asia, it is 71%. This difference is quite large and suggests an environmental or ethnic influence on the prevalence of AFP. This interpretation has been favoured by Foli *et al.* (*20*). While technical factors may explain some of the observed differences, this is not obviously the case for several studies where samples of different geographic or ethnic origin were examined in the same laboratory (*12, 27, 45, 65*). However, evidence for a geographic or ethnic influence on AFP synthesis by tumoral liver is, in our view, still inconclusive. Some factors, examined above, such as age, sex, or tumor weight, may be responsible for these geographic or ethnic differences. In France, for example, the average age of patients with PLC is 63 (*23*) while in Senegal it is 38 (*46*). In many statistics coming from nontropical areas, sex incidence is quite different from African or Asian series, the predominance of males being reduced (the ratio is between 1/1 to 4/1 in Europe or America while 5/1 to 10/1 is commonly observed in statistics from Africa or Asia). The time of blood examination is also of importance since a late sample is more likely to be positive than an early one: Patients in the tropics very often attend at a very late stage of the disease. It is still possible that genetic factors play only an indirect role in AFP production, *e.g.*, by influencing the evolution of the disease. Tumoral growth seems faster in Africans. Alpert *et al.* (*9*) reported that tumors weighed during postmortem examination were 500 to 1,000 g heavier in Africans than in U.S. patients or Caucasian patients from South Africa. Thus, the influence of genetic or ethnic factors on AFP production is a hypothesis that, in our view, needs more documentation before being accepted.

The experimental results of Stanislawski *et al.* (*61*) suggested that etiological factors may influence AFP production. This worker showed that, in the rat, hepatomas induced by 3-methyl-4-dimethylazobenzene often produced AFP while those induced by aflatoxin-B_1 did not.

Such experiments are not transposable to human PLC, where the etiological agent is still unknown. However, the recent finding of high prevalence of the hepatitis-associated antigen (HAA) in the sera of patients with PLC has given a new strength to the hypothesis of an oncongenic role for the hepatitis virus. Vogel *et al.* (*66*), in a series of 45 cases, found a definite correlation between the presence of HAA and AFP, while Masseyeff *et al.* (*39*), in a larger series of 209 cases, were unable to confirm this finding.

Factors involved in the biosynthesis of AFP can be investigated at the cellular level. There is a large body of evidence that AFP is produced by the tumor itself. The disappearance of AFP after tumor removal (*11*, *40*), the demonstration by immunofluorescence of AFP in cancerous liver cells (*25*, *49*), and *in vitro* production of AFP by tumor cells in culture (*2*, *53*) are convincing proofs.

Studies by immunofluorescence were undertaken in cooperation with Abelev's group. One aim of these experiments was to verify whether all tumor cells were producing AFP or only some of them. One drawback of this immunofluorescence technique is that it does not indicate whether or not a protein found in a cell has actually been produced by the cell or whether it has passively entered the cell. This is likely to occur if tissue fixation has been delayed, especially when cells have fragile membranes, like hepatocytes. Our studies were made using the controls suggested by Engelhardt *et al.* (*19*). Since hepatocytes do not synthesize IgG, they must not be positive in immunofluorescence using an anti-IgG serum. Staining then means that their membrane has been damaged. A positive staining with anti-AFP serum is thus not significant. This technique has been applied to consecutive cuts, one being stained with anti-IgG, the next with anti-AFP. Thus, the only cells accepted as specifically positive are those which are AFP-positive and IgG-negative.

The results were quite unexpected (*60*). Only a small proportion (5%) of cancer cells were found to synthesize AFP. Of course, the method of analysis tends to underestimate the number of cells actually producing AFP, but even if IgG-positive cells are counted, the proportion of AFP-positive cells does not exceed 10–15%.

The cell arrangement is characteristic: They form sorts of sleeves around capillaries of tumor sinuses. The intensity of fluorescence is very heterogeneous, but usually the brighter cells are located close to the capillary.

A different pattern was obtained in 2 metastases in the lungs. The majority of cells were AFP-positive and the intensity of fluorescence was less heterogeneous. However, the cells located near vessels were still more fluorescent. No morphological difference was observed between AFP-positive and AFP-negative cells.

Thus the main conclusion reached as a result of this work is that only a small proportion of tumor cells produced AFP and that the only difference between positive and negative cells lies in their environmental conditions, the former being located around vessels.

Dynamics of AFP Production

We were interested in the dynamics of AFP production for theoretical and practical reasons. One of the practical questions is, does AFP detection allow an early diagnosis of PLC, early enough to offer a possibility of surgical cure?

The observation of currently attending patients is unlikely to solve this question, since PLC is an insidious disease and tumors are frequently quite large when patients report the first symptoms. Thus, it was decided to follow up a sample of susceptible population with the AFP Ouchterlony test. This was done in Senegal on approximately 9,000 male workers, 3 times a year for 2 years (*64*). Nine cases of PLC were identified during this period, 6 of which were AFP-positive. Of these cases, 3 were found in apparently healthy people: In fact, liver tumors could be found. It was only in 1 case that the tumor was small and limited enough to permit surgical removal. However, 1 month after partial hepatectomy, the patient died from extensive metastases. The rather pessimistic conclusion of these experiments is that the gel immunodiffusion test is usually positive, too late to give a chance for curative treatment. However, a more sensitive test may permit a different conclusion.

Some patients with a clinically demonstrable tumor, AFP-negative on hospital admission, became positive after 1 to 2 months. This observation, made in 3 patients out of 14 in our series, is interesting since it raises the question of the cellular origin of this protein. It may be produced either by the existing tumoral cells becoming less differentiated, or by new cancerous cells, these latter cells being either daughter cells of the existing cancerous cells or new cancerous cells arising from noncancerous surrounding hepatocytes. The last hypothesis is not unlikely, since the observation of liver cancer patients in Senegal often gives the impression of a cancerous disease beginning at nearly the same time in different parts of the liver. Thus, the idea of the emergence of new cancerous clones, starting from less differentiated cells, seems acceptable. However, it is still impossible to prove it.

The wide dispersion of AFP levels observed in different patients is an indication of the absence of a mechanism resulting in regulation of AFP biosynthesis.

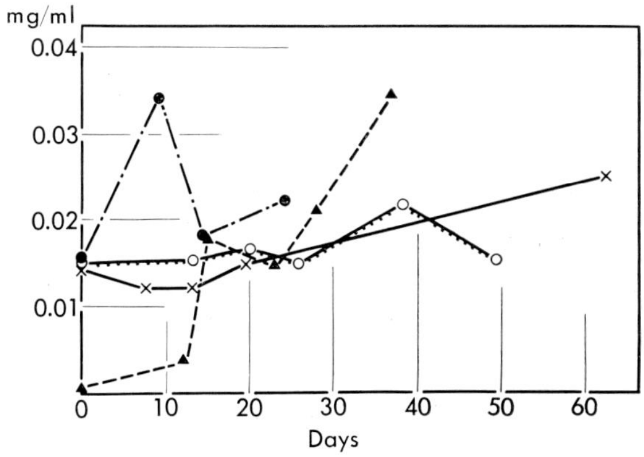

FIG. 3. Evolution of serum AFP levels in 4 patients with PLC

A study of the evolution of AFP level in some patients confirms this hypothesis, but with some restrictions.

In our series, AFP level has been assayed in 10 patients over a period of several months (Figs. 3–5) (*37*). The levels tend to increase. This was also the conclusion of Purves *et al.* (*52*), who give quantitative data. The average increase of AFP level is +27% per month. We agree with the conclusion of these workers that AFP level does not rise at the same speed that the tumor grows. This fact may be taken as being in favour of the existence of a homeostasis mechanism, though imperfect.

However, the opposite conclusion may be derived from Fig. 5, which shows the existence of important and transient peaks in some patients. The causes of

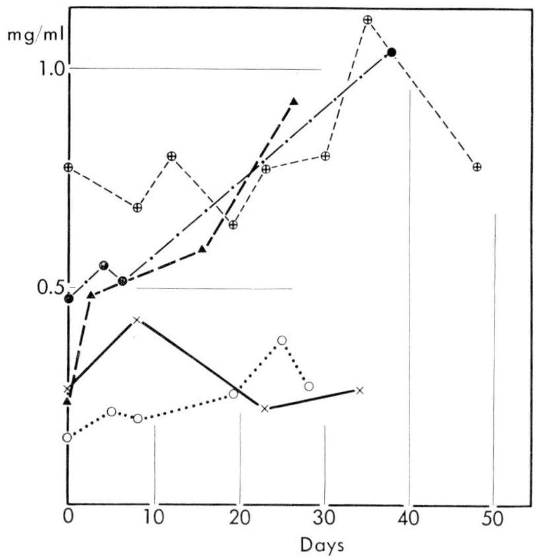

FIG. 4. Evolution of serum AFP levels in 5 patients with PLC

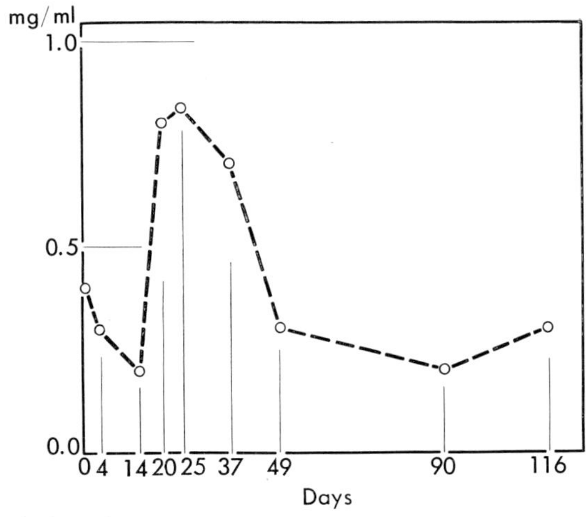

FIG. 5. Evolution of AFP level in a patient with PLC, showing a temporary increase of this protein

this temporary increase of AFP are unknown: Sudden necrosis of AFP-producing cells whose intracellular content is released into the blood stream, or predominant growth of AFP-producing clones followed by necrosis and fibrosis of the corresponding area.

In conclusion, the existence of a mechanism of regulation of AFP level in PLC patients seems unlikely on grounds of (1) the very large dispersion of individual levels. One might admit that the setting of this feedback mechanism would be unique for each individual patient, and (2) the existence of temporary peaks in some patients.

Abelev (*2*) has observed in mice a correlation between the level of AFP and the growth rate of tumors. Thus, the possibility is raised of a similar correlation in man. In this hypothesis, a high AFP level would appear as a grave factor. From our data (*40*) no such correlation can be established. Purves *et al.* (*50*) reach the same negative conclusion, but Alpert *et al.* (*8*) state that " AFP-negative patients appeared to have a longer survival, whereas the strongly AFP-positive patients all died within 4 months. However, there was no statistically significant difference between the groups when the data were subjected to computer analysis and when the number of survivors was compared at a 30-day interval."

α-Fetoprotein in Diseases Other than PLC

Other diseases where AFP is found with high frequency and in relatively large amounts (*i.e.*, detectable by immunodiffusion) are the TRB's. The cellular origin of this production is not known. However the most likely hypothesis is that these tumor cells are differentiated in multiple directions, some of which are related to fetal hepatocytes. Thus, they are AFP producers. We have no personal experience of this disease and we shall not consider it.

In all other diseases, AFP is only exceptionally found by immunodiffusion methods. The only exceptions already published are found in Table IV. Several cases concern tumors of the digestive tract. In all cases, with the exception of a single case (*15*), metastatic involvement of the liver was found.

These findings deserve some comment:

1) It is always very difficult to eliminate the simultaneous occurrence of PLC. An interesting example is given by Purves and Geddes (*51*), who have recently found a patient with a serum AFP level of 0.02 mg% suffering from a primary esophageal cancer. However, careful postmortem examination revealed two small primary liver carcinomas, only 0.5 cm in diameter.

2) No work has been yet published showing the localization of AFP synthesis, for example, using the fluorescent antibody test. It is not known whether the primary tumor or the liver metastasis produces AFP.

3) Most papers on the above subject do not include quantitative data. From the available information, it seems that in such cases the AFP level is rather low. This would be compatible with the hypothesis of production by a small, hidden, primary tumor.

4) However, Gitlin (*24*) has recently reported that AFP was synthesized by the gastrointestinal tract of 6 out of 9 human embryos. Thus, this would be in agree-

TABLE IV. Diseases Other than PLC and TRB Where AFP Has Been Demonstrated in Plasma, Using Immunodiffusion Methods

Nature of the disease	Number of cases	Postmortem examination	Ref.
Tumors of the gastro-intestinal tract			
Gastric cancer (linitis plastica)	1	Yes	(*37*)
Gastric cancer (linitis plastica)	1	Yes	(*16*)
Gastric cancer (carcinoma)	1	Yes	(*21*)
Gastric cancer (carcinoma)	2	No	(*21*)
Gastric cancer (adenocarcinoma) +prostatic carcinoma	1	Yes	(*42*)
Gastric cancer (adenocarcinoma)	1	No	(*30*)
Gastric cancer (carcinoma)	1	Yes	(*10*)
Gastric cancer (carcinoma)	1	Yes	(*15*)
Gastric cancer (adenocarcinoma)	1	Yes	(*15*)
Gastric cancer (adenocarcinoma)[a]	1	Yes	(*15*)
Pancreatic adenocarcinoma	1	Yes	(*37*)
Pancreatic adenocarcinoma	1	Yes	(*13*)
Pancreatic adenocarcinoma	1	Yes	(*15*)
Colonic carcinoma	1	Yes	(*13*)
Noncancerous hepatic diseases			
Viral hepatitis	1	No	(*12*)
Viral hepatitis	1	No	(*32*)
Viral hepatitis	1	No	(*22*)
Viral hepatitis	5	No	(*58*)
Infant hepatitis and hepatic disorders	17	No	(*35*)
Indian childhood cirrhosis	26	No	(*43*)
Hemochromatosis	1	No	(*21*)
Other diseases			
Down syndrome	1	No	(*7*)

[a] This case was the only one showing no secondary liver tumor.

ment with the association of AFP production with at least some gastrointestinal carcinomas.

5) It would be interesting to know whether these represent strictly exceptional cases or marginal cases of a more general phenomenon of low-rate production of AFP in gastrointestinal carcinomas, demonstrable only with high sensitivity methods such as radioimmunoassay.

In fact, use of radioimmunoassay has definitely proven that the normal individual has a minimal quantity in his blood. According to Ruoslahti and Seppälä (*54*), this quantity amounts to 2–16 g/ml. We have also found that in normal adults AFP is in the range 1–5 ng/ml (*38*).

Conversely, hepatic diseases induce a rise in this level. We have tested 17 patients with viral hepatitis and found that they have highly variable serum levels (from subnormal to higher than 1,000 ng/ml). We also found that 52 patients with liver cirrhosis had slightly elevated levels (8 ng/ml on an average).

It is highly probable that systematic investigation will show that serum AFP is raised in several other pathologic circumstances. Some preliminary findings of Abelev (*3*) indicate that other hepatic diseases, and some malignant blood diseases, may induce a slight rise in AFP level. Radioimmunoassays performed in our laboratory confirm this latter view.

However, it should be kept in mind that the range of levels observed in these diseases is very different from that observed in PLC, which is currently 1,000 to 10,000 times higher than in viral hepatitis or cirrhosis. It is likely that in the latter disease AFP rise represents only a stimulation of the mechanism of AFP production of the normal individual, which seems to be controlled by a homeostatic mechanism, while in PLC this mechanism is obviously overwhelmed.

Mechanism of AFP Biosynthesis

The mechanism of AFP production in the adult is still obscure. Our lack of knowledge on the biochemical processes of differentiation considerably hinders elaboration of any hypothesis.

It is evident that, in the adult, PLC is a single disease in which a mass production of AFP is observed with plasmatic rates of several mg/ml. In TRB, rates are much lower. As far as hepatitis or cirrhosis are concerned, they exceptionally give a level demonstrable by conventional methods of immunodiffusion.

High sensitivity methods such as radioimmunoassays have to be used in such cases. As a matter of fact, the inventory of diseases inducing a slight increase in the rate of AFP production is not yet complete. According to our recent results, several nontumoral hepatic diseases may also increase the AFP production rate. In any event, the observed rates in the normal individual as well as during these different diseases are much lower than those observed in some liver cancers. It seems that the process of AFP biosynthesis is very different in cancerous diseases (PLC and TRB) than in other circumstances (hepatic diseases and normal individual).

It is generally accepted that certain PLC's are not producers of AFP. However, (1) we may speculate whether all PLC's could not finally synthesize AFP provided that the tumor became big enough. This is a simple extrapolation of Table III. In fact the patient very often dies before reaching this stage of the disease. (2) It would be better to consider the problem of AFP production in relation to the whole question of protein biosynthesis by the hepatic cell. Preliminary experiments by Rioche in our laboratory have shown that liver cancer cells in culture incorporate labeled amino acids in various protein patterns according to different patients. Six proteins have been investigated (albumin, AFP, haptoglobin, transferrin, β_2-glycoprotein I, fibrinogen). Preliminary results show that some tumor cells synthesize all 6 proteins, while others synthesize only some of them. One culture did not incorporate labeled amino acids into proteins in spite of active multiplication.

Similar facts have been noted by Becker (*14*) on the rat experimental hepatoma. It is therefore possible that the mechanism which regulates AFP production is dependent on a more general phenomenon which induces the secretion of proteins by the hepatocyte.

It is now more and more evident that the statement expressed in the last century, that embryonic and cancerous cells look much alike is confirmed from the biochemical point of view.

In several kinds of cancer, " isoenzymes " of fetal type or more or less feto-specific antigens have been demonstrated. According to the most popular hypothesis, the cancerization phenomenon simultaneously induces a certain degree of dedifferentiation or, more precisely, of retrodifferentiation.

However, this hypothesis leaves unexplained the fact that tumors with no AFP production do exist, and inside productive tumors many cells are not productive. The link between cancerization and AFP production is not obligatory. Apparently, there is no greater link between classical morphologic signs of cell dedifferentiation and AFP production.

Some workers have suggested that cancerization may essentially result from the alteration of the part of the genome which regulates structural gene function. The same part is certainly also responsible for differentiation phenomena. Thus, alterations responsible for cancer could extend to relatively near zones responsible for phenotypic expression. This extension of gene lesion would not be obligatory: It would only result from the proximity of the DNA segments concerned. However, this hypothesis supposes a hereditary transmission of this alteration-inducing dedifferentiation, as shown by AFP synthesis. In fact, the only evidence is the grouping of cells producing AFP in liver tumors. This is also clearly seen in metastatic nodules, which show homogeneous fields of AFP-producing cells, as observed by Gusev *et al.* (*25*) by immunofluorescence. This can be taken as evidence for the existence of cellular clones producing AFP.

However, another classical hypothesis should be considered. According to this theory, liver cancer originates from stem cells remaining undifferentiated, scattered in the hepatic mass. Such an origin was supported by Lacassagne (*33*) on the basis of cytological evidence. We should admit that these cells are more liable to cancerization than others: This would explain the high proportion of PLC with no AFP synthesis.

In agreement with Pierce (*47*), if we consider that the normal evolution of a tumor is towards a differentiation similar to the normal differentiation, it must be inferred that the majority of tumor cells would repress their AFP synthesis, as this occurs in the normal embryo. This is compatible with the histological aspects described by Gusev *et al.* (*25*), as mentioned above. Why undifferentiated stem cells can persist in an adult liver is not presently explicable, but the same problem comes up in an identical way for organs such as skin or intestinal mucosa where the existence of a layer of non-differentiated stem cells is a well-known fact.

The definite effect of age on AFP-positivity rate is in agreement with this idea, for it is logical that the number of stem cells " dormant " in liver decreases with age. This hypothesis would have the merit of explaining the persistence of AFP synthesis in trace amounts, as shown by radioimmunoassay in the normal individual, recently demonstrated by Ruoslahti and Seppälä (*54*), and confirmed in our laboratory. This would be linked to the persistence of stem cells. The increase in AFP level which is observed in hepatitis and (to a lesser degree) in cirrhosis could be explained by a regeneration process which would induce not only a multiplication of differentiated liver cells, but also of stem cells and consequently an increased AFP synthesis. Hepatic regeneration caused by a partial hepatectomy involves a definite AFP production in mice (*2*) and rats (*3*).

The discovery of AFP has stimulated research on conceptual as well as practical aspects of cancerology. The time lapse between laboratory discoveries and the introduction of AFP determination as a routine laboratory test in medicine was notably shortened by close cooperation between scientists, enhanced by the International Agency for Research on Cancer (IARC, Lyon, France). In this case, laboratory work was undertaken in countries where liver cancer is a rare disease. Thus, the role of IARC, which favoured collaboration with the countries where liver cancer is frequent, was especially valuable.

New research on AFP should be directed towards the fundamental field of cellular differentiation. This would help in throwing some light on the mechanisms of differentiation in eucaryotic cells and their relationships with cancerization.

Acknowledgments

Work reported in this paper was supported by grants from the International Agency for Research on Cancer (Lyon, France), Anna Fuller Fund (New Haven, Conn., U.S.A.), and INSERM, Fondation pour la Recherche Médicale Française contre le Cancer, (Paris, France). It was made possible by the cooperation of several clinical investigators. The contribution of Prof. M. Sankalé of Dakar is gratefully acknowledged.

REFERENCES

1. Abelev, G. I. Antigenic structure of chemically induced hepatomas. *Progr. Exp. Tumor Res.*, **7**, 104–157 (1965).
2. Abelev, G. I. Production of embryonal serum α-globulin by hepatomas: Review of experimental and clinical data. *Cancer Res.*, **28**, 1344–1350 (1968).
3. Abelev, G. I. α-Fetoprotein in ontogenesis and its association with malignant tumors. *Adv. Cancer Res.*, **14**, 295–358 (1971).
4. Abelev, G. I., Alpert, E., Hull E. W., Masseyeff, R., de Nechaud, B., Tatarinov, Y., and Uriel, J. Les protéines sériques foeto-spécifiques. Recommendations en vue d'une normalisation de la terminologie. *Bull. OMS*, **43**, 311–312 (1970).
5. Abelev, G. I., Assecritova, I. V., Kraevsky, N. A., Perova, S. D., and Perevodchikova, N. I. Embryonal serum α-globulin in cancer patients: Diagnostic value. *Int. J. Cancer*, **2**, 551–558 (1967).
6. Abelev, G. I., Tsvetkov, V. S., *et al.* Assessment of the use of highly sensitive methods determining α-fetoprotein for the diagnosis of hepatocellular cancer and teratoblastoma. *Bull. Exp. Biol. Med.* (*U.S.S.R.*), **4**, 75–81 (1971).
7. Adinolfi, M., Gardner, B., and Martin, W. Fetal proteins and immunoglobulins. *Atti. Assoc. Genet. Ital.*, **12**, 133–143 (1967).
8. Alpert, E., Hershberg, R., Schur, P. H., and Isselbacher, K. J. α-Fetoprotein in human hepatoma: Improved detection in serum and quantitative studies using a new sensitive technique. *Gastroenterology*, **61**, 137–143 (1971).

9. Alpert, M. E., Hutt, M. S. R., and Davidson, C. S. Primary hepatoma in Uganda. *Am. J. Med.*, **46**, 794–802 (1969).
10. Alpert, E., Pinn V. W., and Isselbacher, K. J. α-Fetoprotein in a patient with gastric carcinoma metastatic to the liver. *New Engl. J. Med.*, **285**, 1058–1059 (1971).
11. Alpert, E., Starzl, T. E., Schur, P., and Isselbacher, K. J. Serum α-fetoprotein in hepatoma patients after liver transplantation. *Gastroenterology*, **61**, 144–148 (1971).
12. Alpert, E., Uriel, J., and de Nechaud, B. α_1-Fetoprotein in the diagnosis of human hepatoma. *New Engl. J. Med.*, **278**, 984–986 (1968).
13. Andrieu, J., Breart, G., Rodier, B., and Robert, P. E. A propos de l'existence de α_1-foetoprotéine en dehors de l'hépatome. *Presse Med.*, **79**, 1596 (1971).
14. Becker, F. F. Neoplasia and the cell cycle. *Fed. Proc.*, **30**, 1736–1741 (1971).
15. Bernades, P., Smadja, M., Rueff, B., Bonnefond, A., Tursz, T., Martin, E., Bognel, C., Barge, J., and Uriel, J. Présence de l'α-foetoprotéine sérique dans quatre cas de cancers digestifs primitifs autres que l'hépatome. *Presse Med.*, **79**, 1585–1587 (1971).
16. Bourelle, J., Metayer, P., Sauger, F., Matray, F., and Fondimare, A. Existence d'α-foetoprotéine au cours d'un cancer secondaire du foie d'origine gastrique. *Presse Med.*, **78**, 1277–1278 (1970).
17. Economopoulos, P., Theodoropoulos, G., and Sakellaropoulos, N. α-Fetoprotein in Greece and France. *Lancet*, **1**, 1337 (1970).
18. Endo, Y., Eto, S., Ino, S., Fujiwara, K., Miyake, K. Kanetaka, T., Yamanaka, M., Suzuki, H., Oda, T., Yoshitoshi, Y., Juji, T., Yokochi, T., and Miura, T. Diagnosis of primary carcinoma of the liver by α-fetoglobulin (in Japanese). *Kanzo (Liver)*, **10**, 143–146 (1969).
19. Engelhardt, N. V., Gusev, A. I., Shipova, J. Ja., and Abelev, G. I. Immunofluorescent study of α-fetoprotein in liver and liver tumors. *Int. J. Cancer*, **7**, 198–206 (1971).
20. Foli, A. K., Sherlock, S., and Adinolfi, M. Serum α_1-fetoprotein in patients with liver disease. *Lancet*, **2**, 1267–1269 (1969).
21. Geoffroy, Y., Boureille, J., Denis, P., Colin, R., and Metayer, P. Bilan d'une recherche systématique de l'α-foetoprotéine dans 224 hépatopathies. *Sem. Hôp. Paris*, **47**, 1281–1285 (1971).
22. Geffroy, Y., Denis, P., Colin, R., Sauger, F., Matray, F., and Fondimare, A. Présence d'α_1-foetoprotéine chez l'adulte au cours d'une hépatite virale traitée par corticothérapie. *Presse Med.*, **78**, 1107–1108 (1970).
23. Girard, M., Planchu, M., and Chapuy, H. Le cancer primitif du foie chez l'adulte européen (à propose de 90 observations). *J. Med. Lyon*, **51**, 773–798 (1970).
24. Gitlin, D. Sites of α-fetoprotein synthesis. *New Engl. J. Med.*, **285**, 1436–1437 (1971).
25. Gusev, A. I., Engelhardt, N. V., Masseyeff, R., Camain, R., and Basteris, B. Immunofluorescent study of α-fetoprotein in liver tumor. *Int. J. Cancer*, **7**, 207–217 (1970).
26. Hirsch-marie, H. and Conte, M. Présence et signification de l'α-foetoprotéine dans le sérum. *Sem. Hôp. Paris*, **46**, 3057–3063 (1970).
27. Hull, E. W., Carbone, P. P., Moertel, C. G., and O'Conor, G. T. Serum α-fetoprotein in U.S.A. *Lancet*, **1**, 779 (1970).

28. Hull, E., O'Gara, R., Carbone, P., and Smith, C. Synthesis of α-fetoprotein by monkey hepatoma cells *in vitro*. *Proc. Am. Assoc. Cancer Res.*, **10**, 41 (1969).
29. Hull, E., Moertel, C., and Carbone, P. Serum α-fetoprotein (AFP) in cancer patients. *Clin. Res.*, **17**, 403 (1969).
30. Kozower, M., Fawaz, K. A., Miller, H. M., and Kaplan, M. M. Positive α-fetoglobulin in a case of gastric carcinoma. *Med. Intel.*, **285**, 1059–1060 (1971).
31. Kresno, S. B., Gandasoebrata, R., and Rümke, Ph. Serum α-fetoprotein in Indonesia. *Lancet*, **1**, 1178 (1970).
32. Kresno, S. B., Gandasoebrata, R., and Rümke, Ph. Serum α-fetoprotein in patients with hepatoma from Djakarta. *Protides Biol. Fluids*, **18**, 243–245 (1971).
33. Lacassagne A. Sur l'histogénèse des carcinomes hépatiques. A propos des foeto-protéines spécifiques. *Bull. Cancer*, **55**, 181–204 (1968).
34. Lin, T. Y. Primary cancer of the liver. Quadrennial review. *Scand. J. Gastroenterol.*, Suppl. **6**, 223–241 (1970).
35. Masopust, J., Rádl, J., and Houštěk, J. Occurrence of α_1-fetoprotein in some infants suffering from hepatopathy. *Protides Biol. Fluids*, **18**, 239–242 (1971).
36. Masseyeff, R. Human α-fetoprotein. *Pathol. Biol.*, **20**, 703–725 (1973).
37. Masseyeff, R., Basteris, B., and Leblanc, L. Use of the α-fetoprotein test for the diagnosis of primary liver cancer. *Protides Biol. Fluids*, **18**, 217–220 (1971).
38. Masseyeff, R. and Bonet, Cl. Unpublished data.
39. Masseyeff, R., Prince, A., Leblanc, L., and Szmuness, W. Detection of HAA in the sera of patients with primary carcinoma of the liver. *Am. J. Dis. Child.*, **123**, 412–413 (1972).
40. Masseyeff, R., Sankale, M., Onde, M., Menye, A., Camain, R., Quenum, C., Maydat, L., Mattern, P., Ancelle, P., and Leblanc, L. Valeur de la recherche de l'α-foetoprotéine sérique pour le diagnostic du cancer primitif du foie. *Bull. Soc. Med. Afr. Noire*, **13**, 537–548 (1968).
41. Mawas, C., Buffe, D., and Burtin P. Influence of age on α-fetoprotein incidence. *Lancet*, **1**, 1292 (1970).
42. Mehlman, D. J., Bulkley, B. H., and Wiernik, P. H. Serum α-fetoglobulin with gastric and prostatic carcinomas. *New Engl. J. Med.*, **285**, 1060–1061 (1971).
43. Nayak, N. C., Malaviya, A. N., Veena, C., and Chandra, R. K. α-Fetoprotein in Indian childhood cirrhosis. *Lancet*, **1**, 68, 69 (1972).
44. Nunez, E., Engelmann, F., Benassay, G., and Jayle, M. F. Identification et purification préliminaire de la foetoprotéine liant les oestrogènes dans le sérum de rats nouveaux nés. *C. R.*, **273**, 242–245 (1971).
45. O'Conor, G. T., Tatarinov, Y. S., Abelev, G. I., and Uriel, J. A collaborative study for the evaluation of a serologic test for primary liver cancer. *Cancer*, **25**, 1091–1098 (1970).
46. Payet, M. and Sankale, M. Les cancers du foie et du pancréas chez le noir africain. *Med. Afr. Noire*, **18**, 215–226 (1971).
47. Pierce, G. Differentiation of normal and malignant cells. *Fed. Proc.*, **29**, 1248–1254 (1970).
48. Portugal, M. L., Azevedo, M. S., and Manso, C. Serum α-fetoprotein and variant alkaline phosphatase in human hepatocellular carcinoma. *Int. J. Cancer*, **6**, 383–387 (1970).
49. Purtilo, D. T. and Yunis, E. J. Localization of α-fetoprotein synthesis in human fetuses and hepatomas. *Fed. Proc.*, **30**, 634 (1971).
50. Purves, L. R., Bersohn, J., and Geddes, E. W. Serum α-fetoprotein and primary cancer of the liver in man. *Cancer*, **25**, 1261–1270 (1970).

51. Purves, L. R. and Geddes, E. W. A more sensitive test for α-fetoprotein. *Lancet*, **1**, 47–48 (1972).
52. Purves, L. R., Macnab, M., and Bersohn, I. Serum α-fetoprotein. I: Immunodiffusion and immunoassay results in cases of primary cancer of the liver. *S. Afr. Med. J.*, **42**, 1138–1141 (1968).
53. Quelin, S., Rioche, M., Bresson, Y., and Masseyeff, R. Synthèse *in vitro* d'α-foetoprotéine par le foie humain cancéreux en culture. *C. R.*, 768–771 (1972).
54. Ruoslahti, E. and Seppälä M. α-Fetoprotein in normal human serum. *Nature*, **235**, 161–162 (1972).
55. Sauger, F., Duval, C., Fondimare, A., Matray, F., and Buffe, D. Systematic α-fetoprotein research in 2,500 sera results. *Protides Biol. Fluids*, **18**, 247–250 (1971).
56. Sauger, F., Duval, C., Fondimare, A., Matray, F., and Buffe, D. Systematic analysis of α-fetoprotein in 5,000 sera. *Rev. Eur. Et. Clin. Biol.*, **16**, 471–473 (1971).
57. Smith, J. B. α-Fetoprotein: Occurrence in certain malignant diseases and review of clinical applications. *Med. Clin. N. Am.*, **54**, 797–803 (1970).
58. Smith, J. B. Occurrence of α-fetoprotein in acute viral hepatitis. *Int. J. Cancer*, **8**, 421–424 (1971).
59. Smith, J. B. and O'Neill, R. T. Fetal gut antigen: A substance in fetal gut and its relationship to gut carcinoma. *Res. Commun. Chem. Pathol. Pharm.*, **2**, 1–15 (1971).
60. Smith, J. B. and Todd, D. Fetoglobin and primary liver cancer. *Lancet*, **2**, 833 (1968).
61. Stanislawski-birencwajg, M., Uriel, J., and Grabar, P. Association of embryonic antigens with experimentally induced hepatic lesions in the rat. *Cancer Res.*, **27**, 1990–1997 (1967).
62. Tatarinov, Y. S. Detection of embryospecific α-globulin in the blood sera of patients with primary liver tumor. *Vopr. Med. Khim.*, **10**, 90–91 (1964).
63. Teres, J., Bertran, A., Mas, A., and Gras, J. α_1-Fetoprotein in Spain. *Lancet*, **2**, 465 (1970).
64. Tuyns, A. J., Leblanc, L., and Masseyeff, R. *Digestion*, in press.
65. Uriel, J., de Nechaud, B., Stanislawski-birencwajg, M., Masseyeff, R., Leblanc, L., Quenum, C., Loisillier, F., and Grabar, P. Le diagnostic du cancer primaire du foie par des méthodes immunologiques. *Presse Med.*, **76**, 1415–1416 (1968).
66. Vogel, C. L., Anthony, P. P., Mody, N., and Barker, L. F. Hepatitis-associated antigen in Uganda patients with hepato-cellular carcinoma. *Lancet*, **2**, 621–624 (1970).

SOME CHEMICAL, EXPERIMENTAL, AND CLINICAL INVESTIGATIONS OF α-FETOPROTEIN

Hidematsu HIRAI, Shinzo NISHI, Hiroyuki WATABE, and Yutaka TSUKADA

*Department of Biochemistry, School of Medicine, Hokkaido University**

α-Fetoproteins (AFP) were highly purified from such sources as sera of human and rat fetuses, and sera and/or ascites of hepatoma patients and hepatoma-bearing rats. The AFP of human was crystallized.

Some physicochemical, chemical, and immunochemical analyses of the purified materials were made. No significant differences in molecular weights (*ca.* 70,000), sedimentation coefficients (4.5S), isoelectric points (4.7), and amino acid compositions were observed between fetal and hepatoma AFP's. Various animal AFP's cross-reacted with each other in the precipitin reaction.

α-Fetoproteins in patient blood of various diseases were determined either by the ordinary immunodiffusion techniques or the radioimmunoassay. The AFP was detected frequently not only in hepatoma but also in hepatitis and cirrhosis patients though in low concentration.

α-Fetoprotein production during hepatocarcinogenesis in rats fed 4-dimethylaminoazobenzene was precisely observed, and it was found that AFP appeared transiently in the blood in an early stage when no cancer cells appeared yet in the liver.

Based on these clinical and experimental observations possible relations between hepatitis and hepatoma were discussed.

Since 1961, we have been investigating tumor-specific antigenic proteins. Our effort was focused mostly on the isolation and chemical characterization of the proteins from cancer cells, and this goal was partially achieved when we isolated a protein from a transplantable rat hepatoma, AH-49. This protein was found specifically in AH-49 hepatoma cells only and was neither in the serum of rats bearing hepatoma nor in fetal rats. The results of these investigation were summarized and reported (7) in " Symposium on Tumor-Specific Antigens " held at Sukhumi, U.S.S.R., in 1965 under the auspices of the UICC and arranged by Zilber and Abelev.

After the symposium, AH-49 hepatoma was sent to Abelev and was proved to be an α-fetoprotein (AFP)-synthesizing tumor strain. In 1968 a comparison was made in our laboratory between this protein and rat AFP and it was shown that these were different proteins.

* Kita-15-jo, Nishi-7-chome, Kita-ku, Sapporo 060, Japan (平井秀松, 西　信三, 渡部博之, 塚田　裕).

The first paper on AFP in Japan was published by Endo (*4*) in 1969, reporting that the prevalence of AFP in primary liver cancer (PLC) patients was 60%. In 1969 in our laboratory human and rat AFP were successfully purified, and a large quantity of specific antiserum against AFP was obtained by immunizing horses. This antiserum was then widely distributed to other institutions and considerable data have been accumulated so far.

The present paper surveys the biochemical, experimental, and clinical aspects of AFP studies, using data obtained primarily in our laboratory.

Chemistry of AFP

1. Preparation of specific antiserum

The first antiserum against human AFP was prepared by the conventional method. Rabbits were immunized with serum of fetuses or hepatoma patients. The antiserum obtained was absorbed with normal adult serum. The absorbed antiserum reacted specifically with AFP. The first antiserum thus prepared was mixed with fetal or hepatoma sera, forming specific antigen-antibody precipitates which were throughly washed, as will be described later. The precipitate itself was a good antigen to immunize horses or rabbits. α-Fetoprotein was isolated from the complex in a pure form which was a very potent antigen. The details of purification will be described later. Several horses were immunized either with the complex or with purified AFP suspended in Freund's complete adjuvant. The precipitin titers of the specific antisera were 128–512.

The antiserum against rat AFP was prepared in the same way. Fetal rat serum, amniotic and ascitic fluids of rats transplanted with ascites hepatoma were the source of AFP.

2. Purification of AFP (9)

Chromatography using ion exchangers such as DEAE- or CM-cellulose was a useful tool but it was not easy to avoid contamination with albumin without reducing the yield of AFP since the physicochemical properties of AFP and albumin are very similar, as described later. Therefore, we used a specific method, *i.e.*, the isolation of AFP from the antigen-antibody complex. The details are as follows:

Several hundred ml of the horse antiserum was used in a single experiment. The flow chart for the purification procedure is shown in Chart 1. Sera or ascites material containing AFP was mixed with the antiserum in the optimal proportion and placed in an ice-box overnight. The antigen-antibody precipitate formed was spun down and washed several times with cold saline. The precipitate was then dissolved in an appropriate amount of 0.1 M glycine-HCl buffer (pH 1.8), giving a clear solution. The solution was neutralized by addition of 0.4 M Na_2HPO_4. The antigen-antibody complex was precipitated again. The complex was spun out and washed. The procedure of dissolution in acid and reprecipitation by neutralization was repeated 3 times to thoroughly wash out contaminants from the AFP and the antibody. Since the molecular weights of AFP and IgG are quite different, these proteins were easily separated by gel fil-

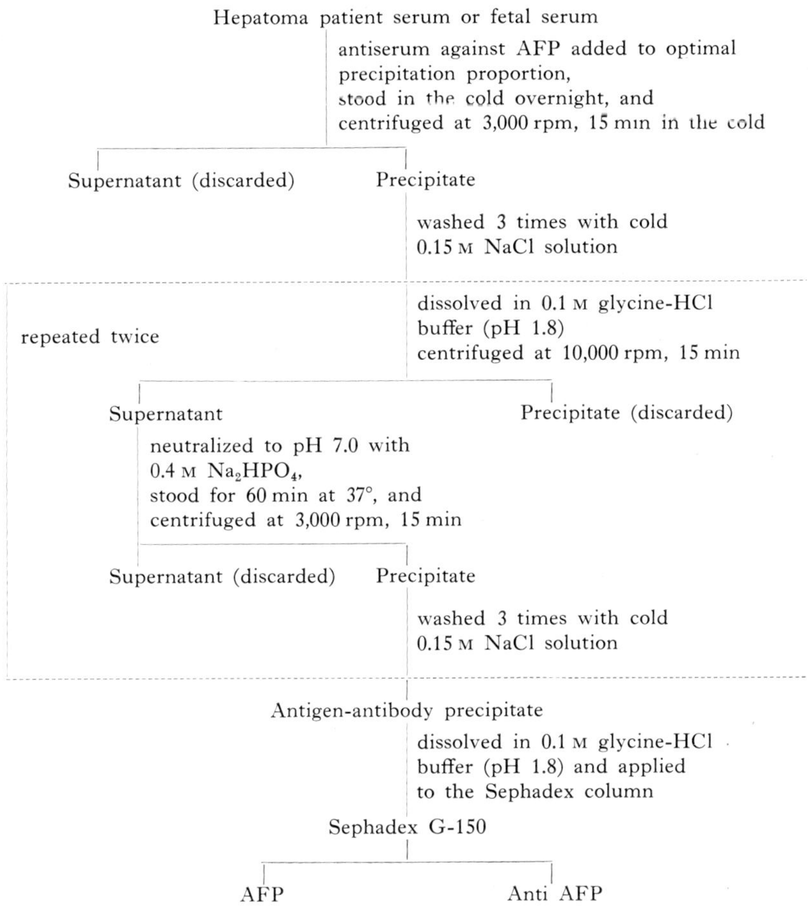

CHART 1. Purification of AFP

tration. A column of Sephadex G-150 was equilibrated with 0.1 M glycine-HCl buffer (pH 1.8), and the dissolved antigen-antibody complex was applied and eluted with the same buffer. The elution pattern indicated 3 peaks, as shown in Fig. 1,A. The 1st peak was antigen-antibody complex or aggregates of denatured antibody, the 2nd was the antibody, and the last peak was AFP. The last fraction was collected and neutralized. In this case no precipitate was obtained on neutralization because the fraction consisted mostly of AFP. This neutralized fraction was applied to a Sephadex column at pH 7.0. The elution diagram, as shown in Fig. 1,B, showed a small peak which was identified as a soluble antigen-antibody complex formed in antigen excess. The main peak was AFP. The AFP thus obtained was practically 100% pure, judged from electrophoresis, such as disc electrophoresis, immunoelectrophoresis, and so on, and also by ultracentrifugation.

Recently, purification was carried out using an immunoadsorbent column (*10*). An IgG fraction purified from the horse antiserum was coupled to Sepharose 6B by means of BrCN, according to the method of Porath (*2*). The immuno-

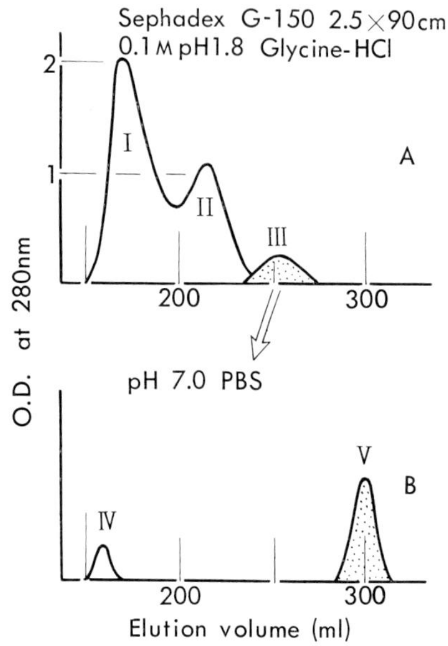

FIG. 1. Gel filtration of dissolved antigen-antibody complex

I: Aggregate of denatured antibody. II: Antibody. III: Crude AFP. IV: Soluble antigen-antibody complex. V: Purified AFP. PBS: Phosphate buffer solution, 0.1 M. Sephadex G-150 2.5 × 90 cm, 0.1 M pH 1.8 glycine-HCl.

adsorbent thus prepared was poured into a column to which samples containing AFP were applied. α-Fetoprotein combined with the adsorbent was then eluted with 0.1 M glycine-HCl buffer (pH 2.8), obtaining a highly purified AFP. The elution of AFP from the adsorbent was easily accomplished at pH 2.8 instead of 1.8, and the time exposure to this acidic environment was much shorter (2–3 hr only) than that required in the complex dissociation method. The yield was about 80%. The elution of AFP was also achieved by 2 M NaI solution at neutral pH although the yield was poorer (60%) than that using the acidic buffer solution.

The immunoadsorbent method thus offers the advantage of avoiding possible denaturation of the protein. Another advantage was that the column could be used repeatedly without any appreciable loss of capacity. The antibody combined with Sepharose appeared to be quite stable under the conditions used.

3. *Crystallization of AFP* (*10*)

To 1–2% solution of the purified AFP, a saturated $(NH_4)_2SO_4$ solution was added to a final concentration of about 2.3 M. After keeping the solution cold for several days, hexagonal crystals appeared, as shown in Photo 1. Apparently strict control of pH was unneccessary: Crystallization occurred in all batches at pH 5–7, though the yield was poor.

4. *Chemical and physicochemical properties of AFP*

Table I shows some chemical characteristics of human and rat AFP. The data for human serum albumin (*15*) are shown for reference. No marked difference was observed between AFP from the sera of human fetuses and hepatoma

TABLE I. Chemical Composition of AFP (%)

	Human		Rat	Human (*15*)
	Hepatoma	Fetus	Hepatoma	Albumin
Nitrogen	14.9	14.7	13.1	16.0
Sulfur	1.8	1.7	2.0	1.5
Carbohydrate	3.4		5.3	0.08
Mannose	0.68 (3)			
Galactose	0.49 (2)			
Glucosamine	0.89 (4)			
Fucose	±			
Sialic acid	1.3 (3)			

Numbers in parentheses indicate mole per 70,000 *g* AFP.
Nitrogen and sulfur were determined at the Element Analysis Center, Hokkaido University. Carbohydrates were analyzed by gas chromatography by the courtesy of Prof. Z. Tamura, Faculty of Pharmaceutical Sciences, University of Tokyo.

patients. The data for rat AFP were also quite similar to those for human AFP. Total carbohydrate content was 3.4%. Recently, Ruoslahti *et al.* (*13*) reported the chemical properties of AFP and the sugar content was 4% containing 3 moles of sialic acid.

Table II indicates some physicochemical properties. The data are very similar to those of human albumin (*15*). The mobilities of human and rat AFP, observed by zone electrophoresis, were just between those of albumin and α_1-globulin, although the mobilities of AFP from some other animal species were quite different.

Table III indicates the amino acid composition. Practically no difference was observed between human fetal and hepatoma AFP. Though in general the data for rat AFP were also similar to those for human AFP, some conspicuous exceptions are evident, *e.g.* methionine, histidine, lysine, *etc.* The data for albumin also appear to be not very different from those for AFP except for several amino acids. Ruoslahti *et al.* (*13*) also reported the amino acid composition of human AFP. Their data show a good agreement with ours except for a few amino acids.

TABLE II. Some Physicochemical Properties of AFP

	Human AFP		Rat AFP	Human (*15*)
	Fetus	Hepatoma	Hepatoma	Albumin
Sedimentation constant $s_{20,w}$ [a]	4.50	4.50	4.76	4.6
Diffusion constant $D_{20,w}$ [b]	6.18		5.68	6.1
Partial specific volume V_{20} [c]	0.726	0.726	0.726	0.733
Molecular weight	64,600		75,100	69,000
Isoelectric point pI [d]	4.7	4.7	4.7, 5.0	4.9
$E^{1\%}_{1cm}$ (278 nm) [e]	5.30	5.26	4.27	5.8

[a] 10^{-13} sec (S). [b] $10^{-7}\cdot cm^2\cdot sec^{-1}$. [c] ml/g. [d] pH. [e] Optical density of a 1% solution in 1 cm cuvette at 278 nm.

TABLE III. Amino Acid Composition of AFP (moles/mole protein)

	Human AFP		Rat AFP	Human (*15*)
	Fetus	Hepatoma	Hepatoma	Albumin
Asx	49	49	60	52
Thr	36	35	33	28
Ser	37	36	38	24
Glx	110	104	103	81
Pro	21	22	32	25
Gly	26	27	31	12
Ala	50	49	58	62
½Cys	22	26	34	17
Val	27	29	27	41
Met	4	6	14	5
Ile	25	26	31	8
Leu	53	54	66	60
Tyr	16	16	16	16
Phe	27	29	25	30
Lys	36	35	54	56
His	12	12	21	15
Arg	17	17	23	23
Trp	2	2	1	1

Asx: Aspartic acid+asparagine. Glx: Glutamic acid+glutamine. Amide of albumin (asparagine+glutamine) is 38 moles.

We have considered whether or not the AFP's from fetuses and hepatoma patients (or hepatoma-bearing animals) are the same protein. However, we could not find any significant difference between these two proteins either chemically or physicochemically, as shown in the above tables.

Immunological Properties of AFP

1. Antigenic identity of fetal and hepatoma AFP

Photo 2 shows precipitin reactions of a rabbit antiserum against human fetal AFP. The lines formed with both fetal and hepatoma AFP fuse well. Photo 3 indicates the reactions of 2 antisera against human fetal and hepatoma AFP. These data indicate that both AFP's are immunologically indistinguishable when Ouchterlony's technique is employed.

The same identity was observed between rat fetal and hepatoma AFP, although the data are not shown here.

2. Cross-reactivity of AFP of various animals

α-Fetoprotein is a protein whose species specificity is rather low. Gitlin and Boesman (*5*) investigated the cross-reactivity of AFP of several mammals using anti-human-AFP rabbit serum, although there are some discrepancies with our results (*11*), indicated as follows.

We have prepared several antisera against human and rat AFP by immunizing

TABLE IV. Cross Reaction of AFP in Several Mammals

Antisera / Antigens	Anti-human AFP			Anti-rat AFP	
	Horse	Rabbit	Rat	Horse	Rabbit
Human	⧻	⧻	⧺	—	—
Horse	⧺	+	+	—	—
Calf	⊥	⊥	+	—	—
Sheep	⊥	⊥	⊥	—	—
Pig	+	+	+	—	—
Rabbit	⧺	+	+	—	—
Dog	⧺	⧺	⧺	—	—
Cat	⧺	⧺	⧺	—	—
Rat	+	+	—	⧻	⧻
Mouse	+	+	—	⧺	⧺

⊥: The reaction was observed only in 5-fold concentrated antigen serum.

horses, rabbits, and rats. Table IV indicates the reactivity of 10 mammalian AFP's with these 3 antisera. The horse and rabbit antisera reacted with all 10, but the rat antisera reacted with 8 out of 10. On the other hand, the antisera against rat AFP reacted only with rat and mouse AFP.

Photo 4 shows the precipitin reaction. Some of the lines fuse with each other, while others show spur formation.

Interestingly, rabbit antisera obtained by immunization with human AFP reacted with rabbit fetal AFP (Photo 4) and horse antisera obtained by immunization with human AFP reacted with horse fetal AFP, thus exhibiting homologous reactions (*12*). The animals are expected to be tolerant to their own AFP but when they are immunized with heterologous AFP this tolerance appears to be circumvented. Homologous immunization, *i.e.*, immunization of rabbits with rabbit AFP and immunization of rats with rat AFP, was also attempted but it was not successful in demonstrating homologous antibody formation. Further investigation of the homologous reaction is in progress using the radioimmunoassay technique.

Quantitative Assay Method for AFP

1. *Radial immunodiffusion technique*

This is a most simple and specific method for routine determination. Mancini's method (*8*) was employed. Horse or rabbit antisera with precipitin titers of 64–128 were diluted, usually 4- to 8-fold, and mixed with a buffered agar for preparing immunoplates. The purified AFP previously described was used as a standard. α-Fetoprotein levels over 10 μg/ml could be determined accurately. α-Fetoprotein between 10 and 1 μg/ml cannot be determined quantitatively by this method since there is a risk of quite erroneous results.

2. *Radioimmunoassay of AFP*

For accurate measurement of amounts less than 10 μg/ml of AFP, we set up a radioimmunoassay using highly purified human or rat AFP labeled with ^{125}I.

Double antibody techniques were employed. This method is sensitive to 2 ng/ml, or 5,000 times better than the radial immunodiffusion technique. The details of the method are described by Nishi and Hirai in this issue.

Some Clinical Aspects of AFP

1. Significance of AFP level in serum of hepatoma patients

Table V summarizes data to October 1970 obtained by the cooperation of 14 institutions in Japan. All data listed here were obtained by the Ouchterlony technique. The occurrence of a positive AFP test (>10 μg/ml) in patients with histologically diagnosed hepatoma was about 80%. Thus, we classified the hepatoma into 2 types, AFP-producing and AFP-nonproducing hepatoma.* Even by the very sensitive radioimmunoassay, about 10% of the patients are still AFP-nonproducing (<20 ng/ml). The clinical and pathological differences between these types of hepatoma are fully discussed in this issue.

The distribution of serum AFP levels was very wide, from 2×10^{-8} to 1×10^{-2} g/ml. A partial explanation of this finding may be that the hepatoma has a mosaic structure consisting of both AFP-producing and AFP-nonproducing cells, and the ratio of the 2 types of cell may be reflected in the serum AFP level. Some experimental data supporting a mosaic structure will be offered in detail by Watabe and Hirai in this issue. The antibody fluorescence technique also demonstrated directly the presence of 2 types of hepatoma cell, as shown elsewhere

TABLE V. Prevalence of AFP in Japan (Data to September 1970)

Reporting institution	PLC	Hepa-toma[a]	Cholan-gioma[a]	Meta-static liver cancer	Liver cir-rhosis	Others	Total
Hokkaido Univ.	38/60	23/30	0/3	1/34	0/35	0/6,099	39/6,228
Sapporo Med. Col.	27/34	23/28	0/0	0/10	0/9	0/8	27/61
Niigata Cancer Center	15/18	14/15	1/1	0/10	0/3	0/149	32/180
Tokyo Univ.	28/43	17/22	0/3	0/56	1/64	3/903	32/1,066
National Cancer Center	51/62	35/45	0/1	2/48	1/73	4/924	58/1,107
Nihon Univ.	10/17	10/17	0/0	0/5	0/30	0/13	10/65
Okayama Univ.	21/30	14/17	0/0	0/24	1/82	0/116	22/252
Yamaguchi Univ.	27/37	21/26	0/4	1/21	3/20	0/45	31/123
Kyushu Univ.	25/34	9/10	0/1	0/6	0/34	0/76	25/150
Others	12/19	12/17	0/1	1/4	0/0	0/34	13/59
	254/354	178/227	1/14	5/218	6/350	7[b]/8,369	272/9,291
	72%	78%					

[a] Cases with histological diagnosis. [b] Teratoma of testis.

* "Nonproducing hepatoma" is not an exact expression. This simply means hepatoma patients with a serum AFP level below 20 ng/ml. The significance of AFP in such low concentrations is still obscure, as discussed later.

in this issue. Therefore, the size of the tumor is not necessarily related to the serum AFP level. However, in some patients with AFP-producing hepatoma, elevation of AFP level may be observed with the growth of the tumor. Here there is a possibility of early diagnosis of hepatoma by detecting AFP in very low concentrations while the tumor is very small. The radioimmunoassay has made it possible to detect such low concentrations.

2. *α-Fetoprotein in hepatitis and liver cirrhosis patients*

By using radioimmunoassay, low concentrations of AFP were detected in many cases of hepatitis and cirrhosis. The details are reported by us elsewhere in this volume. The AFP in hepatitis patients was previously reported by Abelev (*1*), using an immunoradioautographic technique. This important phenomenon will be dealt with later in the discussion section.

3. *Half-life ($T_{1/2}$) of AFP*

We observed several patients who underwent partial hepatectomy for hepatoma. The AFP level decreased after the operation in some cases. In a typical case, AFP in the blood disappeared a month after the operation. From the AFP decay curve we calculated $T_{1/2}$ to be 6.0 days. These data were confirmed by the injection of ^{131}I-labeled AFP into a hepatoma patient (55-year-old male, AFP (+) hepatoma). From the rate of disappearance of radioactivity from the blood, we calculated the half-life of AFP as 6.2 days.

Experimental Studies on AFP

1. *α-Fetoprotein during hepatocarcinogenesis induced in rats by 4-dimethylaminoazobenzene (DAB)*

One of the important observations in our laboratory was the finding of a " primary reaction " in the course of experimental hepatocarcinogenesis in rats. We fed rats with a carcinogenic azo dye, DAB, and followed the appearance of AFP. Under the conditions employed in the experiment (continuous feeding with a synthetic diet containing 0.06% DAB), hepatoma usually developed after 4 months of dye ingestion. Unexpectedly, AFP began to appear in the blood in the 3rd week and increased to a peak at the 6th week. The AFP then decreased and disappeared by the 10th to 11th week. After the 12th week AFP reappeared, accompanied by hepatoma development.

The change of AFP level is shown in Fig. 2. The phenomenon of the early appearance of AFP was designated " primary reaction." In the period of the primary reaction no cancer cells could be observed. The details of the histological changes during the course are fully discussed by Onoe *et al.* in this volume.

Of 22 rats that showed the primary reaction, 20 developed hepatoma. These data indicated an intimate correlation between the appearance of the primary reaction and the development of hepatoma.

Another significant observation was made by Watabe. When the DAB-containing diet was replaced by a normal diet before the 7th week none of the

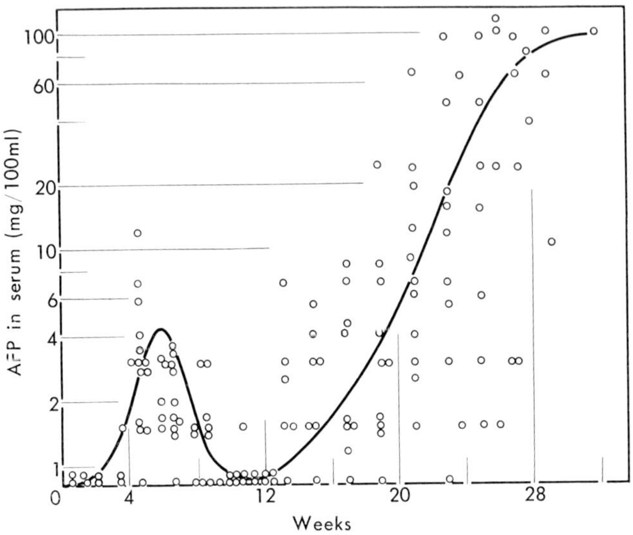

FIG. 2. α-Fetoprotein levels in rat serum during DAB carcinogenesis

Rats were fed synthetic standard diet containing 0.06% DAB for 30 weeks. Blood was collected every week from a tail vein. α-Fetoprotein was determined by Mancini's immunodiffusion method. No. of rats used was 20.

rats developed hepatoma, but when DAB feeding was stopped at the 11th week, hepatoma developed in all rats. This suggests that DAB feeding must continue throughout the period of the primary reaction for the development of hepatoma.

2. *α-Fetoprotein synthesis in cultured rat hepatoma cells*

Several cell lines of rat ascites hepatoma were cultured in the Eagle medium containing 20% newborn calf serum, and AFP and albumin secreted in the medium were determined. The results obtained by Tsukada in our laboratory are shown in Table VI. This experiment indicates that AFP is synthesized directly by hepatoma cells, and also that some strains synthesize AFP while others do not.

TABLE VI. α-Fetoprotein and Albumin Synthesis in Cell Culture

Strain	AFP	Albumin
AH-1091B	+	+
AH-1091C	+	+
AH-66	+	+
AH-49WH	+	+
AH-712	—	—
AH-782	—	—
YS	—	—
LY-176	+	—
LY-5	+	—

AH: Rat ascites hepatoma. YS: Yoshida sarcoma. LY-5: Mutant of YS. LY-176: Mutant of AH-66.

As discussed elsewhere in this volume by Watabe and Hirai, the transplantable ascites hepatoma cell lines we have were established from hepatoma nodules formed in a rat liver. All of these hepatomas in the rat liver synthesized AFP and secreted it into the blood stream, but after the establishment of the transplantable ascites hepatoma cell lines, some of the lines failed to produce AFP. This may probably be explained by the selection of AFP-nonproducing cells during serial transplantation.

This observation provides some of the evidence in support of the postulate of the mosaic structure of hepatoma as discussed previously.

Cloning experiments also confirm this supposition. One cell line, AH-66, is a strong AFP-producing ascites hepatoma. We have established 19 clones from this cell line employing a " single cell cloning " technique. Out of 19 clones, 15 synthesized AFP, but 4 synthesized none or only trace amounts.

DISCUSSION

Regarding the appearance of fetal components in cancer cells, several reports are available. The isozyme patterns of some enzymes are examples. Suda *et al.* (*17*) found that the muscle-type isozyme of pyruvate kinase constitutes the major fraction of this enzyme in the liver of fetal rats, but after birth the liver-type isozyme predominates. However, when hepatoma cells develop in the adult, the fetal-type isozyme (muscle-type) again becomes the major fraction. Essentially the same phenomena were observed in the isozyme patterns of aldolase (*14*, *16*) and hexokinase (*16*) in rat liver and hepatoma.

Gold and Freedman (*6*) reported that an antigenic substance specifically present in fetal digestive tract tissues but not in those of normal adult appeared again in neoplasma of the digestive tract. The substance was soluble in 0.6 M perchloric acid and was identified as a glycoprotein, which was designated by Gold as " carcinoembryonic antigen."

Burtin *et al.* (*3*) and Wada *et al.* (*18*) found some serum proteins which were designated by them as α_2H- and βs-globulins, respectively, which were present in sera of human fetuses or in patients with malignant tumors, but not in sera of healthy adult persons. Perhaps these substances, including the enzymes, the glycoprotein of Gold, and the serum proteins described above should be included together under the designation " carcinoembryonic proteins." The particular antigenic glycoprotein of Gold may be better called " Gold antigen."

The appearance of AFP may be observed in the sera of humans or animals in such situations as (1) hepatoma-bearing humans or animals, (2) hepatitis and liver cirrhosis patients, (3) DAB-intoxicated rats, (4) carbon tetrachloride-intoxicated rats or mice, and (5) partially hepatectomized rats or mice (regenerating liver).

The situations enumerated above more or less implicate injury of liver cells, and the animals (patients) respond to liver damage by regeneration and repair.

Returning to the experiment on DAB carcinogenesis in rats previously described. Administered DAB probably injures the liver cells in the first 3 weeks, and this is followed by regeneration of liver cells. The synthesis of AFP started

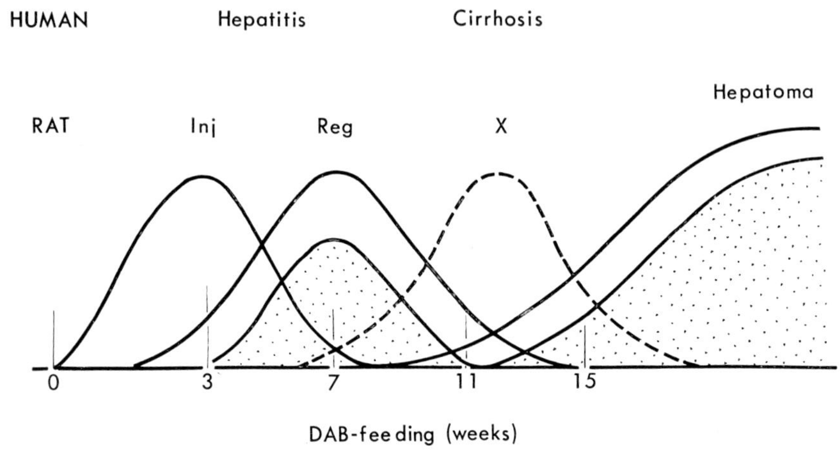

FIG. 3. Hypothetical incident during hepatocarcinogenesis

Inj: Injured liver cells. Reg: Regenerative liver cells. X: Transformed liver cells. Dotted area: Serum levels of AFP.

in the 3rd week, as shown in Fig. 2, presumably being associated with the onset of regeneration. Regeneration is most active in the 6th week but the toxicity of DAB continues to exert an effect on the regenerative cells, resulting in the suspension of AFP synthesis. The carcinogenic action of DAB will eventually cause the transformation of regenerative cells. At the 10–11th week, the synthesis of AFP stops and the transformed cells begin to acquire malignancy.

As described earlier, the administration of DAB must be continued until the 10–11th week, when the primary reaction is completed. This fact may be interpreted as indicating that DAB must act on dividing cells to cause malignant change. Figure 3 shows this speculative sequence of events schematically.

Hepatitis in human patients may correspond to the injury and regeneration phase indicated in Fig. 3. Liver cirrhosis may be placed after the stage of hepatitis. Actually, AFP levels in cirrhotic patients, determined by radioimmunoassay, seemed to be rather lower than in hepatitis patients. Abelev (*1*) could not detect AFP at all in the sera of cirrhotic patients by the immunoradioautograph technique, although it was detectable in sera from hepatitis patients. From these observations, part of the cirrhotic stage in patients may be thought of as corresponding to the 10–11th week phase in the rat experiment.

The transformed cells, designated " X " in Fig. 3, are not identified. Most of the cells in the liver in the 10–11th week of DAB ingestion do not synthesize AFP. The cells appear to be different from either normal regenerating liver cells or hepatoma cells, but are probably readily transformable to malignant cells. It might be possible to find such cells in the cirrhotic livers of patients.

The speculative scheme in Fig. 3, however, does not provide answers to the following questions: (1) Is AFP synthesized in the regenerative cells and in hepatoma cells the same in each case? (2) why do regenerative cells convert readily to malignant cells? and (3) what is the difference between fetal and regenerative liver cells?

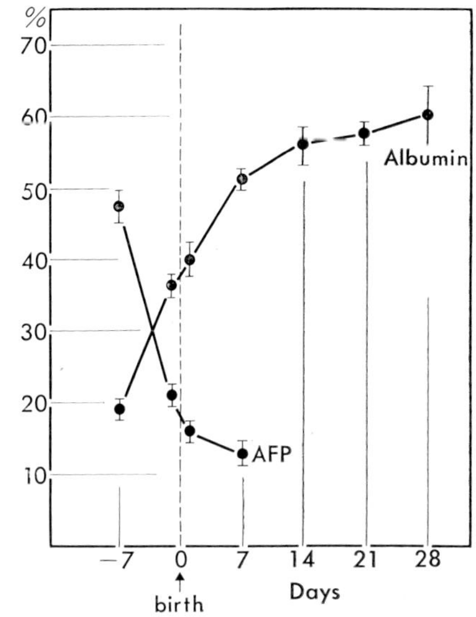

FIG. 4. Change of albumin and AFP in rat serum before and after birth (*19*)
The proteins, measured electrophoretically, are expressed as percent of total serum protein. The AFP was detected until the 28th day by the immunodiffusion method.

Many more clinical, experimental, and histological observations must be accumulated to elucidate the correlation between hepatocarcinogenesis and AFP synthesis.

The physiological role of AFP is not yet known at all, like albumin. Figure 4 indicates the rise and fall of AFP and albumin levels in rats determined by electrophoresis and precipitin reaction by Watabe *et al.* (*19*). A characteristic inverse relationship was observed, similar to that between hemoglobin F and A. This suggests that AFP plays a role in the fetus corresponding to the role of albumin in the adult. The amino acid compositions of AFP and albumin are, however, quite different, as shown in Table III. The proteins might not be related. More precise analysis of the primary structure of these proteins is definitely necessary for their comparison.

The species specificity of AFP is quite low, as shown in Photo 4. This suggests that, phylogenically, it is rather an immature protein. Synthesis of such immature proteins may be one element of the biochemical evidence for the anaplastic feature of cancer cells.

REFERENCES

1. Abelev, G. I. α-Fetoprotein production by normal liver and liver tumors. *Protides Biol. Fluids*, **18**, 203–209 (1971).
2. Axén, R., Porath, J., and Ernback, S. Chemical coupling of peptides and proteins to polysaccharides by means of cyanogen halides. *Nature*, **214**, 1302 (1967).
3. Burtin, P., von Kleist, S., and Buffe, D. Étude sur les antigènes foetauk

humaines. I. Étude immunoélectrophorétique des antigènes du sérum fetal humaine absents du sérum adulte. *Bull. Soc. Chim. Biol.*, **49**, 1389–1398 (1967).
4. Endo, Y., Etoh, S., and Oda, S. Clinical significance of α_1-fetoglobulin (in Japanese). *Naika (Internal Medicine)*, **24**, 24–28 (1969).
5. Gitlin, D. and Boesman, M. Fetus-specific proteins in several mammals and their relation to human α-fetoprotein. *Comp. Biochem. Physiol.*, **21**, 327–336 (1967).
6. Gold, P. and Freedman, S. O. Demonstration of tumour-specific antigens in human colonic carcinomata by immunological tolerance and absorption techniques. *J. Exp. Med.*, **121**, 439–462 (1965).
7. Hirai, H. Specific antigenic protein(s) of rat ascites hepatoma. *In* "Tumor-Specific Antigens (UICC Monograph)," ed. by H. J. Harris, Munksgaard, Copenhagen, Vol. 2, pp. 42–66 (1967).
8. Mancini, G., Carbonara, A. O., and Heremans, J. F. Immunochemical quantitation of antigens by single radial immunodiffusion. *Int. J. Immunochem.*, **2**, 235–254 (1965).
9. Nishi, S. Isolation and characterization of a fetal α-globulin from sera of fetuses and a hepatoma patient. *Cancer Res.*, **30**, 2507–2513 (1970).
10. Nishi, S. and Hirai, H. Purification of human, dog and rabbit α-fetoprotein by immunoadsorbents of Sepharose coupled with anti-human α-fetoprotein. *Biochim. Biophys. Acta*, **278**, 293–298 (1972).
11. Nishi, S., Watabe, H., and Hirai, H. Immunological cross-reactivity of α-fetoprotein of several mammals (in Japanese). *Seibutsu-Butsuri-Kagaku (Physicochem. Biol.)*, **16**, 79–82 (1971).
12. Nishi, S., Watabe, H., and Hirai, H. Production of antibody to homologous α-fetoprotein in rabbits, rats and horses by immunization with human α-fetoprotein. *J. Immunol.*, **109**, 957–960 (1972).
13. Ruoslahti, E., Seppälä, M., Pihko, H., and Vuopio, P. Studies of carcinofetal Proteins. II. Biochemical comparison of α-fetoprotein from human fetuses and patients with hepatocellular cancer. *Int. J. Cancer*, **8**, 283–288 (1971).
14. Schapira, F., Dreyfus, J. C., and Schapira, G. Anomaly of aldolase in primary liver cancer. *Nature*, **200**, 995–997 (1963).
15. Schlutze, H. E. and Heremans, J. F. *In* "Molecular Biology of Human Proteins," Elsevier Publishing Co., Amsterdam-London-New York, Vol. 1, p. 182 (1966).
16. Sugimura, T., Matsushima, T., Kawachi, T., Hirata, Y., and Kawabe, S. Molecular species of aldolase and hexokinase in experimental hepatomas. *GANN Monograph*, **1**, 143–149 (1966).
17. Suda, M., Tanaka, T., Sue, F., Harano, Y., and Morimura, H. Dedifferentiation of sugar metabolism in the liver of tumour-bearing rat. *GANN Monograph*, **1**, 127–141 (1966).
18. Wada, T., Anzai, A., Yachi, A., Takahashi, A., and Sakamoto, S. Incidence of three different fetal proteins in sera of patients with primary hepatoma. *Protides Biol. Fluids*, **18**, 221–226 (1971).
19. Watabe, H., Hirai, H., and Satoh H. α-Fetoprotein in rats transplanted with ascites hepatoma. *GANN*, **63**, 189–199 (1972).

EXPLANATION OF PHOTOS

PHOTO 1. Crystals of human AFP

α-Fetoprotein was purified from a hepatoma patient serum and crystallized in 2.3 M ammonium sulfate solution at pH 7.

PHOTO 2. Ouchterlony test for AFP

Anti-AFP: Horse antiserum against human fetal AFP.

Hepatoma: Serum of a patient with hepatoma.

Hepatitis: Serum of a patient with hepatitis.

Metastasis: Serum of a patient with metastatic liver cancer (original: gastric cancer).

Cirrhosis: Serum of a patient with liver cirrhosis.

Adult: Serum of a healthy adult man.

Fetus: Serum of a human fetus, 5 months gestation.

PHOTO 3. Immunological identity of AFP in sera of human fetus and hepatoma patient

Fetus: Fetal serum. Hepatoma: Serum of a hepatoma patient. Anti-AFP hepatoma: Antiserum of rabbits immunized with AFP of hepatoma patient. Anti-AFP fetus: Antiserum of rabbits immunized with AFP of human fetuses.

PHOTO 4. Cross-reactivity of AFP from various animals

Anti-human AFP serum (aAFP) is placed in the center well and fetal sera of various animals are placed in peripheral wells.

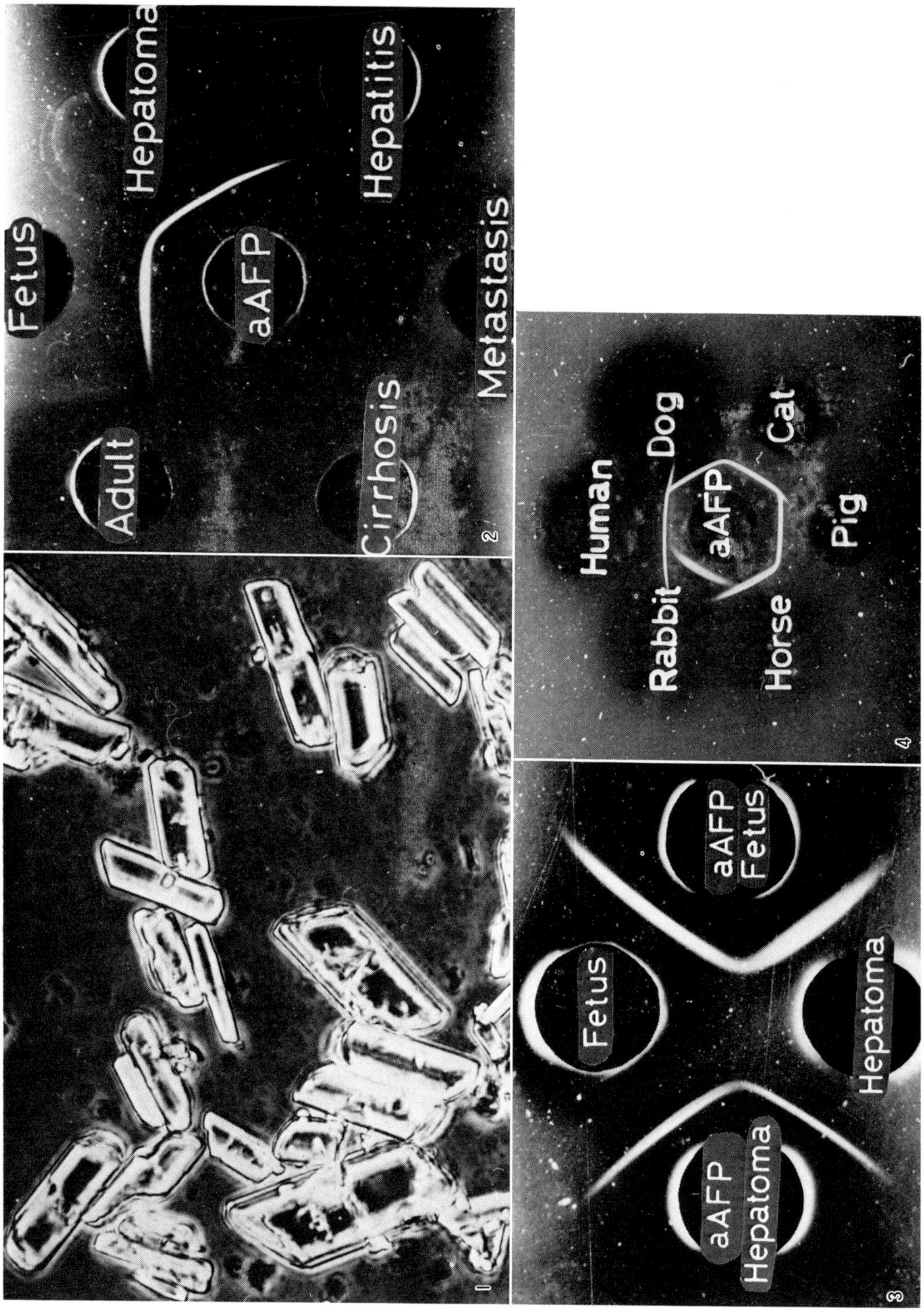
1
2
Fetus
Hepatoma
aAFP
Adult
Cirrhosis
Hepatitis
Metastasis
3
aAFP
Fetus
Fetus
Hepatoma
aAFP
Hepatoma
4
Human
Dog
Rabbit
aAFP
Cat
Horse
Pig

GANN Monograph on Cancer Research 14, 1973

AN OUTLINE OF THE PHYSIOPATHOLOGY OF RAT α-FETOPROTEIN

J. URIEL and B. de NECHAUD
Institut de Recherches Scientifiques sur le Cancer[*1]

The present contribution reviews the major facts of our present knowledge on the physiopathology of rat liver α-fetoprotein (AFP).

The physicochemical, immunological, and biological properties of this fetospecific serum protein are outlined. Special attention is given to the recent discovery of the estrogen-binding activity of AFP of rodents and man, an observation which probably opens a new way to approach the unresolved problem of its physiological significance during ontogenesis and early postnatal life.

The dynamics of the synthesis and secretion of rat AFP in fetuses, newborn, and young animals are presented in detail and discussed in connection with the reappearance of AFP in adult serum during early phase of experimental liver injury and in the course of neoplastic transformation with chemical carcinogens. The liver synthesis and the serum secretion of AFP in adults do not appear as intrinsic of malignancy because waves of secretion can be demonstrated in the absence of any anatomical or histological sign of tumor. Nevertheless, if the specificity of the association between AFP and hepatocellular carcinoma is not absolute, the search for the protein remains of high diagnostic value in both chemical and experimental work.

Since the discovery of fetuin by Pedersen in 1944 (*28*) and its designation as an α-globulin present in fetal calf serum but absent in the serum of adult animals, proteins with fetospecific character have been found in all mammalian fetal sera that have been examined.

These fetospecific serum proteins, like fetal hemoglobin, belong to a general class of biological constituents that we have proposed to designate transitory cell antigens (*40*); they are normal synthetic products expressed during a transient period of the overall process of differentiation and maturation of multicellular organisms.

The interest in the study of serum fetoproteins increased greatly when Abelev and his co-workers reported, in 1963 (*3*), the reappearance of a fetospecific α-globulin, at present known as α-fetoprotein (AFP)[*2] in the blood of mice bearing chemically induced hepatomas.

Analogous associations between AFP and liver tumors were confirmed and

[*1] B.P. No. 8, 94-Villejuif, France.

[*2] The terminology used here is that recommended by WHO (World Health Organization Bulletin, No. 43, 309 (1970)). See also Refs. (*4*) and (*40*).

extended to experimental rat hepatomas by our group in Villejuif (*35*) and to hepatocellular carcinoma in man, first by Tatarinov (*36*), and then by others (*2*, *4*, *31*, *39*). A useful application of these findings has been the development of a serological test for the diagnosis of primary liver cancer in humans, now of well-recognized value (*27*).

Very recently, the discovery of the estrogen-binding properties of AFP from different species (*25*, *37*) has opened a new approach to the unresolved question of its physiological significance during ontogenesis and early postnatal life.

In addition to the abundant literature, several reviews on AFP, particularly of human origin, have been published in the last year (*1*, *21*). The subject will also be extensively treated in this monograph. We will limit our contribution here to an outline of our present knowledge of the physicochemical and biological properties of rat AFP, as well as the kinetics of its secretion and synthesis under physiological and/or experimentally induced pathological situations.

Properties of Rat AFP

1. General

The fetospecific character of rat AFP was first demonstrated by Abelev *et al.* (*3*) and by Stanislawski-birencwajg (*33*) using gel immunodiffusion methods. Rat AFP, as its counterparts in other mammalian sera, possesses several general properties which allow its definition as the first α-globulin to appear in mammalian sera during ontogenic development; the dominant serum protein in early embryonic life. It reappears in the serum of adult animals in several situations, principally in patients or animals with " hepatocellular carcinoma " (WHO Bulletin, No. 13, 309 (1970)).

The recent demonstration (*25*, *37*) of specific binding ability of AFP for estrogens of rats, mice, and man constitutes an additional general property of these fetospecific proteins.

2. Physicochemical and immunological

Rat AFP, like its counterparts in man and monkeys, has an electrophoretic mobility and a molecular weight similar to that of albumin. These properties make conventional methods of fractionation and isolation, such as salting out, ion-exchange, or gel filtration chromatography, partially inadequate, at least for achieving an efficient purification of the fetoprotein. Thus the isolation must be totally carried out or completed by immunoadsorbents (*16*, *24*, *34*).

Native rat AFP from purified preparations of biological fluids appears homogeneous after agar electrophoresis and immunoelectrophoresis (*34*). Nevertheless, electrophoresis on sieving gels (starch, polyacrylamide, *etc.*) under appropriate conditions shows at least two close but distinct bands in both native and isolated preparations (*cf.* Refs. *5*, *16*, *18*, *42*, and Fig. 1). Although more work and additional information are needed to ascertain its electrophoretic behavior, it can be proposed that such heterogeneity seems not to be due to genetic variants, an explanation given for human AFP heterogeneity. The two electro-

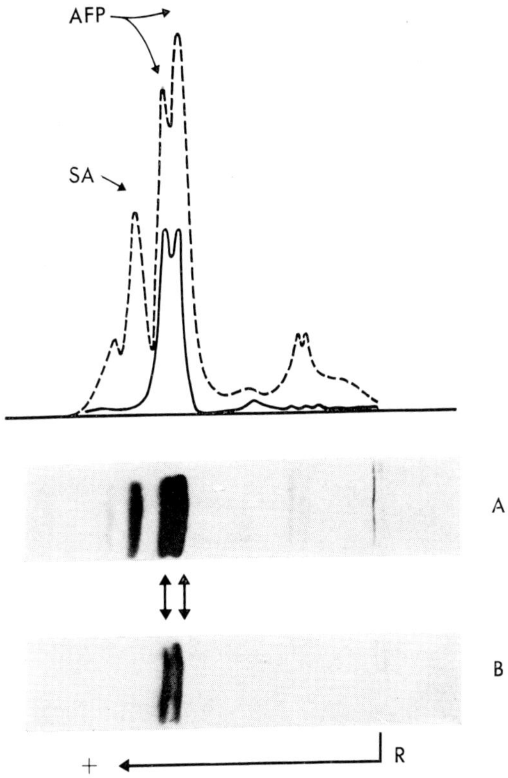

FIG. 1. Electrophoretic separation in acrylamide-agarose gels (11% polyacrylamide; 0.8% agarose) of rat amniotic fluid (A) and a purified preparation of AFP from the same origin

Top: Photometric scanning of electrophoregrams (A), and (B) serum albumin (SA) and AFP bands are indicated by arrows (*5*).

phoretic bands of rat AFP have been observed in pooled as well as in individual samples of amniotic fluid and fetal sera.

Finally, using immuno-autoradiographic techniques, some immunological cross-reactivity has been demonstrated between rat, man, and monkey AFP (*30*). Cross-reactions of different extent have also been observed between other species. It is probable that all types of AFP bear some common antigenic determinants.

3. Biological

Recent studies on the estrogen-binding ability of fetal and newborn rat serum as well as the serum from pregnant rats (*25*, *26*, *32*) have led to the demonstration by immunological methods of the estrophilic properties of AFP (*37*).

Figure 2 shows the immunoelectrophoretic pattern of rat serum fetospecific proteins: AFP, α_M-fetoprotein, and lipoprotein esterase.* After incubation in 4-^{14}C-estradiol, two of the three fetoproteins appear radio-labeled (Fig. 2,B),

* LA-protein, α-macroglobulin, and lipoprotein esterase, respectively, in Stanislawski's terminology (*34*).

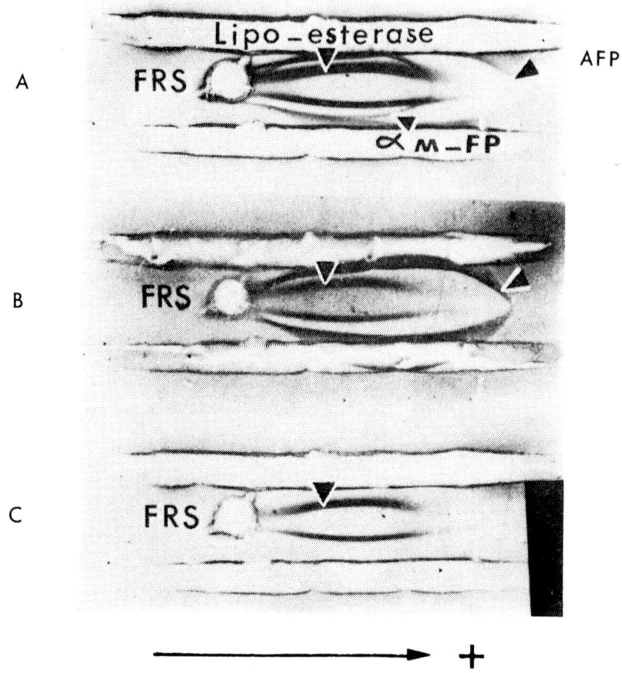

Fig. 2. Immuno-autoradiographic assay for the identification of estradiol-binding fetospecific proteins in fetal serum (FRS)

Immunoelectrophoretic pattern obtained with a rabbit antiserum to feto-specific rat serum proteins. (A) Protein staining (Amido Black). (B) Autoradiograph. (C) Lipid staining (Sudan Black). AFP, α-fetoprotein; α_M-FP, α_M-fetoprotein; lipo-esterase, lipoprotein esterase. From Uriel *et al.* (*37*).

namely, AFP and lipoprotein esterase, the latter easily recognizable by its sudanophilic properties (Fig. 2,C). No estradiol-binding activity was associated with the α_M-fetoprotein.

The experiment illustrated in Fig. 3 shows the binding properties of other serum proteins in fetal and adult rats. An anti-fetal rat serum was used for the immunoelectrophoretic assays. This antiserum revealed, in addition to the three fetoproteins, a large number of other proteins common to adult and fetal rat sera (Fig. 3,A). The immuno-autoradiographic pattern of fetal serum shows the expected radio-labeling of the two fetoproteins (bottom of Fig. 3,B). However, all the other proteins in the immuno-pattern lack the ability to bind estradiol.

Similar results were obtained when 4-^{14}C-estrone, instead of estradiol, was used for the immuno-autoradiographic assays. In mouse and human fetal serum and in the serum of a patient bearing a hepatocellular carcinoma, AFP showed the same estrogen-binding ability. On the other hand, the AFP from the three species examined appears devoid of affinity for testosterone, progesterone, or cortisol.

Rat, human, and mouse fetal and adult lipoproteins bind indiscriminately the five hormones examined, probably due to the lipophilic affinity of steroids. The strength of the association seems, however, much less than that of the estrogen-

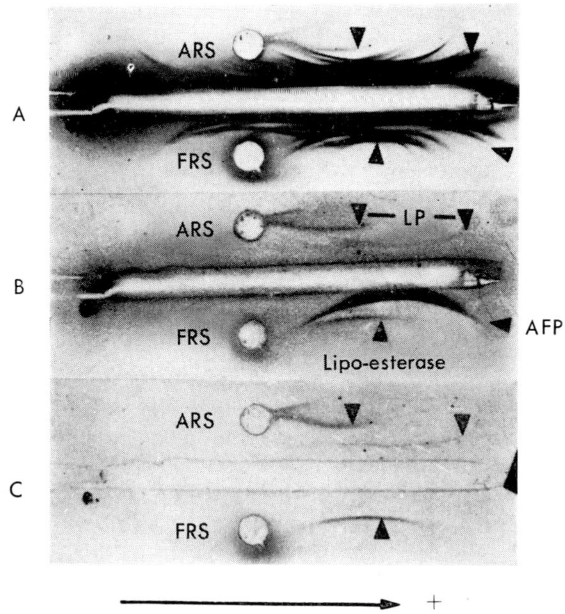

FIG. 3. Immuno-autoradiographic assay for the identification of estradiol-binding proteins in adult and fetal rat sera

Immunoelectrophoretic pattern obtained with a rabbit antiserum to newborn rat serum. (A) Protein staining (Amido Black). (B) Autoradiograph. (C) Lipid staining (Sudan Black). ARS, FRS: Adult and fetal rat serum, respectively. LP, lipoproteins; AFP, α-fetoprotein; lipo-esterase, lipoprotein-esterase. From Uriel *et al.* (*37*).

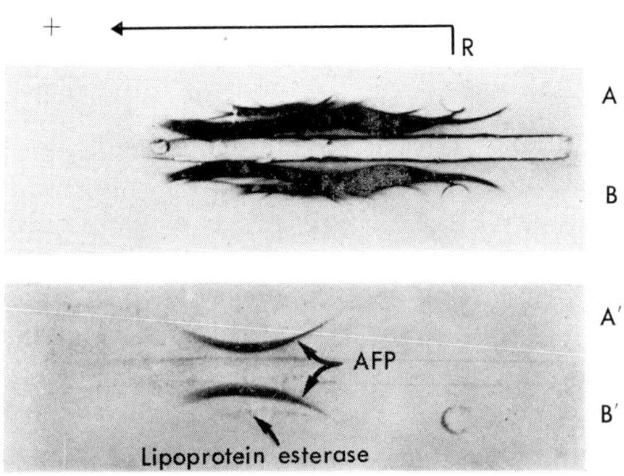

FIG. 4. Estrone-binding ability of newborn rat serum

Aliquots of a serum from a 2-day-old rat were incubated with different amounts of 4-^{14}C-estrone (0.2 and 1 μCi/ml of serum) for 2 hr at 37°. The samples were then subjected to immunoelectrophoresis using a rabbit anti-fetal rat serum. After development of immune precipitates (24 hr), the plate was washed in buffered saline for 24 hr, dried in air under filter paper, and put in contact (2 to 3 weeks) with a Kodak Regulix-HS radiographic film.

Top: Protein staining (Amido Black) of immunoelectrophoretic patterns of samples A and B (0.2 and 1 μCi/ml of serum, respectively). Bottom: Autoradiographs of the same samples.

AFP complex, as can be concluded from the experiment illustrated in Fig. 4, where different concentrations of 4-^{14}C-estrone were added to the same volume of rat fetal serum before the immunoelectrophoretic assay. The lipoprotein esterase appears radio-labeled only after saturation of the estrogen-AFP complex (Fig. 4,B′).

The physiological significance of the estrophilic properties of AFP is still unknown. However, increasing information points to the involvement of steroids in cell differentiation processes. One can propose, for instance, that during ontogenesis and by its estrophilic ability, AFP "protects," in some way, the embryo from maternal estrogens (*25*) or exerts some regulatory effect as an intermediate carrier between free hormones and target cells or tissues. In connection with this, it is interesting to point out that the physiological disappearance of rat serum AFP in young animals closely precedes the onset of sexual maturation.

Much more work, indeed, will be necessary in this promising area before the elucidation of what still appears, at present, as an intriguing property.

Synthesis and Secretion of Rat AFP

The hepatic origin of AFP from rats, mice, man, and other mammals is at present well established.*1 *In vivo* and *in vitro* studies of incorporation of radio-labeled amino acids in AFP synthesized by liver slices (*13*, *43*), liver organ cultures (*20*), or perfused livers (*17*) strongly support this conclusion. Additional evidence is provided by the intracellular localization of AFP using immunofluorescence techniques (*11*, *14*).

1. In ontogenesis and postnatal life

The starting date of embryonic synthesis of rat AFP, like that of other mammals, is unknown. Gitlin and Boesman (*13*) demonstrated that the yolk sac from developing rats incorporates ^{14}C-amino acids in AFP. It is possible, as suggested by Abelev (*1*), that this organ is the initial site of AFP synthesis.

Radioimmunodiffusion assays of serum samples following intraperitoneal injection of radio-labeled amino acids in pregnant rats and newborn animals have enabled us to demonstrate AFP synthesis from the middle of pregnancy to delivery and during postnatal life until arrest of synthesis, which, under physiological conditions, occurs on the 27th day (*8*).

More abundant data are available on AFP secretion into blood and amniotic fluid (*8*, *29*). In Fig. 5, serum levels of AFP and albumin in growing fetuses and newborn animals are plotted. Quantitation was carried out by the electroimmunodiffusion technique of Laurell (*19*) with monospecific antisera. As is shown, AFP increases up to the 18th day of gestation, declines for 24 hr, then increases again to attain the highest level the day before parturition. Newborn levels decrease progressively, disappearing on the thirtieth to thirty-second day.*2 In the same period a stepwise increase of albumin is observed with adult levels at-

*1 For a detailed bibliography see Ref. (*1*).

*2 In our experimental conditions the lowest concentration of AFP that can be estimated is about 200 ng/ml.

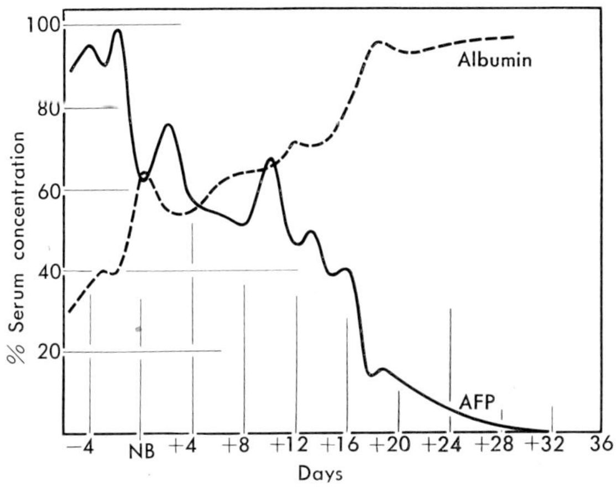

FIG. 5. Serum concentrations of rat albumin and AFP during ontogenesis and postnatal life
NB refers to newborn. Reproduced from Uriel *et al.* (*37*).

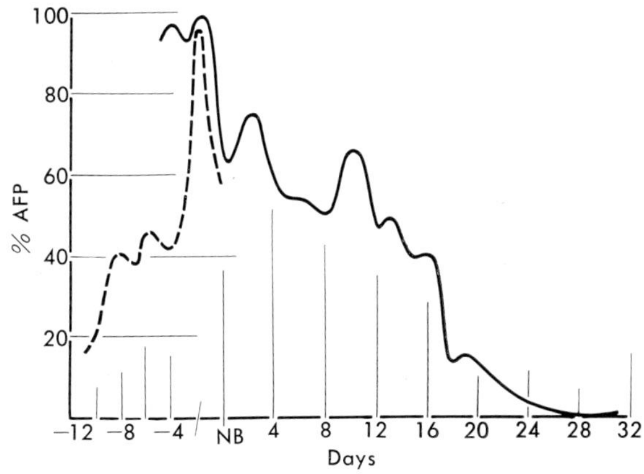

FIG. 6. Comparative curves of AFP secretion in serum and amniotic fluid
——rat AFP in serum; - - - - rat AFP in amniotic fluid.

tained as soon as 3 weeks after birth. The two curves intersect at the end of the first week.

Figure 6 shows comparative curves of AFP levels in serum and amniotic fluid. The serum concentrations of AFP in pregnant rats are represented in Fig. 7. After parturition, the AFP declines rapidly and disappears from the serum 4 to 6 days later. This interval gives an estimation of the half-life of the protein which correlates well with the delay between the time of arrest of AFP synthesis in young animals (27th day) and the time when AFP becomes undetectable in serum (30–32nd day).

2. *In the early phase of experimental liver injury*

As indicated above, the synthesis and secretion of rat AFP follow, under physiological conditions, well-defined patterns. In normal adult mice, a tran-

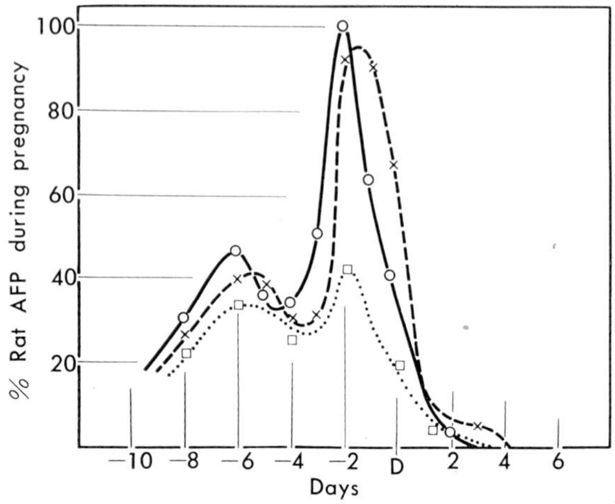

FIG. 7. α-Fetoprotein levels in the serum of three pregnant rats and after delivery (D)

Reproduced from Uriel *et al.* (*37*).

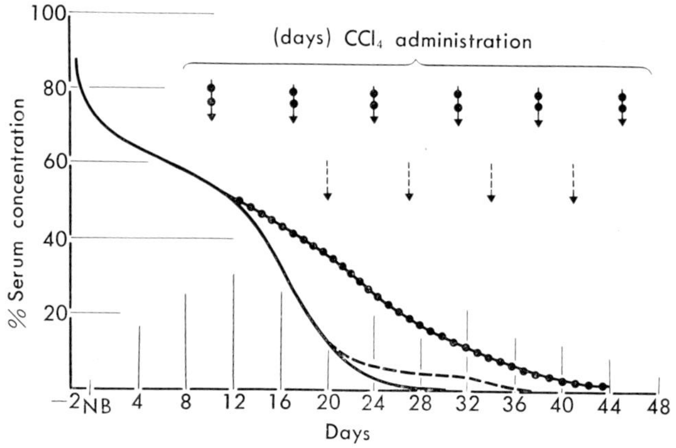

FIG. 8. Serum levels of AFP after serial injections of CCl_4 to rats aged 10 days (●) and 20 days (- - - -) at the beginning of treatment

The continuous line is the reference curve. Each curve represents the average values obtained from 10 animals. Serum samples were taken every 2 days and analyzed for AFP content.

Reproduced from Uriel *et al.* (*37*).

sitory secretion of AFP was demonstrated after partial hepatectomy (*3*) or carbon tetrachloride administration (*7*).

Using immunoautoradiographic methods and three- to fourfold concentrated serum samples* the temporary reappearance of AFP was also observed in adult rats after partial hepatectomy (*30*). Intraperitoneal injections of CCl_4, $CdSO_4$, or D-galactosamine to newborn and young rats change the normal pattern of

* Under these conditions serum concentrations of AFP as low as 50 to 100 ng/ml can be estimated.

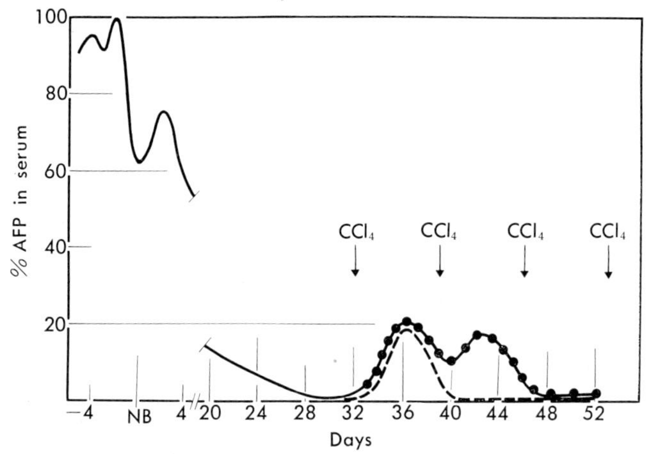

FIG. 9. Reappearance of AFP in the serum of young rats under serial injections of CCl_4 started at 32 days of age
Reproduced from Uriel *et al.* (*37*).

AFP diminution (*8*). Thus, depending on the precocity of the treatment (Fig. 8), the date of disappearance from serum of AFP takes place one to several weeks later than the normal limit of 30 days. On the other hand, if serial injections of CCl_4 at 8–10 day intervals are administered to rats aged between 32 and 50 days (a time when AFP is no longer detectable in serum) one or several waves of AFP secretion can be observed. The AFP was detected 48 hr after the first injection, reached a maximum on the third or fourth day, and disappeared from circulation in approximately 1 week, unless a second injection was given (Fig. 9). Disregarding the number of CCl_4 injections, one or several, but never more than three, waves of AFP were observed. No AFP was detected in serum when CCl_4 treatment was started in rats older than 7 weeks.

On the contrary, more drastic effects were obtained with another hepatotoxin, dimethylnitrosoamine (DMN). One single injection of DMN induces the transitory secretion of AFP in rats until the age of 10 weeks, and serial injections of the same substance delay the disappearance of AFP until the age of 3 months (2 months later than the " physiological " date of AFP disappearance (*9*)).

The explanation of the results outlined above is still unclear, and further work should be done in this area of great interest to elucidate the major problem of AFP association with hepatocellular carcinoma.

The *de novo* synthesis of AFP secreted into blood during acute liver injury has been demonstrated by the incorporation in the protein of ^{14}C radio-labeled amino acids and its inhibition by cycloheximide (*9*). In spite of this, the question remains as to whether this synthesis reflects a true derepression of a switched-off gene or the amplification of some undetectable background of AFP synthesis by normal adult liver.

Experiments on intracellular localization of AFP-synthesizing hepatocytes has proved (*12*) that only a very small proportion of the entire population is involved in AFP production during the acute phase of liver regeneration. Nevertheless, the exact nature and functional state of these AFP-positive cells is unknown. Assuming that liver differentiation and maturation are not processes affecting synchronously the whole population of hepatic parenchymal cells, it has been suggested that the induced secretion of AFP by hepatotoxins is a consequence of the enhanced activity of some incompletely differentiated cell clones (*8*).

3. In neoplastic transformation

The reappearance of AFP in rodents and in humans bearing hepatocellular carcinomas is at present a fact of general acceptance which allows us to consider this protein a " tumor-associated antigen." While the specificity of the association is not absolute (*1*, *21*, *38*), the diagnostic value for primary hepatoma of the presence of AFP in both clinical and experimental situations has been recognized by all workers in the field.

In rats the frequency of the association between AFP and hepatocellular carcinoma varies according to the carcinogen used (Table I), and is, with the exception of aflatoxin B, quite high (*35*). As reported by Stanislawski, this frequency also changes from one group of animals to another, even under analogous experimental conditions. More recent studies suggest, however, some relationship between age and frequency of AFP-positive tumors, the latter being higher in animals who were started on the carcinogenic diet at a younger age (*10*). This point is to be related to observations made in humans, establishing an analogous relationship between age and incidence of serum AFP (*6*, *22*).

TABLE I. Frequency of AFP Appearance in Primary Hepatomas Induced in Rats by Several Carcinogens

Carcinogen		Ref.
DAB[a]	22/28	(*35*)
3′-Me-DAB[a]	78/94	(*35*)
DMN[a]	1/2	(*35*)
Aflatoxin B_1	0/15	(*35*)
Aflatoxin B_1	0/60	(*23*)

[a] DAB=4-dimethylaminoazobenzene; 3′-Me-DAB=3′-methyl-4-dimethylaminoazobenzene; DMN=dimethylnitrosoamine.

On the other hand, a comparison of the histologic variety of hepatoma and the presence of AFP in the serum yielded no clear-cut evidence favoring an association with a well-defined morphologic type of tumor. Moreover, there were cases where one or several tumor nodules of the same liver contained AFP, while others did not (*35*).

In transplantation experiments the pattern of AFP incidence apparently reflects that of the primary tumor. Thus, one line of AFP-positive tumor was followed during 75 generations and 4 other lines during 26 generations. The serum titer of AFP remained constant in the transplanted animals. In contrast, AFP never appeared in the sera of animals transplanted with AFP-negative tumors (*35*).

The specificity of the association between AFP and hepatoma seems excellent although the number of cases studied was relatively low (*35*). α-Fetoprotein was absent from the sera of animals bearing bile duct carcinoma or tumors of nonhepatic origin (*35*).

The dynamics of serum secretion of AFP in animals undergoing neoplastic liver transformation when subjected to carcinogenic diets shows great individual differences. However, as observed by Watabe (*41*) and by ourselves (*10*), a wave of AFP secretion can be demonstrated 2 to 3 weeks after the beginning of the diet and in the absence of any histological or anatomical signs of liver tumor. After a period of time of variable length during which the fetoprotein disappears from the serum, one or several new waves of secretion are detectable, followed in many cases by constant levels of AFP secretion. At this time hepatoma nodules are already present.

Different hypotheses have been proposed to explain the reappearance of AFP in primary hepatoma (*4*, *15*, *40*); it is, however, out of the scope of this paper to discuss them. As a conclusion one can say that many points remain unsolved in the physiopathology of AFP, particularly those concerning its physiological significance during ontogenesis and early postnatal life, and its association with liver carcinoma. Nevertheless, the active work which is at present being pursued in these areas permits us to hope for fruitful developments in the near future.

Acknowledgments
The authors are indebted to Mr. Sheldon Glazer for his assistance in preparing this manuscript.

REFERENCES

1. Abelev, G. I. α-Fetoprotein in ontogenesis and its association with malignant tumors. *Adv. Cancer Res.*, **14**, 295 (1971).
2. Abelev, G. I., Assecritova, I. V., Kraevsky, N. A., Perova, S. D., and Perevodchikova, N. I. Embryonal serum α-globulin in cancer patients: Diagnostic value. *Int. J. Cancer*, **2**, 551 (1967).
3. Abelev, G. I., Perova, S. D., Khramkova, N. I., Postnikova, Z. A., and Irlin, I. S. Production of embryonal α-globulin by the transplantable mouse hepatomas. *Transplant. Bull.*, **1**, 174, (1963).
4. Abelev, G. I. Production of embryonal serum α-globulin by hepatomas: Review of experimental and clinical data. *Cancer Res.*, **88**, 1344 (1968).
5. Aussel, Cl. and Uriel, J. Unpublished results.
6. Bagshawe, A. and Parker, A. M. Age distribution of α-fetoprotein in hepatocellular carcinoma. *Lancet*, **2**, 268 (1970).
7. Bakirov, R. D. Appearance of embryonal serum α-globulin in adult mice after inhalation of carbon tetrachloride. *Byull. Eksp. Biol. Med.*, **2**, 45 (1968).
8. de Nechaud, B. and Uriel, J. Antigènes cellulaires transitoires du foie de rat. I. Sécrétions et synthèse des protéines sériques foetospécifiques au cours du développement et de la régénération hépatique. *Int. J. Cancer*, **8**, 71 (1971).
9. de Nechaud, B. and Uriel, J. Antigènes cellulaires transitoires du foie de rat. II. Effet des inhibiteurs de synthèse sur les foetoprotéines sériques à la fin du premier mois de vie et après intoxication hépatique aiguë. *Int. J. Cancer*, **10**, 58 (1972).

10. de Nechaud, B. and Uriel, J. Antigènes cellulaires transitoires du foie de rat. III. Mode de réapparition de l'α-foetoprotéine au cours de l'hépatocarcinogénèse chimique. *Int. J. Cancer*, **11**, 104 (1973).
11. Engelhardt, N. V., Gusev, A. I., Shipova, L. J., and Abelev, G. I. Immunofluorescent study of α-fetoprotein in liver and liver tumors. *Int. J. Cancer*, **7**, 198 (1971).
12. Engelhardt, N. V., Shipova, L. J., Gusev, A. I., Jazova, A. K., and Ter-Grigorova, E. N. Immunohistochemical detection of α-fetoglobulin on sections of the liver of human embryo and new-born mice. *Byull. Eksp. Biol. Med.*, **12**, 62 (1969).
13. Gitlin, D. and Boesman, M. Sites of serum α-fetoprotein synthesis in the human and in the rat. *J. Clin. Invest.*, **46**, 1010 (1967).
14. Gitlin, D., Ketzes, J., and Boesman, M. Cellular distribution of serum fetoprotein in organs of the fetal rat. *Nature*, **215**, 534 (1967).
15. Grabar, P. Introduction remarks on fetal proteins and their reappearance in tumors. *Protides Biol. Fluids*, **18**, 201 (1970).
16. Gusev, A. I. and Jazova, A. K. Isolation and purification of embryospecific α-globulins of man and animals by the method of preparative disc electrophoresis in polyacrylamide gels. *Biokhimiya*, **35**, 172 (1970).
17. Kekomäki, M., Seppälä, M., Ehnholm, C., Schwartz, A., and Raivio, K. Perfusion of isolated human fetal liver: Synthesis and release of α-fetoprotein and albumin. *Int. J. Cancer*, **8**, 250 (1971).
18. Kirsh, I., Wise, R., and Oliver, I. Post albumin, a foetal specific rat plasma protein. Purification, physicochemical and immunological studies. *Biochem. J.*, **102**, 763 (1967).
19. Laurell, G. B. Quantitative estimation of proteins by electrophoresis in agarose gels containing antibodies. *Annu. Biochem.*, **15**, 45 (1966).
20. Luria, E. A., Bakirov, R. D., Yeliseyeva, T. A., Abelev, G. I., and Fridenstein, A. I. Differentiation of hepatic and hematopoietic cells and synthesis of blood serum proteins in organ cultures of the liver. *Exp. Cell. Res.*, **54**, 111 (1969).
21. Masseyeff, R. Human α-fetoprotein. *Pathol. Biol.*, **20**, 703 (1972).
22. Mawas, C., Buffe, D., and Burtin, P. Influence of age on α-fetoprotein incidence. *Lancet*, **1**, 1292 (1970).
23. Monjour, L. and Mariage, C. Antigènes embryonnaires et aflatoxine. *C. R. Biol.*, **163**, 1288 (1969).
24. Nishi, S. Isolation and characterization of a human fetal α-globulin from the sera of fetuses and a hepatoma patient. *Cancer Res.*, **30**, 2507 (1970).
25. Nunez, E., Engelmann, F., Benassayag, C., and Jayle, M-F. Identification et purification préliminaire de la foetoprotéine liant les oestrogènes dans le sérum des rats nouveau-nés. *C. R.*, **273**, 831 (1971).
26. Nunez, E., Engelmann, F., Benassayag, C., Savu, L., Crepy, O., and Jayle, M-F. Mise en évidence d'une fraction protéique liant les oestrogènes dans le sérum de rats impubères. *C. R.*, **272**, 2396 (1971).
27. O'Conor, G. T., Tatarinov, Y. S., Abelev, G. I., and Uriel, J. A collaborative study for the evaluation of a serologic test for primary liver cancer. *Cancer*, **25**, 1091 (1970).
28. Pedersen, K. O. Fetuin, a new globulin isolated from serum. *Nature*, **154**, 575 (1944).
29. Perova, S. D. (1969). Cited in Ref. (*13*).
30. Perova, S. D. and Abelev, G. I. Embryonal antigens in the serum of the rats. *Vopr. Med. Khim.*, **13**, 369 (1967).

31. Purves, L. R., Macnab, M., and Bersohn, I. Serum α-fetoprotein. I. Immunodiffusion and immunoassay results in cases of primary cancer of the liver. *S. Afr. Med. J.*, **42**, 1138 (1968).
32. Soloff, M. S., Creange, J. E., and Potts, G. O. Unique estrogen-binding properties of rat pregnancy plasma. *Endocrinology*, **88**, 127 (1971).
33. Stanislawski-birencwajg, M. Etude immunochimique d'antigènes embryonnaires du rat. *C. R.*, **260**, 364 (1965).
34. Stanislawski-birencwajg, M. Specific antigens of rat—embryonic serum. *Cancer Res.*, **27**, 1982 (1967).
35. Stanislawski-birencwajg, M. Uriel, J., and Grabar, P. Association of embryonic antigens with experimentally induced hepatic lesions in the rat. *Cancer Res.*, **27**, 1990 (1967).
36. Tatarinov, Y. Detection of embryospecific α-globulin in the blood sera of patients with primary liver tumor. *Vopr. Med. Khim.*, **1**, 90 (1964).
37. Uriel, J., de Nechaud, B., and Dupiers, M. Estrogen-binding properties of rat, mouse and man fetospecific serum proteins. Demonstration by immuno-autoradiographic methods. *Biochem. Biophys. Res. Commun.*, **6**, 1175 (1972).
38. Uriel, J. and de Nechaud, B. La recherche d'α-foetoprotéine en pathologie humaine. *Annu. Inst. Pasteur*, **122**, 829 (1972).
39. Uriel, J., de Nechaud, B., Stanislawski-birencwajg, M., Masseyeff, R., Leblanc, L., Quenum, C., Loisillier, F., and Grabar, P. Antigènes embryonnaires et cancer du foie chez l'homme. Association de l'alpha-foetoprotéine sérique avec l'hépatome primaire. *C. R.*, **265**, 75 (1967).
40. Uriel, J. Transitory liver antigens and primary hepatoma in man and rat. *Pathol. Biol.*, **17**, 877 (1969).
41. Watabe, H. Early appearance of embryonic α-globulin in rat serum during carcinogenesis with 4-dimethylaminoazobenzene. *Cancer Res.*, **31**, 1192 (1971).
42. Wise, R., Ballard, F., and Ezechiel, E. Developmental changes in the plasma protein pattern of the rat. *Comp. Biochem. Physiol.*, **9**, 23 (1963).
43. Wise, R. and Oliver, I. Sites of synthesis of plasma proteins in the foetal rat. *Biochem. J.*, **100**, 330 (1966).

α-FETOPROTEIN IN DISEASES

SERUM α-FETOPROTEIN LEVELS IN PEOPLE SUSCEPTIBLE TO PRIMARY LIVER CANCER IN SOUTHERN AFRICA

L. R. PURVES,*1 C. MANSO, and F. O. TORRES*2

*Life Sciences Division, Atomic Energy Board,*1 and Laboratorio de Quimica Fisiologica, Faculdade de Medicina, Universidade de Lourenco Marques*2*

The negroid peoples of southern Africa have a wide range of susceptibilities to various cancers. In the case of primary liver cancer (PLC) the common factor appears to be geographical, cultural, or nutritional and not genetic. Samples of these populations, including school children and healthy adult males from rural areas working in the mines, were screened with a radioimmunoassay test capable of detecting normal α-fetoprotein (AFP) levels. The more susceptible populations appear to have either bimodal distributions of AFP or greater number of higher AFP results. A link between hepatitis and carcinogenic events, both capable of eliciting AFP production, has therefore been suggested. Arising from studies in southern Africa, various other situations including pregnancy, hepatitis, experimental toxic hepatitis, and liver regeneration have been related to serum AFP levels. It is suggested that the rate of synthesis of normal AFP is a measure of liver cell turnover.

An unusual combination of circumstances, political, economic, and geographical, renders primary cancer of the liver (PLC) very convenient for study in southern Africa.

Primary cancer of the liver is an important category of tumor in many underdeveloped regions of the world. The negroid peoples of Africa are particularly susceptible, and perhaps the highest documented incidence in the world is in Mozambique (*6*). Living alongside the negroid peoples of Africa are other ethnic groups—Indian, Chinese, Arabic, Western European, and Indonesian peoples—sharing the same economic status as the negroid peoples, in some instances, yet lacking their susceptibility to PLC. The factors that seem to categorise the negroid peoples are not only genetic but also their dependence on subsistence economies. A change from this status is, of necessity, integral to economic development.

The prevalence of PLC is not uniform among the negroid peoples of southern Africa. The major variations are as follows:

*1 P. O. Box 2034, Pretoria, South Africa.
*2 Portuguese East Africa.

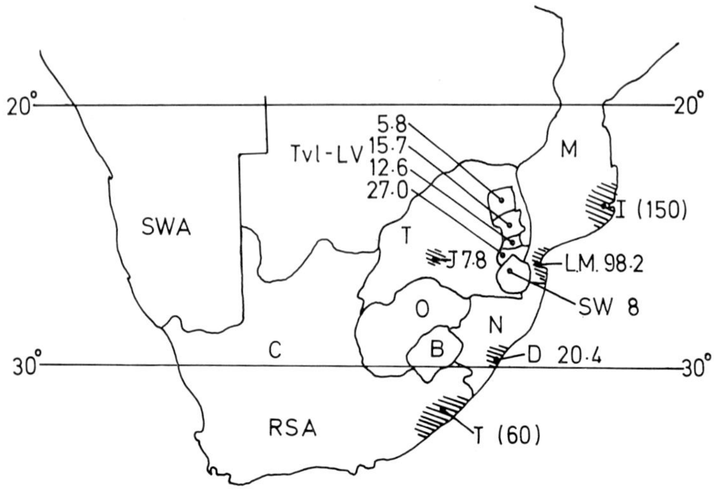

MAP. Geographical range of PLC incidence rates (per 100,000 population *p.a.*)

The incidence rates are given for each area with probable rates in parentheses.
SWA: Southwest Africa.
M: Mozambique with Inhimbane (I) and Lourenco Marques areas (LM).
RSA: Republic of South Africa with provinces of Cape (C), Transvaal (T), Natal (N), and Orange Free State (O), towns of Johannesburg (J), Durban (D), and the area of the Transkei (T).
The Transvaal Lowveld (Tvl-LV) has been further subdivided.
SW: Swaziland.
B: Basutoland.

(1) The lowest incidence appears to be in negroid peoples from the west coast of Africa currently living in America: However, their incidence is higher than for Western Europeans in America (*7*). Genetic factors cannot be the sole reason for this difference however since the American negro has not achieved economic parity although his level of development is very advanced by world standards.
(2) The highest incidence is reputed to be in the Inhimbane province of Mozambique. While precise figures are not available, the incidence appears to be higher than in Lourenco Marques where a recent figure was 98.2/100,000 *p.a.* (*16*). The Inhimbane figure could be 150/100,000 *p.a.*, but this is speculation and is perhaps biased by the fact that economic factors cause more Inhimbane people to seek work in the mines in South Africa than come from the rapidly developing area around Lourenco Marques (*29*).
(3) Many of the independent and semi-independent regions of southern Africa that are as yet underdeveloped depend for a large part of their state revenues on the money earned by their adult males working in the gold, coal, and uranium mines of South Africa. This is an interesting group of people since they represent a fair sample of the healthy, young, adult male negroid population of the rural areas of southern Africa. The labour turnover rate is very high, since although the contract periods are for a year or more, the general practice is to work for about 18 months and perhaps return for 1 or more contracts later. Urbanized

negroid peoples constitute most of the long-term employees as they have acquired special skills through long-term training and education. Many of them now belong to age groups reared entirely in an urban situation. The medical surveillance of the miners is of standard equivalent to that in highly developed countries. All ailments sufficient to impair working ability are treated in the hospital and the miners are highly motivated to report illness early in order to receive therapy. This contrasts markedly with the rural situation.

Although 23.9% of the mine labor force comes from Mozambique, 69% of the PLC cases are from this area, and especially from the Inhimbane area (see above) (*29*). The overall incidence of cancer among the miners is 50.9/100,000 *p.a.* (*29*) of which PLC is the commonest (52.6% or 26.8/100,000 *p.a.*). This situation appears to have existed from the earliest reports available (1929) (*8*). Whether the apparently increasing PLC rate is a reflection of better diagnostic facilities and information retrieval is hard to assess. The present-day overall cancer rates are much higher than those reported in the 1930's (*3*).

(4) In the Transkei, the incidence of PLC is high (possibly 60/100,000 *p.a.*) but it is less frequent (1: 0.7) (*29*) than esophageal cancer though it is not geographically segregated (*31*). This contrasts markedly with the relative rarity of esophageal cancer in Mozambique, 2.6/100,000 *p.a.* (*16*).

(5) In the Lowveld of the Transvaal, PLC incidence is higher but bladder cancer is also prominent (PLC 27.0–5.8, esophageal cancer 4.4, bladder cancer 5.7, all cancers 52.9/100,000 *p.a.*) (*30*).

(6) The urban negroid people of Johannesburg have an incidence of 7.8/100,000 *p.a.* and this figure appears to have decreased (*28*) from an earlier figure of 13.5/100,000 *p.a.* Since political and economic factors have caused the constitution of this population to vary with regard to age, sex and ethnic origin, firm conclusions are hard to draw. Similar factors operate in Natal to a lesser degree so that the incidence of PLC, 20.4/100,000 *p.a.*, is probably a fair reflection of a developing negroid group with close ties to the rural situation (*32*).

(7) The low-lying eastern half of Swaziland contiguous with Mozambique and inhabited by closely related negroid peoples is reputed to have a higher PLC incidence than the western mountainous half (*10*). The overall PLC incidence rate is not very high, however, being about 8/100,000 *p.a.*

(8) The non-negroid peoples of southern Africa have incidence rates comparable with many western populations, *e.g.*, 2.5/100,000 *p.a.*, and in many instances long-standing hepatic disease is antecedent to the tumor.

A note of caution must be introduced in assessing the epidemiological information at present available, since although a pattern is emerging, a number of crucial areas need to be more fully studied, *e.g.*, the Transkei and rural Mozambique. There is little convincing evidence that there are large differences in PLC incidence rates in contiguous geographical areas. The clear definition of such a difference would be crucial in expediting any comparative study of possible etiologic factors.

Just as the epidemiology of Burkitt tumor in Africa has suggested a transmissible agent as a factor in the etiology, so the epidemiology of PLC suggests dietary factors as causative agents. Although other factors must be considered, *e.g.*, marginal nutrition, subclinical hepatitis, bilharziasis (other hepatic flukes are not common), kwashiorkor, viral agents, *etc.*, none weigh as heavily as a dietary factor. Deleterious factors may be present in the food as part of the culinary tradition or as a consequence of inexpertize in mould-free food preservation.

There is no shortage of potential candidate carcinogens but present evidence would not appear to favor any particular agent (*12*) although ease of detection and the experimental demonstration of the carcinogenic potential of these agents in nonprimates has led to undue emphasis, in our opinion, on some (*e.g.*, aflatoxin).

The present epidemiologic/etiologic approach to the PLC problem entails a present-day study of areas selected on the basis of PLC statistics. Since the induction of the cancer process must occur at an earlier phase, this implies that a degree of stability of culinary and agricultural practices is expected. This would be more realistic if the stability was due to a geographical interaction, as has been proposed for the accumulation of nitrosoamines in crops grown on molybdenum-deficient soils (*4*). In the case of a dietary carcinogen, the crucial exposure could be transplacental to the highly susceptible fetus or could occur as a sustained lifelong ingestion. In order to shorten the interval for which the investigator must wait before he can proceed, between induction and the final clinical manifestation, two approaches have been possible: Either (1) to study areas where the disease occurs in children, who do not travel far, or (2) to test the food biologically in experimental animals.

A third, new possibility is to use an early biochemical manifestation of the tumor occurring either in the transformation process, the progressing phase, or the fully evolved subclinical phase. We present evidence that this might be a realizable proposition by using sensitive assays for α-fetoprotein (AFP) (*22*, *25*).

Primary cancer of the liver is an unusual tumor from a number of aspects, and this has led to interesting consequences in interpreting the clinical manifestations. The liver is a very accommodating organ and a tumor causes very little in the way of physiological derangements or morbidity until it has reached an advanced stage. The clinical presentation is usually precipitated by the large tumor causing symptoms in a purely mechanical fashion, *e.g.*, by distending the capsule of the liver, causing pain or rupturing into the peritoneum, or completely infiltrating the residual normal liver. Miners presenting large tumors usually deny any physical discomfort, despite the performance of arduous physical exertion, until just before the presenting symptom. Furthermore, these miners have been through at least 4 medical examinations prior to engagement, conducted by doctors keenly aware of the PLC problem. Just as the prodrome is short, so is the clinical course of the disease, with most patients dying within 3 months of presentation (*18*).

There are no biochemical or other parameters that can distinguish PLC from other causes of hard, tender hepatomegaly in our miners at any stage of the illness, other than the AFP test (discussed later) and hepatic biopsy (*19*). There are, however, many conditions that mimic PLC clinically. In a study on the miners designed to investigate thoroughly all cases in whom the diagnosis of PLC could be reasonably entertained by experienced clinicians, only about 50% were in fact PLC cases. Even with retrospective assays for AFP, only about a further

5% of cases were found to have been missed, using a test giving a positivity rate of 90% for histologically proven PLC cases (*18*, *21*). These figures should emphasize the need for careful diagnostic criteria in field studies. For practical purposes an early stage of PLC does not exist clinically, so that AFP tests of low sensitivity (*e.g.*, Ouchterlony immunodiffusion with a probable lower limit in routine laboratories of 0.5 mg% or 5,000 ng/ml) provide a guide to diagnosis even less efficient than the usual subsequent fact of the patients' demise a few months later.

In areas where the PLC incidence is very high, *e.g.*, in Lourenco Marques, Mozambique, even young children are affected but only occasionally are early tumors seen incidentally at postmortem (*6*, *16*). However, hepatic pathology is demonstrable in a proportion of the healthy population with changes ranging from degrees of hepatomegaly to histological changes suggesting hepatitis of an early or late toxic type and possibly distinguishable from infective hepatitis (*34*, *38*, *39*). Some of these phenomena show progression to a more florid "adenomatous" type of localized hyperplasia associated with cell necrosis (Photo 1). It is possible to collect a series of cases showing intermediate features right up to the unequivocal cancer pattern. Whether this is a real progression of events is highly problematic and the sequence is, of course, extremely difficult to establish in an individual case. Many of the cancer cases (more than 50%) are not associated with cirrhosis (*37*). In some, a vigorous nodular hyperplasia with fibrosis can be seen in the liver near the tumor. This phenomenon has been called " focal cirrhosis " by some of our pathologists and cases showing this phenomenon have distinctive biochemical features including high AFP levels in all the 12 cases studied (*18*, *21*). The cirrhotic process is in many cases clearly a concomitant phenomenon and not antecedent.

The clinical and pathological situation in our cases appears to correlate well with that reported in other negroid populations in Africa but differs from those rare cases in non-negroid people. The main differences apparent to us, in the small number of cases available, are that long-standing hepatic disease was often present, the tumors were smaller, caused symptoms earlier, and the AFP levels were on the average much lower.

Physiology of AFP from Studies in Southern Africa

α-Fetoprotein can be detected in the serum of all healthy people (the average level is about 10 ng/ml; range 1–20 ng/ml (*22*)). The levels in the neonate are very high (average in our series 150,000 ng/ml (*18*)) but young children were about 60% of the adult level. The phenomenon of this apparent age dependence has not been worked out yet. The AFP in fetal serum can reach high levels (*e.g.*, $\times 10^5$ ng/ml) (*9*) and it is not surprising that fetal-maternal plasma exchange can be detected, with maternal sera having values up to 800 ng/ml. The levels during pregnancy can fluctuate markedly and are rarely maintained, but often a drop to levels near normal occurs a few days before the onset of labor, suggesting that the passage of AFP into the maternal circulation is under partial control (*22*, *33*). The AFP level usually rises sharply at birth due to placental disruption but falls rapidly again to near normal. The death and maceration of fetuses cause very high levels of AFP in the maternal circulation (*20*, *22*, *33*). No correlation with maternal AFP has been found yet between the state of the placenta, maternal placental lactogen levels (*26*), or the delivered infant's AFP level.

While information is accruing at a rapid rate, it will be several years before most of the parameters affecting normal AFP levels are known, so that all present interpretations are subject to this qualification.

Although AFP is a secreted protein and does not tend to remain around the cell in the form of a glycocalyx, nevertheless it has many analogies with the carcinoembryonic antigen (CEA) of the gastrointestinal tract (*36*). Normal CEA serum levels might also eventually be established, although this has probably been easier in the case of the liver due to the much larger size of the functioning tissue. We have never found antibodies to AFP in any situation, although the radioimmunoassay technique that we use would register very low antibody levels. This finding, by analogy, would support Burtin's contention that autoimmune antibodies against CEA do not exist (*5*).

α-Fetoprotein in Relation to Proven PLC Cases

1. Biochemical correlations

Since there are no biochemical or other functional parameters capable of distinguishing PLC cases from similar clinical presentations, it is not surprising that the AFP test at the diagnostic level (*21*) (discussed later) does not correlate with any of them. A wide spectrum of parameters has been studied in more than 200 histologically proven cases, using a computer search program (*18*, *19*).

When PLC cases with AFP levels below and above 3,000 ng/ml (Ouchterlony-positive and -negative) were compared, the higher AFP results correlated ($0.01 < P < 0.05$) with a lower mucoprotein, C-reactive protein, and α_1-globulin level, and a higher colloidal red, hemoglobin, and total protein test.

If the PLC cases were divided into 3 groups according to AFP level, some interesting tendencies would be noted (Table I). Although the differences are not large, sufficient cases were studied for the changes to be assessed as being of possible statistical significance ($0.01 < P < 0.05$). It is interesting that the lower

TABLE I. Correlations of Serum Biochemistry with AFP Level

Test	Serum AFP level (mg%)			
	Below 0.1	0.1–20	20–1000	Change from 0 to <20 to >20
Mucoprotein	211	180	167	Decreases
Cholesterol	152	164	198	Increases
Erythrocyte sedimentation rate	33	28	17	Decreases
Serum protein	7.81	8.11	8.25	Increases
α_1-Globulin (%)	10.8	10.2	9.3	Decreases
γ-Globulin (%)	31.4	30.4	31.5	Constant
Hemoglobin	12.7	13.7	15.0	Increases

AFP results were associated with tests usually regarded as indicators of tissue necrosis or the activity of a disease process.

2. Clinical correlations

The AFP results did not assist in predicting the clinical outcome of PLC cases. There were no correlations to be found with age, tribe, weight, survival time, response to therapy, or the presence of bilharziasis, to name a few of the parameters scrutinized. Although the tumors often enlarged rapidly, the average increase in the AFP level was only 65.8% (*21*). One case showed an 8-fold increase. Several cases were below the assay limit when first seen however. It is unusual to find rapidly rising AFP levels even though the range of possible AFP levels in man extends from 1 to 10^7 ng/ml (*21, 22*). Despite diligent searches, no asymptomatic case has yet been found where the AFP level is on the rise; nor do lower AFP values in PLC cases tend to show more rapid increases than higher values (*23*). These findings suggest that the progression of the tumor just before presentation is a rapid process and that the ability of the tumor to synthesize AFP is set at a particular fixed rate at an early stage of the transformation process.

3. Pathological correlations

There was, surprisingly, no correlation of the AFP level with the tumor weight or the weight of the residual liver (*18, 19*). Some minor correlations were noted with a few parameters of possible statistical significance (Table II). Anaplastic and diffuse tumors had the lowest mean AFP levels and, nodular and nodular and poorly differentiated ones the highest.

TABLE II. Correlations of Pathological Anatomy with AFP Levels

Parameter		Mean AFP level (mg%)
Tumor appearance	Massive	24
	Nodular	45
	Diffuse	18
Tumor differentiation	Anaplastic	16
	Poorly differentiated	32
	Well-differentiated	25

Many other features were also scrutinized for correlations (*18, 19*), including the histological patterns, tumor necrosis, and metastases, but none were found. The presence of concomitant cirrhosis has an unexpected effect on AFP levels, since the AFP is synthesized in the tumor (it must be at such high levels). The cirrhosis group was 81% positive on admission whereas the non-cirrhotics were 53% positive. On the other hand, those cases showing the feature of nodular hyperplasia and fibrosis in regions near the tumor, and called "focal cirrhosis," were all AFP-positive on admission.

Although PLC is often assumed to be multifocal in origin the pathologist at postmortem in the fully evolved case has difficulty in demonstrating this. The finding of only a restricted number of AFP variants appearing constantly in the serum of any case over a period of time is also against the multifocal hypothesis (*27*). The AFP variants, 4 or 5 in number, are probably due to enzyme deletions resulting in defective attachment of the sialic acid-containing prosthetic groups.

4. Response to therapy

No effective therapy can be offered yet for PLC and it is unlikely, tumors can be found in the preclinical phase—something that we have not achieved yet, despite the high frequency of the tumor in our gold miners and the large number of sera tested. Nevetheless certain forms of therapy offer palliation; mainly by reducing the size of the tumor and causing subjective improvement. In very few cases could a simultaneous response, judged by shrinkage of the tumor and a fall in AFP level be demonstrated (*17*). The most effective therapy to date has been methotrexate administered by hepatic arterial infusion. Radiation therapy, *e.g.*, telecobalt, is also very effective in causing a fall in the AFP levels, though not improving the patients' survival time (Fig. 2). An attempt is being made now to regulate the dosage of chemotherapeutic agents by following the AFP level.

Diagnostic Criteria for PLC Using the AFP Test

At the level of 3,000 ng/ml (Ouchterlony limit (*21*)) the presence of a tumor is virtually certain. Although the histological type is almost always a PLC, especially in Africa, other tumor types can, on occasion, be positive (*1*, *2*, *14*). For practical clinical purposes no other investigations, besides a confirmatory repeat sample, are necessary for clinical care of the patient. A commonly used routine laboratory test nowadays is crossed electroimmunodiffusion, having many advantages in simplicity and speed (*11*). The routine laboratory lower limit of sensitivity with this technique is probably 500 to 1,000 ng/ml. In this range there is a complete overlap (Fig. 1) between the values found in other clinical situations and the AFP result is only of value if the dynamics of the process are studied. If an increasing AFP level is found over a period of weeks then a tumor is almost certainly present. If the level falls, however, this does not exclude the presence of a tumor. In these cases, other diagnostic criteria have to be used. This applies equally well to the use of even more sensitive tests. About 95% of PLC's have AFP levels above the normal distribution of AFP values and higher AFP values usually develop. The interpretation of our results has, however, always been complicated by the effects of hepatitis due to therapy (Fig. 2).

α-Fetoprotein in Other Illnesses

Besides the appearance of AFP in ill neonates, where the mechanism of AFP synthesis might be a regulatory response of a fully functioning gene (*13*), AFP synthesis occurs in a number of other situations that are being better documented now. Human hepatitis of many types, including infectious hepatitis (*1*), Australia antigen-positive serum hepatitis (*35*), childhood cirrhosis in India (*15*),

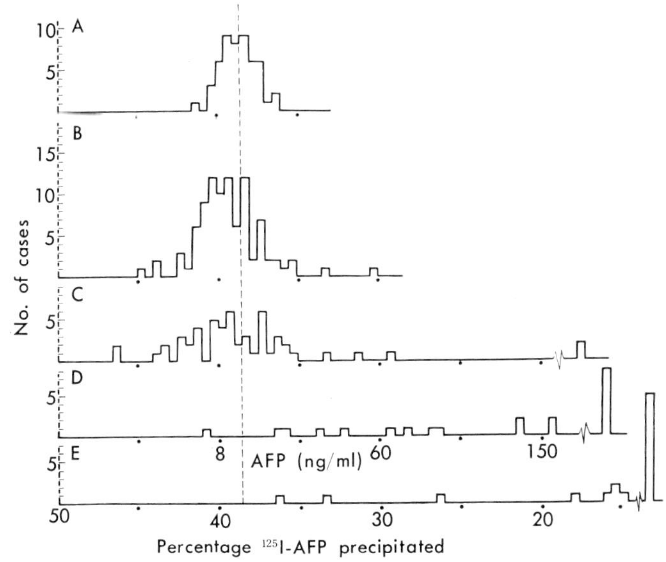

FIG. 1. Serum AFP levels in various categories of miners

A: After a year in the mines. B: New recruits on arrival. C: Ill patients from a medical ward. The diagnosis of PLC was excluded clinically. D: Lowest and E, highest results in each proven case of AFP Ouchterlony-negative PLC. The X-axis has 2 scales; in D, AFP (ng/ml), and E, percentage of ^{125}I-AFP precipitated in the radioimmunoassay. The dotted line is the mean of group A. The broken X-axes indicate cases with serum AFP levels between 150 and 5,000 ng/ml. There is a clear overlap in AFP values between normal new recruits, ill patients, and proven PLC cases. Four PLC cases had AFP levels within the normal range.

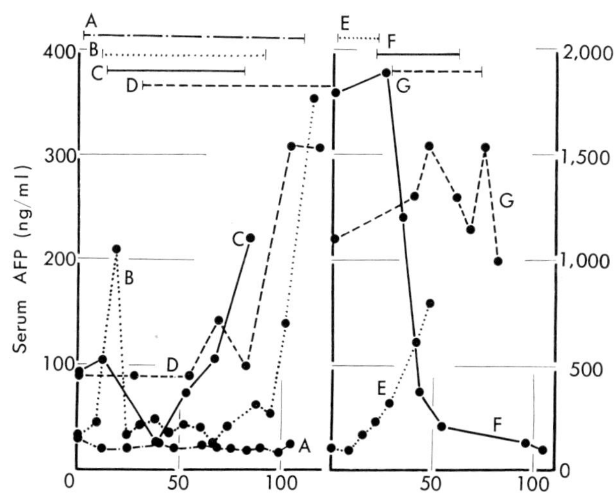

FIG. 2. Response to therapy of PLC cases with low AFP levels

Cases B, E, and F received telecobalt radiotherapy and cases A, C, D, and G received various types of chemotherapy during the intervals indicated.

In some cases the effect on AFP levels is dramatic. Survival time was not prolonged by therapy. Case A had a persistently normal AFP level. Case B is a clear example of an AFP rise due to radiation hepatitis.

toxic hepatitis and probably low grade subclinical hepatitis due to toxins or nutritional factors, can produce increased AFP synthesis, mainly during the regenerative recovery phase. We find that the AFP rise after serum hepatitis is much higher than after infectious hepatitis and seems to last a shorter time. Insufficient cases have been studied yet to explain this in terms of either a more highly synchronized recovery phase in serum hepatitis or merely a different quantitative response. Like in some other parts of Africa (*40*), the incidence of Australia antigen in our cases is higher than in the general population (about 50%) (*26*).

The relation of AFP synthesis to the rate of liver regeneration is a problem needing elucidation. It seems probable that the rate of normal AFP synthesis is closely coupled to liver cell turnover and is not an acute phase type response (*41*). An acute phase protein-type response cannot be ruled out in other situations.

The production of toxic hepatitis in the baboon with diethylnitrosoamine (DENA) (*24*) or carbon tetrachloride causes AFP synthesis at a number of stages: (1) During the initiation of treatment with DENA, AFP rises and falls after 5 months despite continued treatment (Fig. 3).

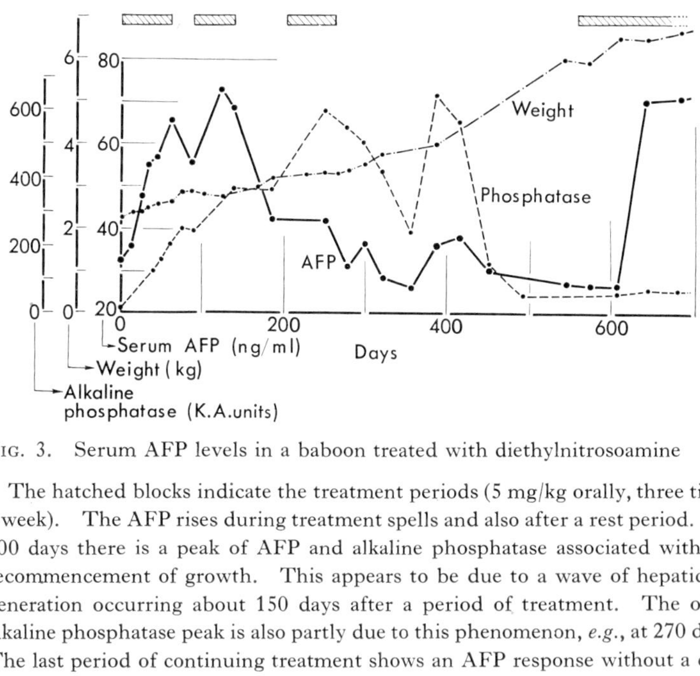

FIG. 3. Serum AFP levels in a baboon treated with diethylnitrosoamine

The hatched blocks indicate the treatment periods (5 mg/kg orally, three times a week). The AFP rises during treatment spells and also after a rest period. At 400 days there is a peak of AFP and alkaline phosphatase associated with the recommencement of growth. This appears to be due to a wave of hepatic regeneration occurring about 150 days after a period of treatment. The other alkaline phosphatase peak is also partly due to this phenomenon, *e.g.*, at 270 days. The last period of continuing treatment shows an AFP response without a concomitant alkaline phosphatase response.

(2) After stopping DENA treatment there is a peak of AFP synthesis at the same time as the recommencement of growth. This delayed escape from DENA toxicity seems to take place after a constant lag period of 4 months.
(3) Subsequent DENA treatment causes AFP responses, but often less dramatic than before.
(4) In some cases, after several spells of treatment, the AFP level continues to rise after DENA treatment has been stopped.

(5) About 12 days after carbon tetrachloride poisoning (one dose intraperitoneally) or hemihepatectomy, the AFP level rises and gradually falls. This corresponds perhaps to the peak of liver cell regeneration.
(6) All these phenomena are more striking in the younger animal.

One general conclusion of importance for the human situation is that it takes a fairly severe hepatic insult to cause rises in AFP levels. Since AFP turnover rate is rapid ($T_{1/2}$ probably 2.5 days (*23*)), raised levels must always be due to continued synthesis and are not due to slowly catabolized residue from past hepatic disease.

α-Fetoprotein Levels in People from Areas of Southern Africa with High PLC Risk

Technical considerations demand at present, for detailed comparisons of the range of AFP levels in populations, that the samples are assayed in batches. Although the radioimmunoassay that we use (*23*) can handle large numbers of samples per day, *e.g.*, 500, there are limitations.

The AFP levels of healthy new recruits to the mines usually show 2 features (Fig. 1). There is slight skewing of the distribution due to cases with levels which are higher than average. Sometimes these cases fall outside the normal distribution completely. After a year in the mines on a balanced diet, the distribution of AFP levels is no longer skewed, suggesting that the process causing raised AFP levels has abated in this time (*22*).

Negroid children in Mozambique show a similar pattern with considerable skewing towards the higher range (Fig. 4). This pattern also contrasts with that of children of other races from the same areas, since they show a lower average value and only a few cases outside the restricted normal range.

If the distribution of AFP levels in newly recruited miners from various re-

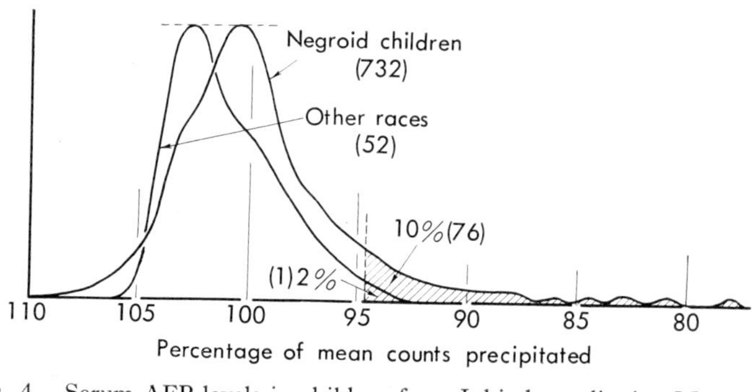

FIG. 4. Serum AFP levels in children from Inhimbane district, Mozambique

There were 732 negroid children and 52 non-negroid (Western European, Indian, and mixed races) in the sample. The former were all on a rural type diet and the latter group were on Western-type diets. The smoothed curves of AFP distribution (for actual data see Ref. *22*) drawn with equal peak heights. The X-axis is the amount of ^{125}I-AFP precipitated in the radioimmunoassay expressed as a percent of the mean negroid result. The true AFP at 80% is equivalent to 4 times the mean AFP. The negroid children showed a higher mean level and had 10% of cases higher than the main range with some very high levels. These children were all clinically well.

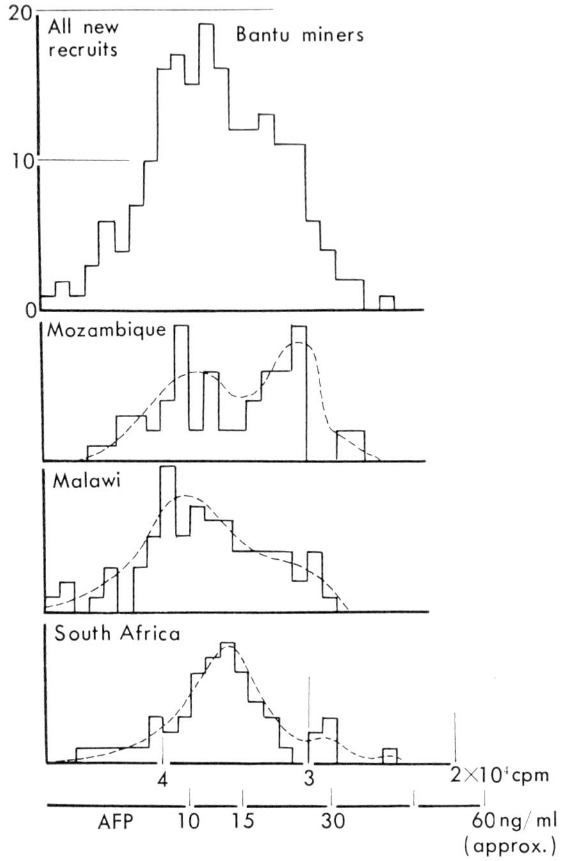

FIG. 5. Serum AFP levels in new recruits to the mines

The vertical scale is indicated in the top graph and the approximate true AFP level at the bottom. The percentage of ^{125}I-AFP precipitated in the radioimmunoassay has been used to plot results along the X-axis. When the overall distribution is broken down into recruits from different areas it is seen that the Mozambique group appears to have a bimodal distribution with the one mode on average 3 times the other in " true " AFP level. The higher mode is less apparent in the Malawi recruits but the highest value is in a South African. The top ten cases were screened clinically but were normal.

gions is plotted (Fig. 5) the Mozambique samples appear to have a bimodal distribution, the South African sample having a unimodal distribution, albeit with a few higher values. The Malawi sample is intermediate. This distribution does seem to follow one's preconceived idea of how AFP distributions might vary in samples from areas with different PLC susceptibilities and might be evidence for a transformation process causing AFP synthesis. Follow-up studies are now in progress, but no case showing progression to a clinically presenting tumor has been found.

Since it appears that a fairly severe insult is necessary to cause AFP rises and that raised AFP levels are due to continued synthesis, it is improbable that the raised levels in adults and children from these areas with high PLC risk are due to a recognized pathogenesis, *i.e.*, either recovery from flagrant hepatitis or established tumors. Either one has to postulate that more trivial events than one expects are capable of stimulating AFP synthesis, or that this AFP synthesis is due to the activities of transformed populations of cells; under suppression, but synthesizing AFP in the autonomous fashion of the cancer cell.

α-Fetoprotein Levels as an Epidemiological Tool

In our opinion, despite the considerable lack of knowledge about the many parameters that could affect AFP levels (these remain to be investigated) there is sufficient evidence available now so that the use of the AFP test in epidemiological/etiologic studies cannot be justifiably ignored. There are no strictures now in the use of a radioimmunoassay either with regard to cost or expertize and there is the advantage of being able to do quantitative assays in large numbers. The technique that we have reported has been in use for 3.5 years and was designed to cater for the problem of low-cost assays in large numbers with a minimum of manipulation (*23*).

Although there are conditions besides PLC capable of causing increased AFP synthesis and no direct link has been established between the AFP synthesis in hepatitic and carcinogenic processes, such a link remains possible. The ability to pinpoint susceptible individuals would be a boon to those seeking the etiologic agents of this form of cancer.

The main topic of this monograph has been AFP and PLC, but we in southern Africa are almost certain that PLC is but one aspect of a problem caused by common agents that are a bane to the developing peoples of Africa and the world. The clinical entities of esophageal cancer, liver cancer, bladder cancer, subclinical liver damage, cirrhosis, cardiomyopathy, and lowered resistance to disease and deprivations could all be due to a similar pathogenesis. The PLC must stand very high on the list of preventable tumors, since a dietary factor is highly likely. This justifies an intense research program now.

Acknowledgments

The following organizations have supported the work resulting in this monograph and we thank them. The Division of Life Sciences of the Atomic Energy Board, South Africa (Director, Prof. C. R. Jansen). The South African Institute for Medical Research (Associate Director, Prof. I. Bersohn). Faculdade de Medicina, Universidade de Lourenco Marques, Mozambique. Director of Medical Services, The Rand Mines Group, South Africa.

REFERENCES

1. Abelev, G. I. α-Fetoprotein in ontogenesis and its association with malignant tumors. *Recent Adv. Cancer Res.*, **14**, 295–358 (1971).
2. Alpert, E., Pinn, V. W., and Isselbacher, K. J. α-Fetoprotein in a patient with gastric carcinoma metastatic to the liver. *New Engl. J. Med.*, **285**, 1058–1059 (1971).
3. Berman, C. Malignant disease in the Bantu of Johannesburg and the Witwatersrand goldmines. *S. Afr. J. Med. Sci.*, **1**, 12–30 (1935).

4. Burrell, R. J. W., Roach, W. A., and Shadwell, A. Esophageal cancer in the Bantu of the Transkei associated with mineral deficiency in garden plants. *J. Natl. Cancer Inst.*, **36**, 201–214 (1966).
5. Collatz, E., von Kleist, S., and Burtin, P. Further investigations of circulating antibodies in colon cancer patients: On the autoantigenicity of the carcinoembryonic antigen. *Int. J. Cancer*, **8**, 298–303 (1971).
6. Doll, R., Payne, P., and Waterhouse, J. Cancer incidence in five continents A report issued by the International Union against Cancer (UICC), (1966).
7. Dorn, H. F. and Cutler, S. J. Morbidity from cancer in the United States. *Public Health Monograph*, **56**, 207 (1958).
8. Fischer, W. O. A preliminary report on 1402 consecutive autopsies on native mine workers. *J. Med. Assoc. S. Afr.*, **3**, 511–516 (1929).
9. Gitlin, D. and Boesman, M. Serum α-fetoprotein, albumin and γG-globulin in the human conceptus. *J. Clin. Invest.*, **45**, 1826–1838 (1966).
10. Keen, P. and Martin, P. Is aflatoxin carcinogenic in man? The evidence in Swaziland. *Trop. Geog. Med.*, **23**, 44–53 (1971).
11. Kohn, J. Method for the detection and identification of α-fetoprotein in serum. *J. Clin. Pathol.*, **23**, 733–735 (1970).
12. Kurata, H., Udagawa, S., Ichinoe, M., Natori, S., and Sakai, S. Field survey of mycotoxin-producing fungi contaminating human foodstuffs in Japan, with epidemiological background. *In* " Mycotoxins in Human Health," ed. by I.F.H. Purchase, Macmillan, London, pp. 101–106 (1971).
13. Masopust, J., Rádl, J., and Houštěk, J. Occurrence of α-fetoprotein in some infants suffering from hepatopathy. *Protides Biol. Fluids*, **18**, 239–242 (1971).
14. Mehlman, D. J., Bulkley, B. H., and Wiernik, P. H. Serum α-fetoglobulin with gastric and prostatic carcinomas. *New Engl. J. Med.*, **285**, 1060–1061 (1971).
15. Nayak, N. C., Malaviya, A. N., Chawla, V., and Chandra, R. K. α-Fetoprotein in Indian childhood cirrhosis. *Lancet*, **1**, 68–69 (1971).
16. Prates, M. D. and Torres, F. O. A cancer survey in Lourenco Marques, Portuguese East Africa. *J. Natl. Cancer Inst.*, **35**, 729–757 (1965).
17. Purves, L. R., Bersohn, I., Geddes, E. W., Falkson, G., and Cohen, L. Serum α-fetoprotein. III. Effects of chemotherapy and radiotherapy on serum α-fetoprotein levels in cases of primary liver cancer. *S. Afr. Med. J.*, **44**, 590–594 (1970).
18. Purves, L. R., Bersohn, I., and Geddes, E. W. Serum α-fetoprotein and primary liver cancer in man. *Cancer*, **25**, 1261–1270 (1970).
19. Purves, L. R. and Bersohn, I. Serum α-fetoprotein. II. Correlation of serum levels with other biochemical parameters in primary cancer of the liver. *S. Afr. Med. J.*, **43**, 1110–1113 (1969).
20. Purves, L. R. and Geddes, E. W. A more sensitive test for α-fetoprotein. *Lancet*, **1**, 47–48 (1972).
21. Purves, L. R., Macnab, M., and Bersohn, I. Serum α-fetoprotein. I. Immunodiffusion and immunoassay results in cases of primary cancer of the liver. *S. Afr. Med. J.*, **42**, 1138–1141 (1968).
22. Purves, L. R., Purves, M., Branch, W. R., Geddes, E. W., Portugal, A. M., and Manso, C. Serum α-fetoprotein. VII. The range of serum values in normal people, pregnant women and primary liver cancer high risk populations. *Cancer* (1972), in press.
23. Purves, L. R. and Purves, M. Serum α-fetoprotein. VI. The radioimmunoassay. Evidence for the presence of α-fetoprotein in the serum of normal people and pregnant women. *S. Afr. Med. J.*, **46**, 1290–1297 (1972).

24. Purves, L. R. Serum α-fetoprotein. VIII. Serum levels during diethylnitrosoamine poisoning of baboons. *Int. J. Cancer*, **10**, 552–556 (1972).
25. Purves, L. R. Surveys for α-fetoprotein among Bantu goldminers. In "Mycotoxins in Human Health," ed. by I.F.H. Purchase, Macmillan, London, pp. 71–73 (1971).
26. Purves, L. R. Unpublished data.
27. Purves, L. R., van der Merwe, E., and Bersohn, I. Serum α-fetoprotein. V. The bulk preparation and some properties of α-fetoprotein obtained from patients with primary cancer of the liver. *S. Afr. Med. J.*, **44**, 1264–1268 (1970).
28. Robertson, M. A., Harington, J. S., and Bradshaw, E. The cancer pattern in Africans at Baragwanath Hospital, Johannesburg. *Brit. J. Cancer*, **25**, 377–384 (1971).
29. Robertson, M. A., Harington, J. S., and Bradshaw, E. The cancer pattern in African goldminers. *Brit. J. Cancer*, **25**, 395–402 (1971).
30. Robertson, M. A., Harington, J. S., and Bradshaw, E. The cancer pattern in Africans of the Transvaal Lowveld. *Brit. J. Cancer*, **25**, 385–394 (1971).
31. Rose, E. F. Interim report on the surveys of cancer of the esophagus in the Transkei. *S. Afr. Med. J.*, **39**, 1098–1101 (1965).
32. Schonland, M. and Bradshaw, E. Cancer in the Natal African and Indian, 1964–1966. *Int. J. Cancer*, **3**, 304–316 (1968).
33. Seppälä, M. and Ruoslahti, E. α-Fetoprotein in normal and pregnancy sera. *Lancet*, **1**, 375–376 (1972).
34. Serrão, D. and Torres, F. O. Surto de hepatite em Mocambique. Estudo histológico por puncão-biópsia. *Actas I. Congr. Nac. Anat. Patol.*, 255–272 (1968).
35. Smith, J. B. Occurrence of α-fetoprotein in acute viral hepatitis. *Int. J. Cancer*, **8**, 421–424 (1971).
36. Thomson, D. M. P., Krupey, J., Freedman, S. O., and Gold, P. The radioimmunoassay of circulating carcinoembryonic antigen of the human digestive system. *Proc. Natl. Acad. Sci. U.S.*, **64**, 161–167 (1969).
37. Torres, F. O. and Gomes de Oliveira, J. J. Carcinoma primitivo do figado. Revisao macroscopica e histologica de 700 casos. *Actas I. Congr. Nac. Anat. Patol.*, 373–390 (1968).
38. Torres, F. O. Punch biopsy of the liver. Its diagnostic value, with special reference to primary cancer of the liver. *S. Afr. J. Med. Sci.*, **29**, 1–10 (1964).
39. Torres, F. O., Purchase, I.F.H. and van der Walt, J. J. The aetiology of primary liver cancer in the Bantu. *J. Pathol.*, **102**, 163–169 (1970).
40. Vogel, C. L., Anthony, P. P., Mody, N., and Barker, L. F. Hepatitis-associated antigen in Ugandan patients with hepatocellular cancer. *Lancet*, **2**, 621–624 (1970).
41. Werner, M. Serum protein changes during the acute phase reaction. *Clin. Chim. Acta*, **25**, 299–305 (1969).

EXPLANATION OF PHOTO

PHOTO 1. Top: Multicentric adenomatous hyperplasia without cirrhosis or tumor in the liver of a man aged 20, dying accidentally. Bottom: Histology of the main nodule shows necrosis, cytoplasmic swelling, vacuolation, and nuclear reaction but no malignant transformation.

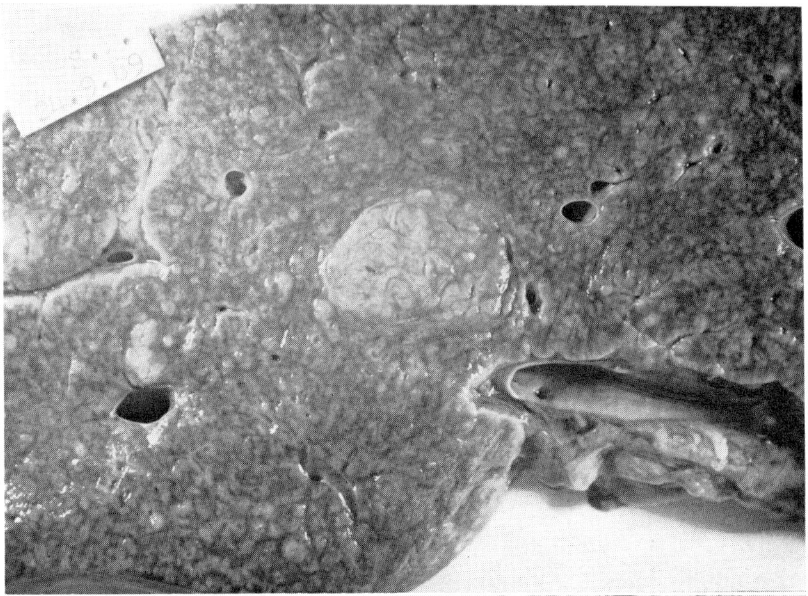

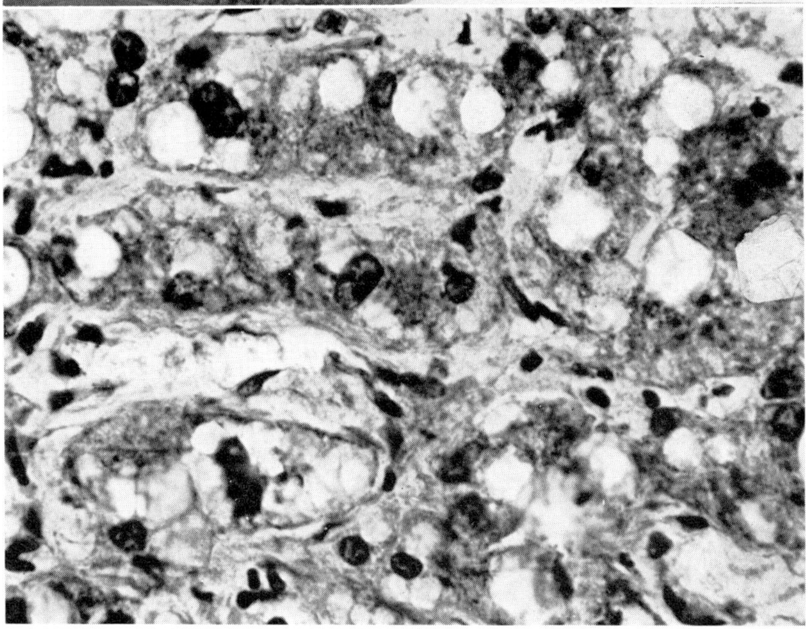

CLINICAL SIGNIFICANCE OF α-FETOPROTEIN
With Special Reference to Primary Cancer of the Liver

Yasuo Endo, Koichi Kanai, Shiro Iino, and Toshitsugu Oda
*First Department of Medicine, Faculty of Medicine, University of Tokyo**

Sera of 52 patients with primary cancer of the liver (PLC) and of 796 with other diseases were tested for α-fetoprotein (AFP) by a double immunodiffusion technique. In 34 cases with PLC histologically proved, 76.4% of the total were AFP-positive. The concomitant presence of liver cirrhosis had no influence on the appearance of AFP. The AFP was detected only in cases with hepatocellular carcinoma and not in cholangiocellular carcinoma. Serum AFP levels, when determined sequentially in the same subject, reflect the clinical status of the illness. Surgical resection of the tumor decreased the levels and recurrence of the tumor, in contrast, increased them prior to the occurrence of other indications.

Further, radioimmunoassay, which is about 1,000 times as sensitive as the double immunodiffusion technique, revealed an increase of serum AFP even in some cases of liver cirrhosis, hepatitis, and pregnancy, as well as some with PLC where the serum AFP levels were too low for detection by the immunodiffusion technique.

The diagnosis of primary cancer of the liver (PLC) (hepatoma) in an early stage is now the most difficult in the field of clinical medicine. The immunological method, using α-fetoprotein (AFP), is now considered a highly specific test for the diagnosis of this disease. α-Fetoprotein is a serum protein specific for the fetus and is not found in the sera of healthy adults, but reappears in the pathological status.

This phenomenon was first demonstrated by Abelev *et al.* (*3*), using transplantable mouse hepatoma. Then the same results for human hepatoma were obtained by Tatarinov (*34*). Abelev (*4*), Uriel *et al.* (*35*), and other workers (*7, 10, 13, 16, 20, 22, 24, 26–28, 30, 32, 33*), carried out a wide survey and the clinical significance of this test is now established. Through further development of radioimmunoassay, the diagnosis of hepatoma even in an early stage is now to be expected.

α-Fetoprotein and Hepatoma

Since the discovery of AFP in the sera of patients with hepatoma (*34*), the clinical usefulness of this test exists in its high specificity for hepatoma, as well

* Hongo 7-3-1, Bunkyo-ku, Tokyo 113, Japan (遠藤康夫, 金井弘一, 飯野四郎, 織田敏次).

TABLE I. α-Fetoprotein in Various Diseases[a]

Diagnosis	No. of cases	Positive cases
PLC	52 (34)	37 (26)
Metastatic liver cancer	60	2[b]
Embryonal cancer	3	3
Other malignant diseases	71	0
Liver cirrhosis	64	1[b]
Hepatitis	192	0
Miscellaneous	385	0
Premature babies	19	19
Healthy	252	0
Total	1,098	62

[a] By double immunodiffusion in agar gel (micro-Ouchterlony method).
[b] Autopsy not performed.
Numbers in parentheses show histologically confirmed cases.

as the high incidence. Table I shows AFP appearance in various diseases. About 70% of hepatomas were positive for AFP by the double immunodiffusion technique. The same positive reaction was also found in 2 cases with metastatic liver cancer, 3 with embryonal cancer, 1 with liver cirrhosis, and 19 premature babies. As for the 2 with metastatic liver cancer, 1 was diagnosed only clinically and the other by open biopsy, and autopsies were not done. There was no evidence to support the existence of hepatoma. The cirrhotic patient with a positive reaction was also diagnosed only clinically. This was an advanced cirrhosis with marked ascites, and died of esophageal bleeding. No autopsy was done. Thus, a definite conclusion was not obtained, but the possibility involving hepatoma was not ruled out in this advanced cirrhotic case.

Out of 34 cases with histologically proved hepatoma, 26 were positive (76.4%) by double immunodiffusion (Table II). All of them were hepatocellular carcinoma and not cholangiocellular carcinoma.

TABLE II. α-Fetoprotein in PLC[a]

Diagnosis	No. of cases	Positive cases	%
Histologically confirmed			76.4
Hepatocellular carcinoma			
Without cirrhosis	9	8	89
With cirrhosis	21	18	85.7
Cholangiocellular carcinoma	4	0	
Clinically or by open biopsy at operation	18	11	
Total	52	37	71.1

[a] By double immunodiffusion in agar gel (micro-Ouchterlony method).

No correlation was observed between the concomitant presence of cirrhosis and appearance of AFP. Purves *et al.* (*29*) reported a slightly higher incidence (but not significant) in PLC with cirrhosis than in that without cirrhosis.

Alpert (5) did not observe such a correlation. No significant difference was observed in our cases. Positive AFP results were found in 85.7% of hepatoma with cirrhosis and in 89% of hepatoma without cirrhosis.

Possibility of an Early Diagnosis of Hepatoma

Clinical interest in the AFP test may exist with regard to the possibility of detecting hepatoma in an early stage. Hepatoma detected by immunodiffusion is usually advanced, but sometimes the AFP test may give indications prior to other clinical signs or laboratory findings.

Table III shows the clinical course of a case with hepatoma accompanying cirrhosis, in which the AFP test showed a positive reaction prior to the clinical manifestation of the tumor. In December 1967, the case was diagnosed as liver cirrhosis with a liver specimen taken at splenectomy. In December 1968, AFP was detected in the serum, but no obvious space-occupying lesion was found on a liver scintigram. There were also no definite signs suggesting a tumor. One year later, in December 1969, liver function tests showed elevated alkaline phosphate (Al-P). Scintiscanning revealed a space-occupying lesion, suggesting a tumor. In this case, AFP was found 1 year prior to the clinical manifestation.

TABLE III. Serum Levels of AFP (I)

	1967 Dec.[a]	1968 Dec.[b]	1969 Feb.	July	Oct.	Nov.	Dec.[c]	1970 Jan.	Feb.
AFP (mg/dl)		4.5	6.2	30.4	65.2	74.5	78.2		124.5
Al-P (BL)		3.0	3.0	2.8	3.3	3.3	4.4	5.1	8.6
GOT		44	36	34	52	56	74	69	65
GPT		24	26	20	39	35	42	30	29

T.T., 40-year-old male, PLC with liver cirrhosis.
[a] Splenectomy, esophageal transsection. [b] No obvious space-occupying lesion. [c] Space-occupying lesion.

Table IV shows the clinical course of a patient with hepatoma, a 68-year-old female. She was admitted to hospital because of liver enlargement and ascites. The diagnosis was liver cirrhosis. The liver scintigram obtained in December

TABLE IV. Serum Levels of AFP (II)

		1971 Jan. 25	Nov. 10	Dec. 16	1972 Jan. 24	Feb. 17[a]	Mar. 15
AFP	Double diffusion			—	—		—
	Radioimmunoassay (ng/ml)			1,300	1,330		270
Al-P (KA)				14.5	9.8		9.7
GOT		167	98	81	107		68
GPT		27	42	28	41		24

S.T., 68-year-old female, hepatocellular carcinoma with liver cirrhosis.
[a] Selective infusion of anticancer drugs into A. hepatica.

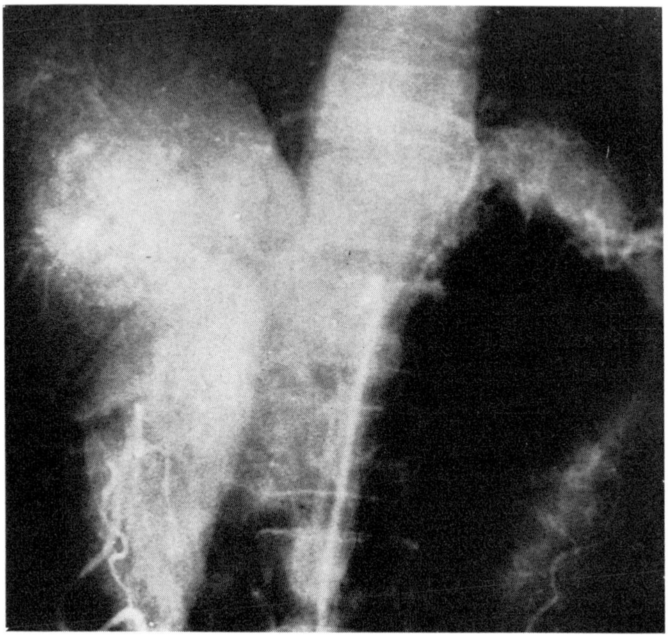

FIG. 1. Angiography (S.T.)

showed no space-occupying lesion. α-Fetoprotein was negative by immunodiffusion, but was positive by radioimmunoassay (1,300 ng/ml). Hepatic angiography revealed a tumor at the right lobe (4.5×4.5 cm in diameter) (Fig. 1). In this case, it may be said that radioimmunoassay gave a clue for the detection of the tumor in an early stage.

It might be thought that the size of the tumor has an influence on the appearance of AFP, with increasing levels of serum AFP paralleling the tumor growth. However, in fact several cases were found in which no AFP was detected, even in a huge hepatoma. Table V shows such a case. This is a 57-year-old male with a large hepatoma, already checked in December 1965. By open biopsy carried out in January 1968, hepatocellular carcinoma was diagnosed. The AFP test was negative at that time. The size of the tumor gradually increased. After

TABLE V. Serum Levels of AFP (III)

	1966	1967			1968		1969	
	July[a]	June	Sept.[b]	Dec.	Jan.[c]	Sept.[d]	Jan.[e]	Feb.[f]
AFP				—	—		+ (15.2 mg/dl)	
Al-P (BL)		6.6	8.2	10.0	12.8		9.2	10.4
GOT		29	38	60	50		200	720
GPT		16	25	48	32		34	58
T. Chol.		256	188				132	128

J.H., 57-year-old male, hepatocellular carcinoma.
[a] Abnormal liver function test. [b] Liver tumor (8 cm at mid.). [c] Selective infusion of anticancer drugs into A. hepatica. [d] Ascites. [e] Jaundice. [f] Liver tumor (15 cm at mid.).

TABLE VI. α-Fetoprotein and Histological Features of PLC

Histological features	No. of cases	Positive cases	Negative cases
Hepatocellular carcinoma			
Mainly trabecular	13	13	0
Mainly solid	3	2	1
Mainly anaplastic	1	0	1
Mainly tubular	1	0	1
Cholangiocellular carcinoma	4	0	4

about 1 year, AFP became positive. This case suggests no correlation exists between the size of the tumor and the appearance of AFP. Some other factors such as the histological features of the tumor may be involved. α-Fetoprotein is likely to appear in trabecular type PLC. One anaplastic case was negative (Table VI).

Serum AFP Levels after Tumor Resection

Surgical intervention of the tumor may result in a decrease or complete disappearance of AFP from the serum. Figure 2 shows a case subjected to resection of the tumor. Serum AFP decreased just after the operation and after 3 weeks, AFP was not detectable by the single radial immunodiffusion technique. However, 5 months later, the patient complained of general malaise and visited the hospital again, and AFP was found to be strongly positive again.

Chemotherapy also diminishes the levels of serum AFP. Figure 3 demonstrates decreased AFP after the infusion of anticancer drugs into A. hepatica by a chronofuser. However, this case also died of an aggravation of the illness.

These facts might suggest that the serum AFP levels parallel the clinical status of the illness. Improvement decreases, and aggravation increases the level even in the same patient. α-Fetoprotein also serves as an index for early detection of recurrence after removing a tumor.

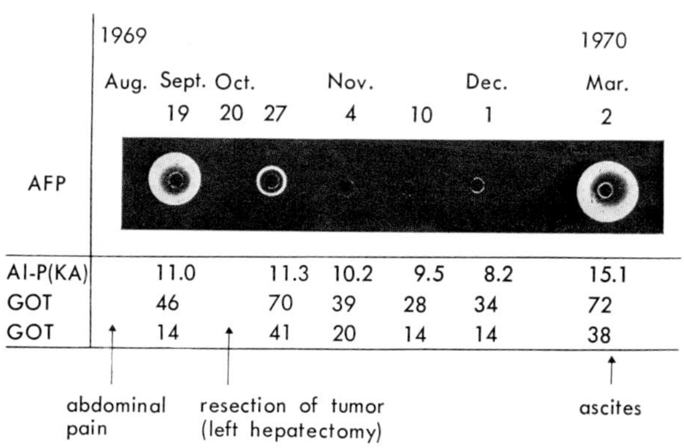

FIG. 2. Serum levels of AFP (IV)
(single radial immunodiffusion)
Y. H., 45-year-old male, hepatoma with liver cirrhosis.

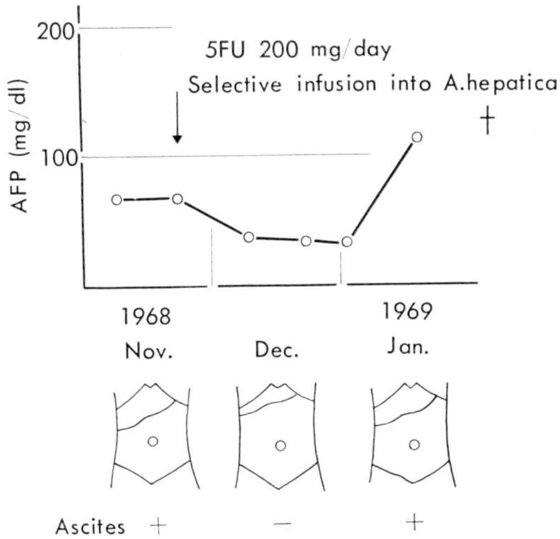

FIG. 3. Serum levels of AFP (V)
K. K., 52-year-old male, PLC with liver cirrhosis.

The site of serum AFP production is the liver cells in the fetus (*2*, *12*, *15*, *18*) and the tumor cells in PLC (*2*, *3*, *8*, *11*, *21*). These facts were confirmed through experiments using radioactive amino acids or immunofluorescence techniques. We also found the production of AFP in the fetal liver, tumor cells of the rat (AH-66), and rat hepatoma tissues produced by administrating 3′-methyl-4-dimethyl-aminoazobenzene (3′-Me-DAB) (to be published).

There was no correlation between the appearance of AFP and the liver function test. In hepatoma, a dissociation of GOT and GPT was generally seen clinically, *i.e.*, the increase in GPT is rather low compared with that of GOT. No relation, however, was found between AFP appearance and GOT/GPT ratio in hepatoma patients.

α-Fetoprotein and Various Diseases Other than Hepatoma

α-Fetoprotein was also found in cases with embryonal carcinoma of the testis or ovary. Abelev reported 35 cases with teratoblastoma which were AFP-positive, but in seminoma it was negative (*4*). We have investigated 3 embryonal carcinoma, the details of which will be discussed elsewhere (Tsuchida *et al.*).

Metastatic liver cancer is usually negative for AFP (*4*, *23*, *32*), but there have been several reports (*6*, *9*, *14*, *19*, *21*, *25*) of metastatic liver cancer showing a positive reaction to AFP. We have observed 2 such cases. One was diagnosed by an X-ray examination for gastric cancer, and a large liver tumor was thought to be a metastasis from the gastric cancer; the other one was adenocarcinoma (probably of gastric origin) as shown by histological examination.

Such cases, positive for metastatic liver cancer, reported by other workers were mostly of gastric origin. As to liver cirrhosis and hepatitis, these will be discussed in the following section.

Radioimmunoassay for AFP

In 20–30% of the total with hepatoma, AFP was found to be negative by the double immunodiffusion technique (micro-Ouchterlony method). Whether it is in fact negative or positive is of interest, and a much more sensitive method is therefore needed. The newly devised radioimmunoassay is 1,000 times more sensitive than double immunodiffusion. This may determine the above problem and may also serve as an early diagnostic technique.

The system of AFP radioimmunoassay is as follows: Iodination of AFP; AFP was purified by gel filtration using AFP-anti-AFP complex (generously provided by Drs. Hirai and Nishi). The iodination procedure was carried out according to the method of Hunter (*17*) using ^{125}I and chloramine-T. The purification of ^{125}I-AFP was done by passing through a column of Sephadex G-75. For the iodination, 5 μg of AFP and 1 mCi of $Na^{125}I$ were used. The double antibody method was then applied. Anti-AFP antiserum was prepared by immunizing a rabbit with hepatoma patient ascites emulsified with

^{125}I-AFP	0.1 ml (6,000–8,000 cpm)
Anti-AFP antiserum (rabbit)	0.1 ml (diluted 1 : 30,000 in final)
Patient's serum or standard	0.1 ml
Standard diluent*	0.7 ml
mixed and incubated for 48 hr at 4°, then added with	
Normal rabbit serum	0.1 ml (diluted 1 : 100)
Anti-rabbit γ-globulin (goat)	0.1 ml (diluted 1 : 10)
mixed and incubated for 24 hr at 4°	

Total radioactivity counted by well-type scintillation counter (total), centrifuged (3,000 rpm for 30 min), radioactivity of the precipitate (bound) counted, and ratio of bound/total (B/T) radioactivity calculated from the standard curve

* 0.1 M Tris buffer (pH 7.5): Physiological saline (1 : 1 v/v).

CHART 1. Assay system for AFP by radioimmunoassay

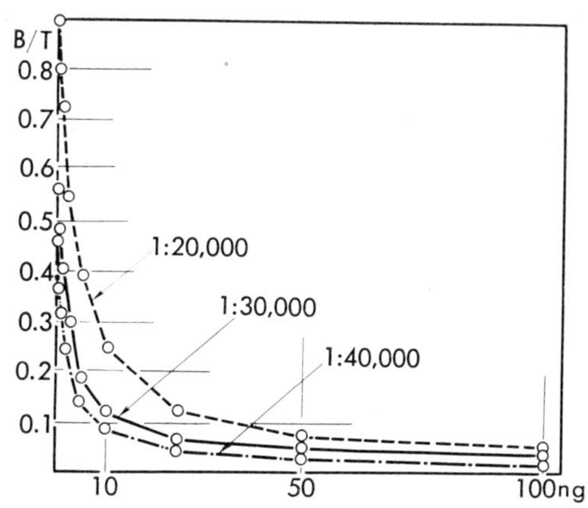

FIG. 4. Dilution of anti-AFP antiserum (optimum dilution: 1 : 30,000 in final)

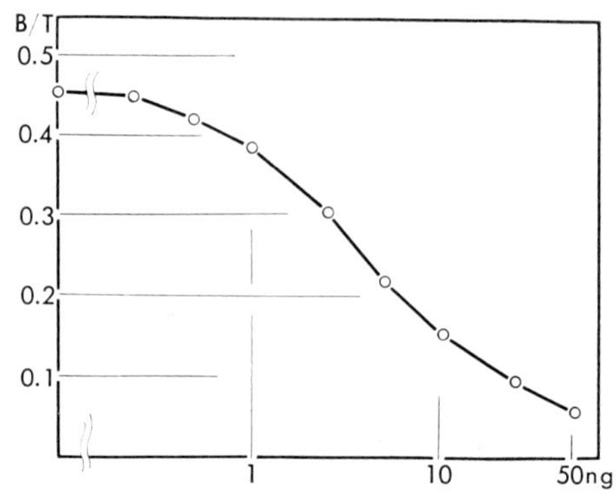

FIG. 5. Standard curve of AFP (radioimmunoassay)

Freund's complete adjuvant, and the nonspecific antibodies were absorbed with pooled normal serum. Anti-rabbit γ-globulin goat serum was purchased from Dainabot Radioisotope Laboratories, Tokyo, Japan. The assay system is listed in Chart 1. The dilution of anti-AFP antiserum was settled to be 40% in B/T ratio, and optimum final dilution is 1: 30,000 (Fig. 4). The optimum incubation times for the 1st and 2nd reactions were determined through preliminary experiments. The standard curve was made using purified AFP diluted by horse serum (Fig. 5). No cross-reaction was seen with human albumin and transferrin by this assay system (Fig. 6). The results are shown in Figs. 7 and 8.

In healthy adults, AFP was less than 10 ng/ml. In pregnant women, increased AFP was found in the 3rd trimester. In other diseases, other than liver diseases, AFP levels were less than 10 ng/ml. Slight increase of AFP (10–50 ng/ml) was observed in acute hepatitis (6 out of 26) and in chronic hepatitis (7 out of 37). However, in the case of liver cirrhosis, about a half (14 out of 26) showed elevated serum AFP levels with a range from 10 to 500 ng/ml.

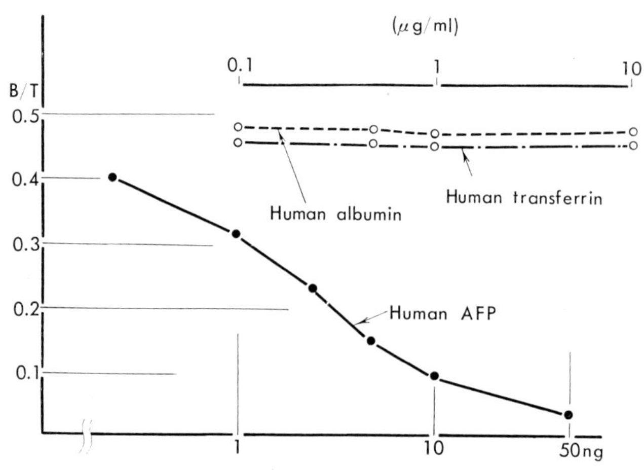

FIG. 6. Cross-reaction of anti-AFP antiserum with human albumin and human transferrin (radioimmunoassay)

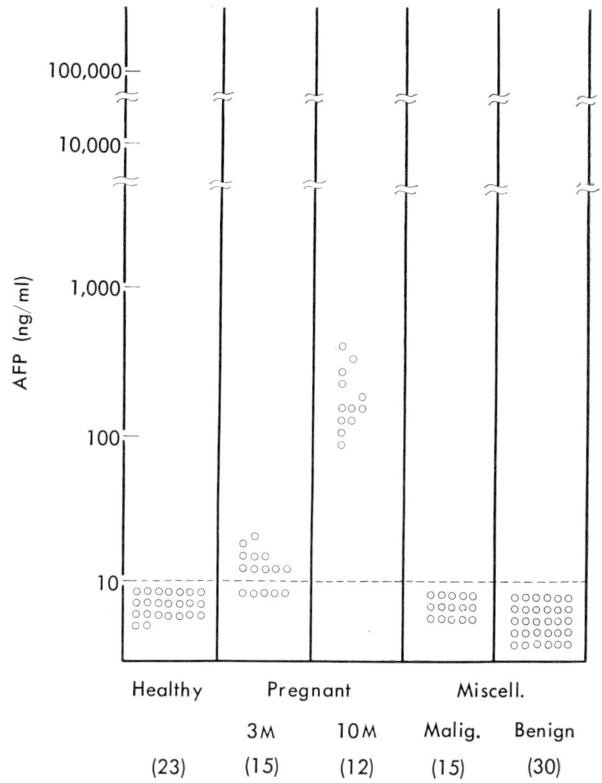

FIG. 7. Serum levels of AFP (radioimmunoassay)

Using radioimmunoassay, 8 of 9 immunodiffusion-negative (below 10 μg/ml) cases of PLC showed increased AFP. The range of the distribution of AFP levels ranged from 170 to 4,000 ng/ml. In one case, AFP was below 10 ng/ml (Table VII).

α-Fetoprotein was considered specific for hepatoma and embryonal cancer, but it has been found in some cases with various types of pathological status (*1*) (hepatitis, liver cirrhosis, and metastatic liver cancer) and in pregnancy, when a

TABLE VII. Radioimmunoassay of AFP in PLC (immunodiffusion-negative cases)

Name	Age (yrs.)	Sex	AFP (ng/ml)	Cirrhosis	Diagnosis
M.I.	42	Male	4,000	+	Autopsy
K.M.	55	Male	2,500	+	Autopsy
E.S.	56	Male	650	—	Open biopsy
S.I.	78	Male	400	+	Autopsy
S.H.	65	Male	380	+	Scintigram
H.U.	40	Male	350	+	Autopsy
T.S.	64	Male	250	+	Autopsy
T.S.	55	Male	170	+	Autopsy
M.N.	65	Female	10	+	Open biopsy

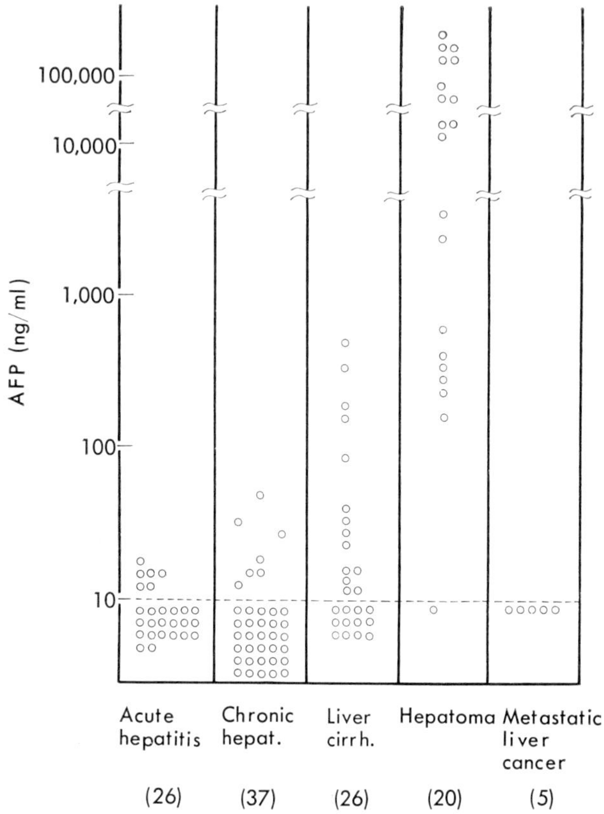

FIG. 8. Serum levels of AFP (radioimmunoassay)

much more sensitive technique was applied. We could not detect AFP in a healthy person by our technique. However, Rouslahti and Seppälä (*31*) found AFP in normal subjects using their sensitive radioimmunoassay technique. α-Fetoprotein might therefore exist in a healthy adult too, in a very minute quantity.

Concluding Remarks

We briefly discussed the clinical significance of AFP in the diagnosis of hepatoma. This method proved to be highly specific for hepatoma (of the histologically confirmed cases, 76.4% were positive). By means of radioimmunoassay, AFP can be detected even in minute quantities, providing a powerful diagnostic tool in clinical medicine. Radioimmunoassay may be useful technique for the detection of hepatoma, and may also serve as an aid in the field of experimental carcinogenesis.

Acknowledgments

This study was supported by a Grants-in-Aid for Scientific Research from the Ministry of Education and from the Ministry of Health and Welfare, Japan.

REFERENCES

1. Abelev, G. I. α-Fetoprotein in ontogenesis and its association with malignant tumors. *Adv. Cancer Res.*, **14**, 295 (1971).
2. Abelev, G. I. Antigenic structure of chemically induced hepatomas. *Progr. Exp. Tumor Res.*, **7**, 104 (1965).
3. Abelev, G. I., Perova, S. D., Khramkova, N. I., Postonikova, Z. A., and Irlin, I. S. Production of embryonal α-globulin by transplantable mouse hepatoma. *Transplantation*, **1**, 174 (1963).
4. Abelev, G. I. Production of embryonal serum α-globulin by hepatomas. Review of experimental and clinical data. *Cancer Res.*, **28**, 1344 (1968).
5. Alpert, E., Hershberg, R., Schur, P. H., and Isselbacher, K. J. α-Fetoprotein in human hepatoma: Improved detection in serum and quantitative studies using a new sensitive technique. *Gastroenterology*, **61**, 137 (1971).
6. Alpert, E., Pinn, V. W., and Isselbacher, K. J. α-Fetoprotein in a patient with gastric carcinoma metastatic to the liver. *New Engl. J. Med.*, **285**, 1058 (1971).
7. Alpert, M. E., Uriel, J., and de Nechaud, B. α_1-Fetoglobulin in the diagnosis of human hepatoma. *New Engl. J. Med.*, **278**, 984 (1968).
8. Basteris, B. Etude par immunofluorescence de la production d'α-fetoprotéine par les cellules hépatiques foetales ou tumorales. Thèse de Doctorat en Médecine (Marseille) (1970).
9. Bourreille, J., Metayer, P., Sauger, F., Matray, F., and Fondimare, A. Existence d'α-fetoprotéine au cours d'un cancer secondaire du foie d'origine gastrique. *Presse Med.*, **78**, 1277 (1970).
10. Endo, Y., Etoh, S., Iino, S., Fujiwara, K., Miyake, K., Kanetaka, T., Yamanaka, M., Suzuki, H., Suzuki, H., Oda, T., Yoshitoshi, Y., Juji, T., Yokochi, T., and Miura, T. Diagnosis of primary liver cancer by demonstrating α-fetoglobulin in the serum (in Japanese). *Kanzo (Liver)*, **10**, 143 (1969).
11. Engelhardt, N. V., Gusev, A. I., Shipova, L. J., and Abelev, G. I. Immunofluorescent study of α-fetoprotein in liver and liver tumors. I. Technique of α-FP localization in tissue sections. *Int. J. Cancer.*, **7**, 198 (1971).
12. Engelhardt, N. V., Shipova, L. J., Gusev, A. I., Jazova, A. K., and Tergrigorova, E. N. Immunohistochemical detection of f-globulin in the liver sections of human embryo and newborn mice. *Bull. Exp. Biol. Med. (U.S.S.R.)*, **12**, 62 (1969).
13. Foli, A. K., Sherlock, S., and Adinolfi, M. Serum α-fetoprotein in patients with liver disease. *Lancet*, **2**, 1267 (1969).
14. Geffroy, Y., Metayer, P., Denis, P., Colin, R., Sauger, F., and Fondimare, A. α-Fetoproteine et cancer secondaire du foie. *Presse Med.*, **78**, 1896 (1970).
15. Gitlin, D. and Boesman, M. Sites of serum α-fetoprotein synthesis in the human and in the rat. *J. Clin. Invest.*, **46**, 1010 (1967).
16. Hirai, H. Embryonal α-globulin and hepatoma (in Japanese). *Sogo Rinsho (Clinic All-Around)*, **19**, 891 (1970).
17. Hunter, W. M. *In* "Handbook of Experimental Immunology," ed. by D. M. Weir, Blackwell Scientific Publications, Oxford and Edinburgh, p. 602 (1967).
18. Kekkomäki, M., Seppälä, M., Ehnholm, C. C., Schwartz, A. L., and Raivio, K. Perfusion of isolated human fetal liver. Synthesis and release of α-fetoprotein and albumin. *Int. J. Cancer*, **8**, 250 (1971).
19. Kitaoka, K., Hattori, S., and Mukojima, T. α-Fetoprotein and metastatic liver cancer—with special reference to gastric cancer (in Japanese). *Igaku-no-Ayumi (The Stride of Medicine)*, **79**, 129 (1971).

20. Kithier, K., Houstek, J., Masopust, J., and Rádl, J. Occurrence of a specific fetal protein in a primary liver carcinoma. *Nature*, **212**, 414 (1966).
21. Kozower, M., Fawaz, K. A., Miller, H. M., and Kaplan, M. N. Positive α-fetoglobulin in a case of gastric carcinoma. *New Engl. J. Med.*, **285**, 1059 (1971).
22. Kresno, S. B., Gandasoebrata, R., and Rümke, P. Serum α-fetoprotein in patients with hepatoma from Djakarta. *Protides Biol. Fluids*, **18**, 243 (1971).
23. Masopust, J., Kithier, K., Rádl, J., Koutecky, J., and Kotál, L. Occurrence of α-fetoprotein in patients with neoplasms and non-neoplastic diseases. *Int. J. Cancer*, **3**, 364 (1968).
24. Masseyeff, R., Sankale, M., Onde, M., Menye, A., Camain, R., Quenum, C., Magdat, L., Mattern, P., Ancelle, I., and Leblanc, L. Valeur de la recherche de l'α-fetoprotéine sérique pour le diagnostic du cancer primitif du foie. *Bull. Soc. Med. Afr. Noire*, **13**, 537 (1968).
25. Mehlman, D. J., Bulkley, B. H., and Wiernik, P. H. Serum α_1-fetoglobulin with gastric and prostatic carcinoma. *New Engl. J. Med.*, **285**, 1060 (1971).
26. Mukojima, T., Shimodaira, K., Hattori, S., Hasegawa, H., and Kitaoka, K. The diagnosis of primary cancer of the liver by α_1-fetoglobulin (in Japanese). *Kanzo (Liver)*, **11**, 325 (1970).
27. O'Conor, G., Tatarinov, Y. S., Abelev, G. I., and Uriel, J. A collaborative study for the evaluation of a serological test for primary liver cancer. *Cancer*, **25**, 1091 (1970).
28. Okita, K. Clinical significance of α-fetoprotein in the diagnosis of primary liver cancer (in Japanese). *Kanzo (Liver)*, **11**, 194 (1970).
29. Purves, L. R., Bersohn, I., and Geddes, E. W. Serum α-fetoprotein and primary cancer of the liver in man. *Cancer*, **25**, 1261 (1970).
30. Purves, L. R., Machab, M., and Bersohn, I. Fetoglobulin and primary liver cancer. *Lancet*, **2**, 634 (1968).
31. Ruoslahti, E. and Seppälä, M. Studies of carcinofetal proteins. III. Development of a radioimmunoassay for α-fetoprotein. Demonstration of α-fetoprotein in serum of healthy human adults. *Int. J. Cancer*, **8**, 374 (1971).
32. Smith, J. B. and Todd, D. Fetoglobulin and primary liver cancer. *Lancet*, **2**, 833 (1968).
33. Sankalé, M., Masseyeff, R., Camain, R., Quenum, C., Ancelle, J. P., and Leblanc, L. Le diagnostic du carcinome primitif du foie par la mise en évidence dans le sérum d'une α_1-globuline embryonnaire. *Presse Med.*, **76**, 2047 (1968).
34. Tatarinov, Y. S. Content of embryo-specific α-globulin in the blood serum of human fetus, newborn and adult man in primary cancer of the liver. *Vopr. Med. Khim.*, **11**, 20 (1965) (*Fed. Proc.*, **25**, 344 (1966)).
35. Uriel, J., de Nechaud, B., Stanislawski-birencwajg, M., Masseyeff, L., Leblanc, L., Quenum, C., Loisillier, F., and Grabar, P. Le diagnostic du cancer primaire du foie par des methodes immunologiques. *Presse Med.*, **76**, 1414 (1968).

GANN Monograph on Cancer Research 14, 1973

RADIOIMMUNOASSAY OF α-FETOPROTEIN IN HEPATOMA, OTHER LIVER DISEASES, AND PREGNANCY

Shinzo NISHI and Hidematsu HIRAI
*Department of Biochemistry, School of Medicine, Hokkaido University**

The sera of 92 hepatoma patients and 664 patients with other diseases were tested for α-fetoprotein (AFP) by precipitin reaction in gels. The AFP was detected only in 70% of the hepatoma cases and in 2 cases of metastatic liver cancer patients, but in no other diseases nor in healthy adults. The serum levels showed a very wide distribution from 10 to 3,750 μg/ml.

A radioimmunoassay was developed which is 500 times more sensitive than the precipitin reaction. In 11% of the hepatoma patients, AFP could not be detected (under 20 ng/ml) even by the sensitive method, but a high prevalence of AFP was demonstrated in hepatitis, cirrhosis, other liver diseases, and in pregnancy.

Prevalence of AFP in Hepatoma Detected by the Ouchterlony Test

In 1964, Tatarinov (*27*) reported the reappearance of α-fetoprotein (AFP) in the sera of patients suffering from hepatoma. The association was confirmed by many other investigators (*1, 4, 6, 8, 13, 15, 16, 19, 21, 26–28*) as highly specific for hepatoma, with the exception of embryonal carcinomas (*1, 8, 15, 16*) of testicle and ovary. However, in these reports there seem to have been some disagreements about the prevalence of AFP in the sera of patients with hepatoma: The highest value was near 90% (*13*), the lowest, near 30% (*6, 8*). Such factors as race (*6, 8*), age (*16*), and sex (*8, 19*) have been suggested as the cause of the difference. Precipitin reactions in gels, such as the Ouchterlony test, and the single radial immunodiffusion method of Mancini, were used to detect the protein in these studies.

In the authors' laboratory, AFP tests have been performed by the Ouchterlony method since 1969. Serum samples were obtained from 756 patients admitted to the Hokkaido University Hospital or several other hospitals in the northern part of Japan. These patients were diagnosed or suspected to have primary liver cancer (PLC), various other liver disorders, and other malignancies. AFP was detected in the sera of 61 out of 92 patients with hepatoma (66%), some of which were diagnosed only clinically. Among them, the sera of 39 out of 56 patients, histologically confirmed as hepatoma cases gave positive tests (70%). On the other hand, all 6 patients with histologically confirmed cholangioma gave negative tests. The sera of 334 patients with other definitely diagnosed miscellaneous

* Kita-15-jo, Nishi-7-chome, Kita-ku, Sapporo 060, Japan (西 信三, 平井秀松).

TABLE I. Occurrence of AFP

Hepatoma	39/56	70%
Cholangioma	0/6	
Metastatic liver cancer	2/50	
Non-liver cancer	0/58	
Hepatitis	0/43	
Liver cirrhosis	0/42	
Other liver and biliary tract diseases	0/31	
Miscellaneous	24[a]/470	
Healthy adults	0/5,998	

[a] Probable hepatoma 22, probable metastatic liver cancer 2. (>10 μg/ml)

diseases gave negative tests with only 2 exceptions. These positive patients both had diagnosis of adenocarcinoma of the stomach with metastasis to the liver at autopsy. Embryonal carcinomas were not included in the cases tested. The sera of 324 patients with some obvious disorders, though the definite diagnoses were obscure because of failure of follow-up or lack of sufficient evidence, gave negative tests. The sera of 5,998 blood donors at Hokkaido Blood Bank were also tested but gave negative results. These results are summarized in Table I.

Serum AFP concentrations were determined by the single radial immunodiffusion method using purified and lyophilized AFP as the standard (*17*). The determined levels, taking the maximum value during the course of the disease in each patient, showed a wide distribution from 3,750 to 10 μg/ml, the lower limit of sensitivity of the Ouchterlony test, with the mode around 65 μg/ml, as shown in Fig. 1. All 6 children with hepatoma gave positive tests and the

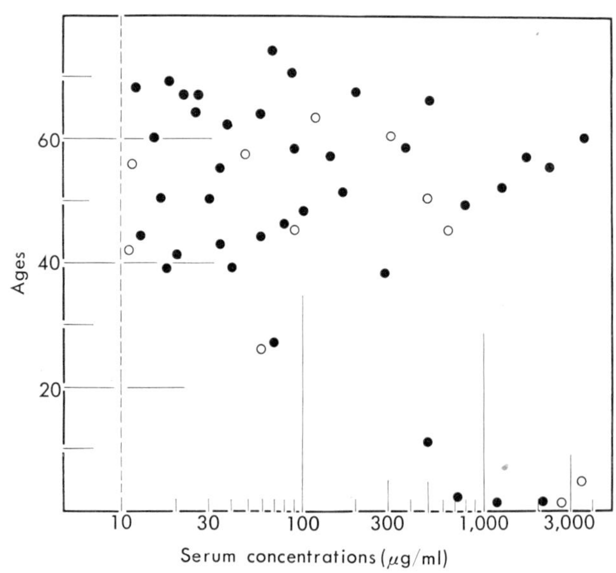

FIG. 1. Serum AFP concentration of hepatoma patients, determined by single radial immunodiffusion

● male; ○ female.

serum levels were quite high, from 500 to 3,450 μg/ml. These data agree with a previous report (*16*). In adult cases, either age or sex difference effects on the prevalence of AFP and on the serum concentration were difficult to discern. The AFP concentration increased with progress of the disease but in some patients, in spite of advanced tumors, serum levels were very low or hardly detectable.

Some correlation was found between histological features of the tumor and the serum AFP concentrations (*24*). The serum AFP decreased with effective treatment (*11*). Some of these data are presented elsewhere in this monograph. The prevalence of AFP in Japanese patients reported by others (*3*, *5*, *7*, *10*, *12*, *14*, *18*, *29*) is essentially the same as reported here. However, the prevalence in Japan (70–80%) is significantly higher than those reported for England (40%) (*6*) and USA (38%) (*8*) but not markedly different from those reported for patients in South Africa (78%) (*21*), Dakar (80%) (*19*), Singapore (72%) (*19*), Hong Kong (59%) (*26*), U.S.S.R. (79%) (*1*), and Indonesia (86%) (*13*).

The wide variations of serum AFP levels in hepatoma patients reported both in the present study and in Purves' study (*21*) suggest that the sensitivity of the technique is critical for the detection of positive cases, because the serum levels of a considerable number of the patients are near the limit of sensitivity and to discuss the difference in prevalence of AFP in hepatoma patients further, quantitative studies with more sensitive methods seem necessary.

Development of the Radioimmunoassay Technique

The appearance of AFP is confirmed to be highly specific for hepatoma, and it is also found less frequently in certain other malignancies when the precipitin reaction in agar gel is used for detection. In mice, AFP appears with regeneration of the liver after CCl_4 intoxication (*1*). A more sensitive technique is desirable to evaluate the specificity of the association of AFP with malignancies, to determine the AFP levels in those hepatoma patient sera for which the Ouchterlony test is negative, and to aid in making an earlier diagnosis of malignancies and other disease states associated with increased serum AFP. A radioimmunoassay for AFP using the double antibody technique was developed for these purposes.

Radioiodination of AFP: α-Fetoprotein was isolated from an antigen-antibody complex by gel filtration at low pH, as previously described (*17*). The purified preparation was labeled with ^{125}I by the chloramine T method of Hunter (*9*). The ^{125}I-labeled AFP was separated from free radioactive iodine by gel filtration. $Na^{125}I$ (1.4 mCi) was reacted with 73.1 μg of AFP and ^{125}I-labeled AFP with a specific activity of 16.6 μCi/μg was prepared.

Antisera: The radioimmunoassay was carried out by a double antibody method using rabbit antiserum to human AFP and goat antiserum to rabbit γ-globulin (Dainabot Radioisotope Laboratories, Tokyo, Japan). The rabbit antiserum was prepared by injecting 1 mg of AFP emulsified in Freund's complete adjuvant weekly, 5 times.

Assay system: The test is based on the competition of labeled and unlabeled AFP for a limited amount of antibody (rabbit) to AFP. A definite amount of

1% HoSA in PBS, pH 7.0, $\mu = 0.15$	0.5 ml
Sample or standard serum	0.1 ml
Labeled AFP, *ca.* 10,000 cpm	0.1 ml
Rabbit anti-AFP (×30,000)	0.1 ml
Normal rabbit serum (×100)	0.1 ml
4°, 24 hr	
Goat anti-rabbit γ-glob. (×10)	0.1 ml
4°, 24 hr	
3,000 rpm, 15 min	
Count precipitate	

CHART 1. Radioimmunoassay of AFP by a double antibody technique

labeled AFP is mixed with the sample to be tested and reacted with the antibody. In the reaction, a mixture of 2 antigen-antibody complexes results, labeled antigen-antibody and unlabeled antigen-antibody. The complexes are separated from the unreacted antigen by precipitating with the 2nd antibody (goat) to the 1st antibody (rabbit γ-globulin). The amount of antigen in the sample is estimated from the amount of labeled antigen in the precipitate.

The assay was carried out as shown in Chart 1. Diluent (1% horse serum albumin in 0.01 M phosphate in saline, pH 7.0, μ=0.16) (0.5 ml), sample serum or standard serum (0.1 ml), labeled AFP (0.1 ml) (about 10,000 cpm), rabbit anti-AFP (diluted 1: 30,000) (0.1 ml), and normal rabbit serum (diluted 1: 100) (0.1 ml) were mixed in a tube (12×105 mm) and incubated for 24 hr at 4°. After the 1st incubation goat antiserum against rabbit γ-globulin (diluted 1: 10)

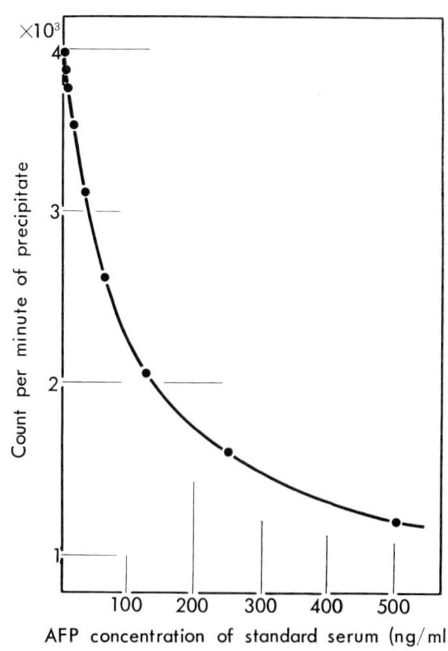

FIG. 2. Standard inhibition curve

(0.1 ml) was added to the mixture and allowed to react for 24 hr at 4°. After centrifugation, the supernatant was removed and the radioactivity of the precipitate was measured in a well-type scintillation counter. The antiserum dilutions and the incubation periods were determined by preliminary experiments. The dilution of the first antiserum was adjusted to combine with 40% of the labeled AFP and the amount of the second antiserum was sufficient to precipitate all of the rabbit γ-globulin including the antigen-antibody complex in the system.

Standard serum was prepared by diluting hepatoma patient serum of a known AFP concentration with normal human serum from which AFP, if any, was removed by passing through an immunoadsorbent column of horse antibody to human AFP. The immunoadsorbent was prepared by coupling the antibody to Sepharose activated with BrCN by the method of Porath *et al.* (*20*). By addition of the standard serum (AFP concentration 500, $500\times(1/2)$, $500\times(1/4)$, . . . $500\times(1/256)$ ng/ml), the precipitation of the labeled AFP was characteristically inhibited. A standard curve is shown in Fig. 2.

Serum AFP Levels of Hepatoma Patients with the Negative Ouchterlony Tests

Sera of 39 patients with histologically confirmed hepatoma giving persistently negative results in the Ouchterlony tests ($<10^4$ ng/ml) were examined by radioimmunoassay. These sera were from 17 among 56 patients described in the 1st section and from 22 additional hepatoma patients giving negative tests in our laboratory or in several other institutions. The serum concentrations were 500–10^4 ng/ml in 13 patients, 500–20 ng/ml in 13 patients, and <20 ng/ml in 13 patients. In the positive cases (>20 ng/ml), 11 from the 17 cases (Table I) were included and among the 56 hepatoma cases 89% were positive. These data are shown in Table II and Fig. 3. In these determinations, values above 20 ng/ml were highly reliable.

TABLE II. Occurrence of AFP

			(%)
Hepatoma		49/56	89
Hepatitis, acute		14/27	52
Hepatitis, chronic		14/35	40
Liver cirrhosis		18/38	47
Metastatic liver cancer		2/8	
Miscellaneous liver disease		11/35	31
Miscellaneous cancer		3/36	8
Heart disease		0/12	
Lung disease		0/9	
Others		0/9	
Pregnancy	1st trimester	0/13	
	2nd, 3rd trimester	18/18	100

(>20 ng/ml)

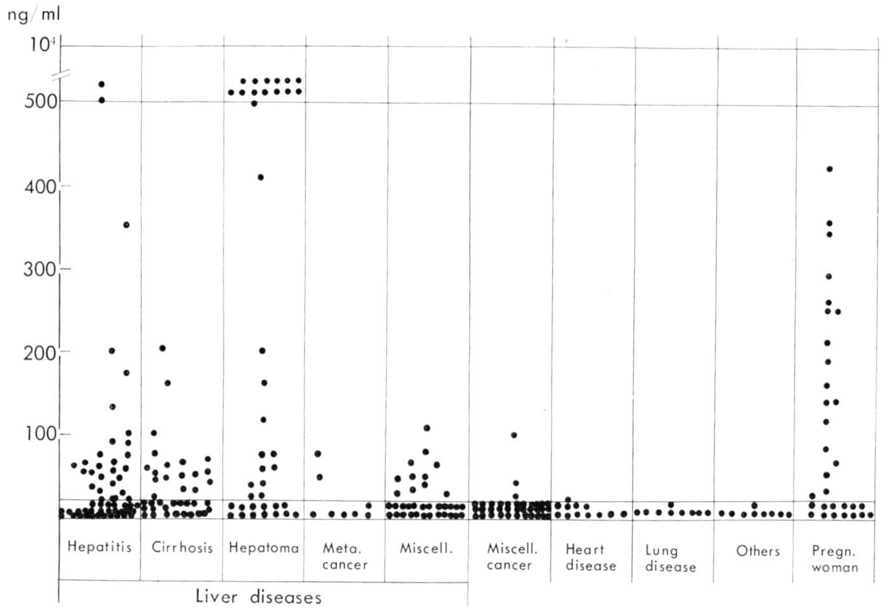

FIG. 3. Serum AFP concentrations of Ouchterlony-negative hepatoma patients, other diseased patients, and pregnant women determined by radioimmunoassay

Serum AFP Levels of Patients with Diseases Other than Hepatoma and of Pregnant Women

α-Fetoprotein was also demonstrated by radioimmunoassay in hepatitis, cirrhosis, metastatic liver cancer, miscellaneous liver diseases, heart diseases, lung diseases, other diseases, and pregnancy. The data are shown in Table II and the serum levels are shown in Fig. 3. The highest value in hepatitis was 800 ng/ml. The peak of AFP concentration during pregnancy was in the 3rd trimester.

In addition to these examinations, sera obtained for routine liver function tests from 430 hospitalized patients were also tested by radioimmunoassay. Among them, AFP was detected in the sera of 55 patients (400–20 ng/ml) as listed in Table III. Some abnormal results in the liver function tests were found in 33 out of

TABLE III. Diagnoses of 55 AFP-positive Cases

Diagnosis	No. of cases
Hepatoma	1
Chronic hepatitis	12
Serum hepatitis	3
Cirrhosis	4
Other liver and biliary tract diseases	8
Other malignancy	8
Psychoneurotic diseases	2
Pregnancy	5
Babies	2
Miscellaneous	10

55 AFP-positive cases (60%). Among 430 patients, 83 had more or less abnormal liver function. Thirty-two out of the 83 cases with abnormal liver function showed AFP in their sera. These data may suggest that regenerating liver cells produce AFP in humans, as had been observed in mice (*1*).

The present results are compatible with the data of Abelev *et al.* (*2*) who reported that AFP was detected in infectious hepatitis (in 12%), metastatic liver cancer (in 13 out of 23), and pregnancy (in 98% after the 15th week). These investigators employed aggregate-hemagglutination or immunoradioautography, which are more sensitive than the Ouchterlony test. Similar results were also reported for serum AFP concentration during pregnancy by Seppälä and Ruoslahti (*25*).

α-Fetoprotein is thus not specific only for hepatoma, but is also detected in patients with hepatitis, cirrhosis, and some other liver diseases and in pregnant women when a sensitive method such as that described here is used. However, the serum levels in the majority of hepatoma patients are considerably higher than those observed in hepatitis and other clinical states. For the early diagnosis of hepatoma, radioimmunoassay may be useful, since in most cases the serum AFP level is thought to increase rapidly as the hepatoma develops. Such increases were observed in 2 patients who died with hepatoma. In case I, the serum concentration increased from 31 ng/ml (April, 1969) to 102,000 ng/ml (August, 1970), and in case II, from 1,000 ng/ml (April, 1971) to 200,000 ng/ml (August 18, 1971). Purves and Geddes (*22*) reported that a 0.5-cm diameter hepatoma nodule was found at autopsy in a patient who died of esophageal cancer whose serum AFP level was 300 ng/ml.

Recently, AFP was found in the sera of healthy adults (around 10 ng/ml) by Ruoslahti and Seppälä (*23*) and Purves and Geddes (*22*). We have not measured levels below 20 ng/ml because the reproducibility of our present assay system is insufficient to measure AFP in such low concentrations. A slight modification of the present method is necessary to demonstrate the presence of AFP in healthy adults.

Acknowledgments

The authors thank Drs. Y. Kasai, M. Mito, J. Uchino, A. Tamaki, S. Shibata, K. Nagase, F. Kondo, F. Dake, C. Sekiya, and K. Yokoo of the Hokkaido University Hospital, and Dr. K. Itoh, Hokkaido Blood Bank, for collecting blood samples, and Dr. H. B. Hamilton, Atomic Bomb Casualty Commission, for reading this manuscript.

REFERENCES

1. Abelev, G. I. Production of embryonal serum α-globulin by hepatomas: Review of experimental and clinical data. *Cancer Res.*, **28**, 1344–1350 (1968).
2. Abelev, G. I., Tsvetkov, V. S., Biryulina, T. I., Elgort, D. A., Olovnikov, A. M., Gusev, A. I., Jazova, A. K., Perova, S. D., Pubtsov, I. V., Shaborina, S. V., Kantorovich, B. A., Tur, V. M., Khazanov, A. I., and Levina, D. M. Assessment of the use of highly sensitive methods of determining α-fetoprotein for the

diagnosis of hepatocellular cancer and teratoblastoma. *Byull. Eksp. Biol. Med.*, **4**, 75–81 (1971).
3. Akai, S. and Kato, K. Serum α-fetoprotein-positive stomach cancer. *GANN Monograph on Cancer Research*, **14**, 149 (1973).
4. Alpert, M. E. α_1-Fetoprotein in human hepatoma. *Clin. Res.*, **17**, 461 (1969).
5. Endo, Y., Kanai, K., Iino, S., and Oda, T. Clinical significance of α-fetoprotein—with special reference to primary cancer of the liver. *GANN Monograph on Cancer Research*, **14**, 67 (1973).
6. Foli, K., Sherlock, S., and Adinolfi, M. Serum α-fetoprotein in patients with liver disease. *Lancet*, **2**, 1267–1268 (1968).
7. Hasegawa, H., Mukojima, T., Hattori, S., Sano, R., and Hirota, T. Embryonal carcinoma and α-fetoprotein—with special reference to hepatoblastoma. *GANN Monograph on Cancer Research*, **14**, 129 (1973).
8. Hull, E. W. Serum α-fetoprotein in the U.S.A. *Lancet*, **1**, 779 (1970).
9. Hunter, W. M. The preparation of radioiodinated proteins of high activity. Their reaction with antibody *in vitro*: The radioimmunoassay. *In* "Handbook of Experimental Immunology," ed. by D. M. Weir, Blackwell Scientific Publications, Oxford and Edinburgh, pp. 602–654 (1967).
10. Ishii, M. Radioimmunoassay of α-fetoprotein. *GANN Monograph on Cancer Research*, **14**, 89 (1973).
11. Kasai, Y. and Mito, M. 14th Symposium on α-fetoprotein and hepatoma. Jap. Cancer Association, Dec. 1971, Tokyo.
12. Kosaka, A. 14th Symposium on α-fetoprotein and hepatona, Jap. Cancer Association, Dec. 1971, Tokyo.
13. Kresno, S. B., Gandasoebrata, R., and Rümke, Ph. *Lancet*, **1**, 1178 (1970).
14. Kuroyanagi, Y. Results in the treatment of hepatocellular carcinoma—with special reference to α-fetoprotein. *GANN Monograph on Cancer Research*, **14**, 107 (1973).
15. Masopust, J., Kithier, K., Rádl, J., Koutecky, J., and Kotál, L. Occurrence of fetoprotein in patients with neoplasms and non-neoplastic diseases. *Int. J. Cancer*, **3**, 364–373 (1968).
16. Mawas, C., Buffe, D., and Burtin, P. Influence of age on α-fetoprotein incidence. *Lancet*, **1**, 1292 (1970).
17. Nishi, S. Isolation and characterization of a human fetal α-globulin from the sera of fetuses and a hepatoma patient. *Cancer Res.*, **30**, 2507–2513 (1970).
18. Nishioka, M., Ibata, T., Miyazato, K., Okita, K., Hironaga, K., and Fujita, T. Immunofluorescence studies on α-fetoprotein in hepatoma tissue. *GANN Monograph on Cancer Research*, **14**, 205 (1973).
19. O'Conor, G. T., Tatarinov, Yu. S., Abelev, G. I., and Uriel, J. A collaborative study for the evaluation of a serologic test for primary liver cancer. *Cancer*, **25**, 1091–1098 (1970).
20. Porath, J., Axen, R., and Ernback, S. Chemical coupling of proteins to agarose. *Nature*, **215**, 1491–1492 (1967).
21. Purves, L. R., Bersohn, I., and Geddes, E. W. Serum α-fetoprotein and primary cancer of the liver in man. *Cancer*, **25**, 1261–1270 (1970).
22. Purves, L. R. and Geddes, E. W. A more sensitive test for α-fetoprotein. *Lancet*, **1**, 47–48 (1972).
23. Ruoslahti, E. and Seppälä, M. Studies of carcino-fetal proteins. III. Development of a radioimmunoassay for α-fetoprotein. Demonstration of α-fetoprotein in serum of healthy human adults. *Int. J. Cancer*, **8**, 374–383 (1971).

24. Sasaki, K., Miyakawa, A., Mito, M., and Kasai, Y. Histology of hepatoma in man with regard to α-fetoprotein. *GANN Monograph on Cancer Research*, **14**, 199 (1973).
25. Seppälä, M. and Ruoslahti, E. Radioimmunoassay of maternal serum alpha-fetoprotein during pregnancy and delivery. *Am. J. Obstet. Gynecol.*, **112**, 208–212 (1972).
26. Smith, J. B. and Todd, D. Fetoglobulin and primary liver cancer, *Lancet*, **2**, 833 (1968).
27. Tatarinov, Yu. S. Presence of embryospecific α-globulin in the serum of patients with primary hepatocellular carcinoma. *Vopr. Med. Khim.*, **10**, 90–91 (1964).
28. Uriel, J. Antigénes embryonaires et cancer du foie chez l'homme: Association de l' α-fetoprotéine sérique avec l'hépatome primaire. *C.R.*, **265**, 75–78 (1967).
29. Wada, T., Anzai, T., and Yachi, A. Immunochemical studies on antigenic components common to carcinoma and fetus, and their diagnostic significances—with special reference to connection with α-fetoprotein. *GANN Monograph on Cancer Research*, **14**, 157 (1973).

GANN Monograph on Cancer Research 14, 1973

RADIOIMMUNOASSAY OF α-FETOPROTEIN

Masaru ISHII
*Second Department of Internal Medicine, School of Medicine, Kobe University**

The isolation of α-fetoprotein (AFP) from AFP-positive ascites by using a technique of immune absorption against adulterant protein was performed and a radioimmunoassay for AFP based on a coprecipitation-inhibition technique using the 2-antibody method was developed. This assay was able to detect reproducibly 15.6 ng of AFP per ml of serum.

A survey using this assay revealed the presence of AFP, not only in patients with primary hepatocellular cancer (PHC), but also in patients with other liver diseases and pregnant women. The presence of AFP in patients with hepatitis or cirrhosis could be demonstrated at the beginning of the improvement of the illness, and thereafter the AFP level was progressively reduced. On the other hand, AFP levels in patients with PHC increased quite rapidly with the progress of the disease.

Abelev *et al.* (*3*) demonstrated in 1963 that transplantable mouse and rat hepatomas synthesize and secrete into the blood an embryospecific α-fetoprotein (AFP). In 1964, Tatarinov (*11*) reported the presence of AFP in the sera of patients with primary hepatocellular cancer (PHC). Thereafter, Abelev *et al.* (*1*), Uriel *et al.* (*12*), and many other workers confirmed the observations of Tatarinov on the diagnosis of PHC. Simultaneously, it was found that AFP also appeared in the serum of patients with malignant teratoblastomas (TRB) of the testis and ovary. At the present time, AFP, originally reported only in fetal serum, is known to be a highly specific indicator of PHC.

The technique of agar gel immunoprecipitation has been used for the detection of AFP, but the sensitivity is relatively low. Attempts have been made to develop highly sensitive methods of AFP determination for the diagnosis of PHC. Recently, highly sensitive methods—aggregate hemagglutination, immunoradioautography, and radioimmunoassay—were established and the detection of AFP using those methods led to the discovery of a lack of specificity for PHC.

Abelev *et al.* (*3*) and Bakirov (*4*) found a temporary appearance of AFP in the sera of adult mice with regenerating liver after partial hepatectomy or inhalation of CCl_4 vapor. Liver regeneration has recently been suggested as a cause of AFP formation in viral hepatitis from the similarity of AFP dynamics during this disease with that of mice with regenerating liver.

The isolation of human AFP was achieved by Nishi (*9*) in 1970, followed by Gusev and Jazova, and the present author and his collaborators in 1971.

* 12 Kusunoki, 7-chome, Ikuta-ku, Kobe 670, Japan (石井 勝).

Isolation of Human AFP

Nishi obtained pure human AFP by precipitation with a corresponding antibody, and described that the purified AFP had $s_{20}=4.50\,S$ and a molecular weight of 65,000.

We isolated pure AFP from the AFP-positive ascites of a patient with PHC by the scheme shown in Chart 1. Crude AFP was first obtained from the ascites by a procedure of Rivanol-ammonium sulfate fractionation. Proteins contained in the crude AFP are albumin, AFP, and some α_1-globulins. The crude AFP was partially purified by 3 cycles of preparative polyacrylamide gel disc electrophoresis in order to remove most of the albumin. The result of separation after the 3rd cycle of electrophoresis is shown in Fig. 1. The partially puri-

AFP-positive ascites
  | Rivanol-ammonium sulfate fractionation
Crude AFP
  | preparative disc electrophoresis
Partially purified AFP
  | absorption by anti-human serum protein rabbit γ-globulin
  | preparative disc electrophoresis
Purified AFP

CHART 1. Scheme of isolation of AFP

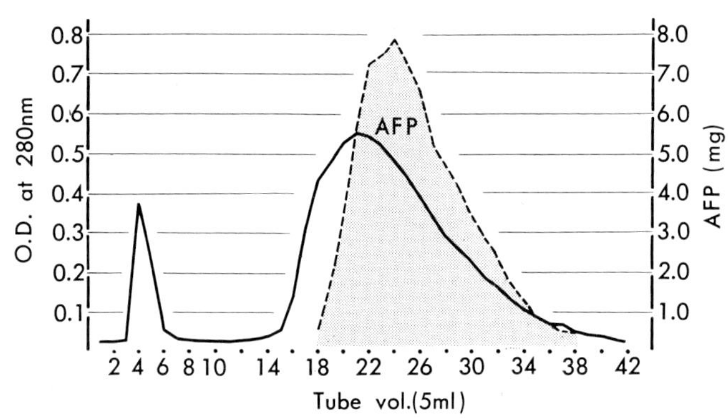

FIG. 1. Separation of AFP by preparative polyacrylamide gel disc electrophoresis

The apparatus of Gordon and Luis was employed. The electrophoresis was carried out in 5 ml of 2.5% polyacrylamide upper gel and 65 ml of 7.5% lower gel using Tris-HCl buffer (pH 9.5) at 4°. Partially purified AFP (109 mg) obtained by 2 cycles of preparative polyacrylamide gel disc electrophoresis was used. A current of 50 mA was passed and the elution buffer flow rate was 60 ml/hr. Each fraction consisted of 5 ml. The concentration curve of protein in the elution stream was obtained by UV absorption at 280 nm. The amount of AFP in each fraction was determined by the method of single radial immunodiffusion
——— absorbance at 280 nm; - - - - amount of AFP in 5 ml.

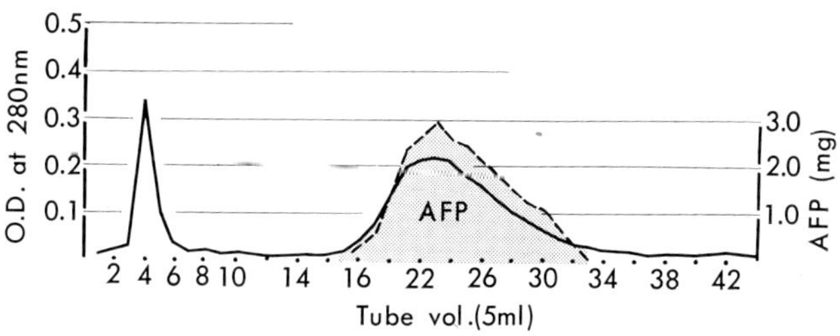

FIG. 2. Separation of AFP by preparative polyacrylamide gel disc electrophoresis after removal of adulterant protein using immune absorption

Electrophoresis was carried out under the same condition as in Fig. 1. ——— absorbance at 280 nm; ---- amount of AFP in 5 ml.

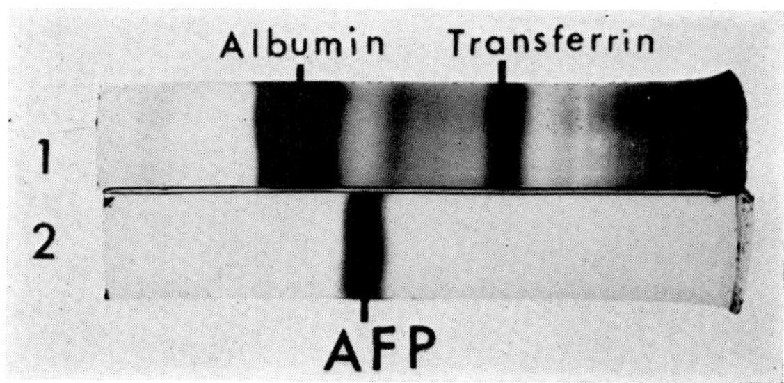

FIG. 3. Disc electrophoretic patterns of purified AFP and normal human serum
1: Normal human serum. 2: Purified AFP.

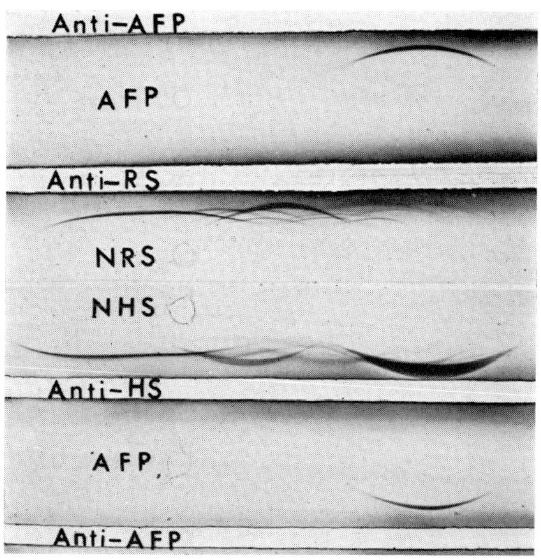

FIG. 4. Immunoelectrophoretic patterns of purified AFP against anti-human serum protein rabbit antiserum and anti-AFP rabbit antiserum

AFP: Purified AFP. NHS: Normal human serum. NRS: Normal rabbit serum. Anti-AFP: Anti-AFP rabbit antiserum. Anti-HS: Anti-human-serum protein rabbit antiserum. Anti-RS: Anti-rabbit serum protein goat antiserum.

fied AFP contained a high concentration of AFP, a low concentration of albumin, and a very small concentration of some α_1-globulins. Following this partial purification, the adulterant proteins were eliminated by a technique of immune absorption using anti-human-serum albumin rabbit γ-globulin and anti-human serum protein rabbit γ-globulin. Next, a preparative disc electrophoresis procedure was carried out to separate AFP from surplus rabbit γ-globulin. The result is shown in Fig. 2. By this method, highly pure AFP was obtained from AFP-positive ascites with a good yield of 15%. The disc electrophoretic pattern of purified AFP revealed a single band, as shown in Fig. 3 and the immunoelectrophoretic pattern (shown in Fig. 4) showed no precipitin line against anti-human serum protein rabbit antiserum and anti-rabbit serum protein goat antiserum, but did show a precipitin line against anti-AFP rabbit antiserum. The protein content of the purified AFP was determined by the method of Lowry-Folin.

Determination of AFP

From the requirement for high sensitivity and specificity for AFP detection, the immunochemical methods—immunoelectrophoresis and agar gel immunoprecipitation using a specific anti-AFP antiserum—are ordinarily employed.

A comparison of sensitivity among these methods was made by us (*7*), using standard purified AFP and the sera from 107 patients with PHC, including 62 histologically diagnosed cases. The results are shown in Table I. The methods of single radial immunodiffusion and immunoelectro-osmophoresis had the highest sensitivity, of 0.3 mg of AFP/dl of serum (3 μg/ml), and by these methods AFP could be detected in 72 out of 107 (67%) cases.

TABLE I. Comparison of Sensitivity and Detection of AFP in PHC by Various Immunoassay Methods

Methods	Sensitivity		PHC-positive cases	Total	(%)
Immunoelectrophoresis	5 mg/dl	Qualitative	41	107	38
Micro-Ouchterlony	1 mg/dl	Qualitative	59	107	55
Electroimmunodiffusion	1 mg/dl	Quantitative	59	107	55
Immunoelectroosmophoresis	0.3 mg/dl	Qualitative	72	107	67
Single radial immunodiffusion	0.3 mg/dl	Quantitative	72	107	67
			(H: 43	62	69)
Radioimmunoassay	15.6 ng/ml	Quantitative	99	107	93
			(H: 57	62	92)

H: Histological diagnosis.

This level of sensitivity appeared, however, not to be sufficient for clinical investigations. Recently, highly sensitive methods—aggregate hemagglutination by Olonikov and Tsvetkov in 1969 and Abelev (*2*) in 1971, indirect immunoradioautography by Abelev *et al.* (*2*) in 1971, and radioimmunoassay by Purves *et al.* (*10*) in 1970, we (*6*) in 1971 and Nishi *et al.* in 1971—have been established.

The AFP radioimmunoassay developed by us is discussed below. A specific anti-AFP antiserum was prepared by immunizing rabbits with purified AFP, and labeled ^{131}I-AFP was produced by the following method. Two hundred μg of purified AFP was radioiodinated with 1 mCi of ^{131}I by the method of Hunter and Greenwood (*5*). Labeled ^{131}I-AFP was separated from residual unreacted ^{131}I by gel filtration using Sephadex G-75 column chromatography. The ^{131}I-AFP of a rather low specific radioactivity of 8 mCi/mg of AFP was obtained, while prepared ^{131}I-AFP of specific activity 20 mCi/mg resulted in a small loss of antigenicity against the antibody.

The radioimmunoassay was based on the coprecipitation-inhibition technique using anti-AFP antiserum, ^{131}I-AFP, and the 2 antibody method of Morgan and Lazarow (*8*) to separate the bound and free ^{131}I-AFP. The first reaction mixture consists of 0.1 ml of test serum or standard AFP, 0.1 ml of a 1: 5,000 dilution of anti-AFP rabbit antiserum, 0.1 ml with 9.4 ng of ^{131}I-AFP, and 0.6 ml of 0.05 M phosphate saline buffer at pH 7.5, containing 1% bovine serum albumin in each tube. The above mixture was incubated at 4° for 48 hr. At the end of this period, 0.1 ml of a 1: 50 dilution of normal rabbit serum as a carrier protein, and 0.1 ml of a 1: 10 dilution of anti-rabbit-γ-globulin goat antiserum as the 2nd antibody were added to the 1st reaction mixture in each tube, and then a 2nd reaction was carried out at 4° for 24 hr. After this incubation, each tube was centrifuged at 4,000 rpm for 40 min. The ^{131}I-AFP content of the precipitate was determined in a welltype scintillation counter.

The standard curve as shown in Fig. 5 was obtained. It is a weak point of the 2 antibody method that test serum occasionally inhibits the second reaction. As a result, a quantitative value obtained from the standard curve might reveal

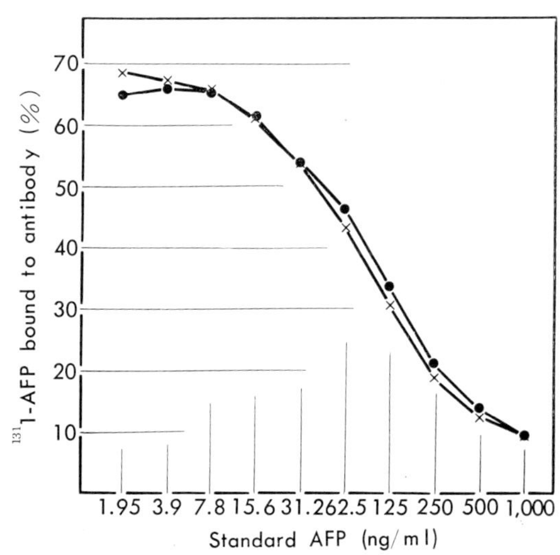

FIG. 5. Standard curve of radioimmunoassay
× standard curve obtained employing only each standard AFP;
● standard curve obtained by addition of AFP-free normal human serum to standard AFP.

an apparently higher level than the actual value. From this point of view, the following experiment was performed. When the separation of the bound and free ^{131}I-AFP in the 1st reaction solution of normal adult serum, as well as in standard AFP samples, was carried out by DEAE-Sephadex A-50 column chromatography, no AFP could be detected in the serum. The standard curve obtained on addition of 0.1 ml of this normal serum to each AFP standard was nearly coincident with a standard curve prepared employing only the AFP standards, excluding the reverse portion at levels under 7.8 ng of AFP per ml. From the above results, no inhibition effect of the test serum on the 2nd reaction could be recognized in this assay system.

Furthermore, the specificity of this assay method for AFP in human serum was examined by a dilution test on the serum of an AFP-positive patient with PHC. The standard curve obtained on dilutions of the serum produced a dose-response line parallel to that of a standard curve prepared employing AFP standards. This assay was found to possess satisfactory specificity for AFP in human serum.

The sensitivity of this assay at present allows reproducible detection of 15.6 ng of AFP/ ml of serum. A radioimmunoassay using ^{125}I-AFP gave the same result as that with ^{131}I-AFP.

Clinical Implications of Radioimmunoassay

Sera from 18 normal subjects, 576 patients with various types of diseases, and 37 pregnant women were available for the study of AFP levels by radioimmunoassay. Table II and Fig. 6 show the results. The presence of AFP was demonstrated in none out of 18 normal subjects, 99 out of 107 (93%) cases of PHC, 38 out of 139 (27%) cases of liver cirrhosis, 47 out of 136 (35%) cases of hepatitis, none out of 21 cases of other liver diseases, 1 out of 14 (7%) cases of gall

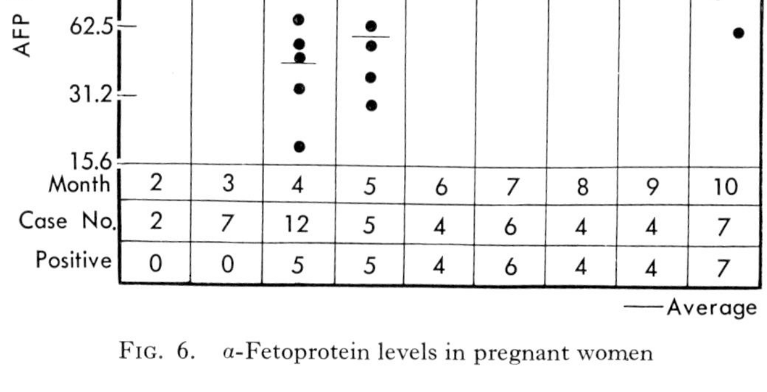

FIG. 6. α-Fetoprotein levels in pregnant women

TABLE II. α-Fetoprotein in Patients with Various Diseases by Radioimmunoassay

Diseases	Case No.	Positive	%
Normal subjects	18	0	0
Liver diseases;			
PHC	107 (62)	99 (57)	93 (92)
Cirrhosis	139 (41)	38 (14)	27 (36)
Hepatitis:	136 (47)	47 (25)	35 (53)
Fulminant	1 (1)	1 (1)	
Subacute	14 (6)	10 (4)	71 (67)
Acute	39 (8)	10 (3)	26 (38)
Chronic	82 (32)	26 (17)	32 (53)
active form	(19)	(11)	(58)
inactive form	(13)	(6)	(46)
Other liver diseases	21 (6)	0 (0)	0
Gall bladder and bile duct disease	14	1	1
Malignant diseases;			
Gastric cancer	42	8	19
Liver metastasis	21	5	25
Duodenal cancer	1	1	0
Colon and rectal cancer	15	2	13
Liver metastasis	6	1	17
Pancreatic cancer	10	2	20
Liver metastasis	9	2	22
Gall bladder and bile duct cancer	9	1	11
Liver metastasis	7	0	0
Other malignant diseases	32	6	19
Liver metastasis	11	3	27
Benign diseases	50	2	4
Pregnancy	37	27	
Total	821	292	

( ): Histological diagnosis.

bladder and bile duct diseases, 9 out of 55 (16%) cases of malignant diseases without metastatic liver cancer, 11 out of 54 (20%) cases of metastatic liver cancer, 2 out of 50 (4%) cases of other benign diseases, and 27 out of 37 pregnant women.

The distribution of AFP levels in cases other than 79 cases of PHC, a case of gastric cancer with liver metastasis, 2 cases of gastric and testicular cancer without liver metastasis, 2 cases of subacute hepatitis, a case of teratoma, and a case of congenital bile duct atresia extended below 1,000 ng of AFP/ml of serum.

The relationship between AFP dynamics and transitions of transaminase activity (GPT) levels in serum during the course of the disease was investigated for 6 patients with PHC, a patient with cirrhosis, and 5 patients with hepatitis, with the results shown in Figs. 7 and 8. The AFP in the sera of patients with hepatitis or cirrhosis could first be detected at the beginning of an improvement of the illness, *i.e.*, in the decreasing phase of transaminase activity, and thereafter the AFP levels fell to undetectable levels as the transaminase activity levels were

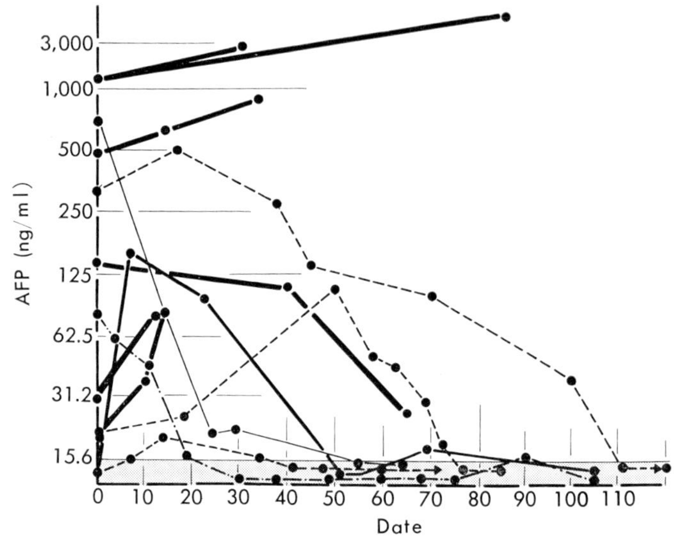

FIG. 7. α-Fetoprotein dynamics in patients with hepatitis, cirrhosis, or PHC during their disease

——— acute hepatitis; - - - - chronic hepatitis, active form; ——— chronic hepatitis, inactive form; •—•—• liver cirrhosis; ▬▬▬ PHC.

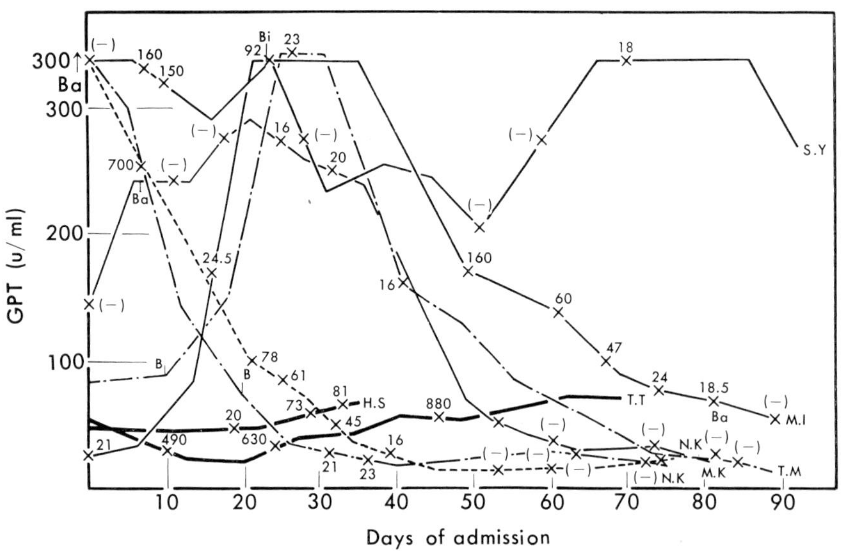

FIG. 8. Relationship between AFP levels and transaminase activity levels (GPT) in patients with hepatitis, cirrhosis, or PHC during their disease

•—•—• acute hepatitis; ——— chronic hepatitis; - - - - liver cirrhosis; ——— PHC. × determination of AFP. AFP level; ng/ml. B: Biopsy of liver. Ba: Chronic hepatitis, active form. Bi: Chronic hepatitis, inactive form.

reduced. On the other hand, AFP levels in sera from 5 out of 6 patients with PHC increased over a short term, having no relation with the transaminase activity levels.

Recently, Abelev (*2*) reported that a survey using a highly sensitive method of indirect immunoradioautography for AFP detection revealed the presence of AFP in 23 out of 176 (13%) patients with infectious and serum hepatitis, none out of 54 patients with cirrhosis, none out of 33 patients with chronic hepatitis, and 1 out of 41 patients with other liver diseases. These results agree with those of the author and others. From these results, it was concluded that the specificity of AFP for PHC was far from being absolute. On the other hand, the presence of non-AFP-producing PHC had been made incontrovertible by the use of radioimmunoassay for AFP detection since the report of the author and others (*6*) in 1971.

α-Fetoprotein tests by the single radial immunodiffusion method for 70 normal adult subjects and 736 patients with various types of diseases revealed the presence of AFP in 72 out of 107 patient with PHC (their AFP levels increased with the progress of the illness), a patient with gastric cancer, a patient with testicular cancer, a patient with teratoma, and a patient with congenital bile duct atresia. From these results, AFP levels higher than 3,000 ng (3 μg) of AFP/ml of serum and the transition from AFP levels lower than that level during the course of the disease seem to present diagnostic implications for PHC.

Abelev (*2*) suggested, based on the similarity of AFP dynamics during hepatitis, and in mice and rats with regenerating liver, that AFP formation in hepatitis was caused by liver regeneration. However, we failed to find obvious differences regarding liver regeneration between AFP-positive and AFP-negative cases from microscopic observations on liver biopsy samples from patients with hepatitis or cirrhosis with and without AFP in their serum.

I proposed the following hypothesis for the synthesis and dynamics of AFP. A reversible genetic change caused by abnormal cell metabolism after liver impediment might induce a temporary synthesis of AFP in hepatitis or cirrhosis apart from the effect of liver regeneration. On the other hand, an irreversible genetic change resulting from cell cancerization might induce continuous synthesis of AFP in PHC.

The presence of AFP in 5 out of 12 women at 4 months' gestation and all women past 5 months' gestation was recognized. This result supported the results of Foy *et al.*, who found the presence of AFP in 7 out of 20 women past 30 week's gestation. Although it had been reported by Gitlin and Boesman that the concentration of AFP in fetal serum was low and falling after 3–5 month's gestation, AFP levels in maternal serum increased with the stage of gestation, particularly up to 8 months.

I suppose that the source of AFP in the serum of pregnant women originates in the transport of fetal serum due to changes in the placental permeability to AFP.

REFERENCES

1. Abelev, G. I., Assecritova, I., Kraevsky, N., Perova, S., and Perevodchikova, N. Embryonal serum α-globulin in cancer patients: Diagnostic value. *Int. J. Cancer*, **2**, 551–558 (1967).
2. Abelev, G. I. α-Fetoprotein in ontogenesis and its association with malignant tumors. *Adv. Cancer Res.*, **14**, 295–358 (1971).
3. Abelev, G. I., Perova, S., Khramkova, N., Postnikova, Z., and Irlin, I. Production of embryonal α-globulin by transplantable mouse hepatoma. *Transplantation*, **1**, 174–180 (1963).
4. Bakirov, R. Appearance of embryonic serum α-globulin in adult mice after intoxication with carbon tetrachloride inhalation. *Bull. Exp. Biol. Med. (U.S.S.R.)*, **65**, 45–47 (1968).
5. Hunter, W. M. and Greenwood, F. C. Preparation of ^{131}I-labeled human growth hormone of high specific activity. *Nature*, **194**, 495–496 (1962).
6. Ishii, M., Ikehara, H., Tozawa, T., Inoue, E., and Shinko, T. Radioimmunoassay of α-fetoprotein and clinical significance (in Japanese). *Igaku-no-Ayumi (The Stride of Medicine)*, **79**, 77–79 (1971).
7. Ishii, M., Ikehara, H., Tozawa, T., Inoue, E., and Shinko, T. The methods of determination for α-fetoprotein and clinical significance. Reported at the 7th Congress of the Japanese Hepatology Society, July 1971.
8. Morgan, C. R. and Lazarow, A. Immunoassay of insulin: Two antibody system. *Diabetes*, **12**, 115–126 (1963).
9. Nishi, S. Isolation and characterization of a human fetal globulin from the sera of fetuses and a hepatoma patient. *Cancer Res.*, **30**, 2507–2513 (1970).
10. Purves, L. R., Bersohn, I., and Geedes, E. W. Radioimmunoassay of α-fetoprotein. *Proc. S. Afr. Assoc. Pathologists*, 67 (1969).
11. Tatarinov, Y. Presence of embryonal α-globulin in the serum of a patient with primary hepatocellular carcinoma. *Vopr. Med. Khim.*, **10**, 90–94 (1964).
12. Uriel, J., de Nechaud, B., Stanislawski-birencwajg, M., Masseyeff, R., Leblanc, L., Quenum, C., Loisillier, F., and Grabar, P. Antigénes embryonaires et cancer du foie chez l'homme: Association de l' α-foetoprotéine sérique avec l'hépatome primaire. *C. R.*, **265**, 75–78 (1967).

GANN Monograph on Cancer Research 14, 1973

CLINICAL SIGNIFICANCE OF α-FETOPROTEIN ESPECIALLY IN THE TREATMENT OF HEPATIC CANCER*1

Katsuhiko SUGAHARA, Akiyoshi KASHII, and Nobuhiro KAWANO
*Department of Surgery, Faculty of Medicine, University of Tokyo**2

The importance of α-fetoprotein (AFP) is reviewed from the standpoint of hepatic surgery. Serial changes of serum AFP before and after resection of primary hepatocellular cancer (PHC) were examined in 5 cases in 1970. In 2 out of 5 cases, AFP was negative. In 2 cases with positive AFP, a marked initial fall of AFP after removal of the hepatoma was followed by higher values in accordance with the recurrence. Histologically, both tumors were hepatomas of the trabecular type, with atypism of Edmondson's grade II in the degree of cellular differentiation. In another case with hepatoma of same histological type, AFP remained negative over a period of 3 months after hepatectomy. The recurrence of the tumor was already suspected on the basis of biochemical findings and a hepatoscintigram in the stage with negative AFP.

In cases of resected hepatoma with intense production of AFP, the concentration of serum AFP could serve as a suitable parameter to detect the recurrence of cancer and as a good guide for reoperation or anticancer chemotherapy. There seems to be some correlation between the production of AFP and the histological type, with the degree of cellular differentiation of the hepatoma, and the AFP value may be closely related to the size of the tumor.

The early diagnosis of hepatoma is still very difficult, although recent progress in several diagnostic methods has made it possible to detect the site of cancer in the upper abdomen. Considering the history of hepatoma cases retrospectively, uncertain upper gastrointestinal symptoms are often noticed. A screening method to detect the presence of hepatic malignancy at an early stage, when the patient complains only of uncertain symptoms, might make radical resection of the lesion possible, for a more favorable prognosis.

Since 1964, it has been reported that serum α-fetoprotein (AFP) which is specific to the fetus is also found in the sera of a large proportion of patients with primary hepatocellular cancer (PHC) (*10*) and embryonal teratoblastoma (TRB). Following the introduction of the quantitative single radial diffusion method by Mancini *et al.* (*8*), which is precise and highly sensitive in the measurement of

*1 This work was supported by grants in aid of cancer research from the Ministry of Health and Welfare

*2 Hongo 7-3-1, Bunkyo-ku, Tokyo 113 (菅原克彦, 柏井昭良, 河野信博).

AFP, we measured serial changes in AFP before and after resection of hepatoma in 5 cases in 1970.

The above cases are reported herewith along with a review of the clinical value of AFP determination, with reference to clinical, histopathological, and radiological findings.

Method

In 1970, we experienced 5 cases of hepatoma and conducted follow-up studies before and after the operations using anti-AFP serum prepared with extract from fetal tissue as the antigen. α-Fetoprotein (AFP) was estimated qualitatively by the double diffusion micro-Ouchterlony method. Using this technique, the sample showed a positive reaction in the presence of 1 mg/dl of AFP, making this method useful as a routine clinical screening test for hepatic tumors. When a positive result was obtained, the serum was further evaluated quantitatively with Mancini's single radial diffusion method (*8*). Routine liver function tests, selective celiac angiography, and liver scintiscanning (^{198}Au colloid and ^{67}Ga citrate) were performed in each case.

Case Presentation

Case 1 was a 14-year-old boy with an epigastric mass. Scintiscanning revealed a space-occupying lesion in the left hepatic lobe. Left hepatectomy was carried out successfully. Histological diagnosis was a thin trabecular-type hepatoma with atypism of Edmondson's grade I (*5*). α-Fetoprotein remained negative throughout the clinical course. The patient is still alive now, 22 months after the operation.

Case 2 was a 62-year-old female complaining of an epigastric mass. Selective angiography and scanning of the liver showed a space-occupying lesion in the left lobe, which was removed successfully. Gross appearance of the specimen was a massive type. Histological diagnosis was a trabecular-type hepatoma with atypism of Edmondson's grade II. Tumor emboli were also noticed in the portal tributaries.

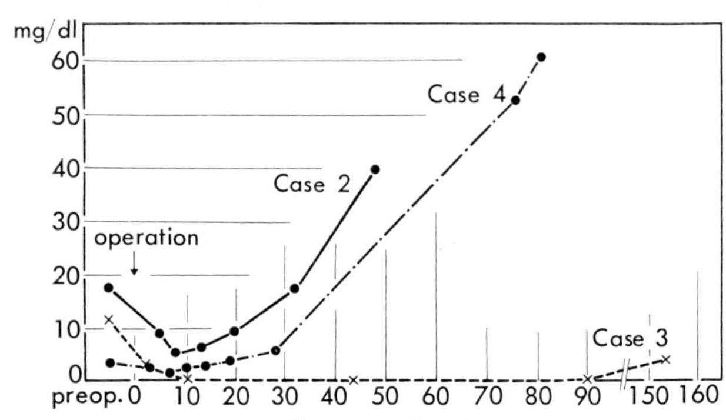

FIG. 1. Serial measurement of AFP before and after resection of PHC

A hepatoscintigram which was taken 30 days postoperatively showed, for the first time, a cold nodule, 3×3 cm in size, in the area of the cut edge. At this stage, the concentration of AFP had already increased to 17.0 mg/dl, 3.3 times higher than the lowest value (Fig. 1). On the 48th postoperative day the AFP value was 39.4 mg/dl and the tumor was 5×6 cm in size in the residual lobe in the liver scan. The patient expired 60 days after the operation.

Case 3 was a 50-year-old male with an abdominal mass in the left upper quadrant. By super-selective angiography and scanning, it was diagnosed as a tumor in the left lobe, and was removed uneventfully. This patient had hepatoma associated with postnecrotic liver cirrhosis. The histological diagnosis was a trabecular-type hepatoma with atypism of Edmondson's grade II. α-Fetoprotein turned out to be negative 2 weeks after hepatectomy (Fig. 1). α-Fetoprotein was still negative 3 months postoperatively despite a positive finding suggesting recurrence in the liver scan. It was noticed that alkaline phosphatase level in the serum had already risen to 15 K-A units. Two months later, the patient was readmitted with jaundice and ascites. AFP was 3.5 mg/dl and the abdominal mass was palpable. The patient died after several episodes of bleeding from esophageal varices. The autopsy showed that local recurrence had occupied over 90% of the remaining right lobe of the liver, weighing 1,710 g.

Case 4 was a 40-year-old male with an abdominal mass in the right upper quadrant. Selective angiography and scintiscanning revealed a space-occupying lesion in the left lobe, which was removed successfully. The histopathological diagnosis of the tumor was a trabecular-type hepatoma with atypism of Edmondson's grade II. Three weeks after surgery, AFP increased as shown in Fig. 1, in spite of a normal alkaline phosphatase value and bilirubin level in the serum. The alkaline phosphatase level began to increase 60 days after the operation and jaundice appeared. A hepatoscintigram taken at this period suggested the recurrence of the tumor, reaching 5×6 cm in size in the residual lobe. One

TABLE I. Summary of 5 Cases

Case No.	Age (yrs.)	Sex	AFP value (mg/dl)			Size of tumor in scintigram		Survival
			Preop.	Postop. (days)		Preop.	Postop. (days)	
1	14	Male	0			5×4		Alive 22 months
2	62	Female	17.2	8.5 (5) 5.1 (8) 6.0(13) 9.4(20)	17.0(32) 26.1(39) 39.4(48)	6×6	3×3(30) 6×5(48)	Died 2 months
3	50	Male	11.0	3.0 (3) 0 (11) 0 (44)	0 (90) 3.5(153)	10×8	5×5(90)	Died 5 months
4	40	Male	3.4	2.3 (3) 1.2 (7) 2.4(10) 2.8(14)	3.9(19) 5.9(28) 52.5(76) 60.2(81)	7×6	6×5(60)	Died 3 months
5	62	Male	0			4×3		Alive 15 months

TABLE II. Histology of 5 Cases

Case No.	Histological type	Edmondson's grade	Liver cirrhosis	Weight of resected specimen (g)
1	Thin trabecular	I	—	200
2	Trabecular	II	—	620
3	Trabecular	II	+	750
4	Trabecular	II	—	700
5	Trabecular	II partially III	—	250

month later, the patient died from hepatic insufficiency, 10 days after readmission.

Case 5 was a 62-year-old male with a mass in the left upper quadrant. A tumor of 2×3 cm in size was palpable, and scintiscanning using ^{67}Ga revealed a 4×3 cm hot nodule. α-Fetoprotein was negative. Successful left lobectomy was performed. On histological examination the tumor consisted of a trabecular-type hepatoma with atypism of Edmondson's grade II and partially grade III. The patient is still alive 15 months after surgery. These cases are summarized in Tables I and II.

DISCUSSION

1. Correlation between AFP and hepatoma

Since Tatarinov (*10*) reported the presence of AFP in the sera of patients with hepatoma, close attention has been directed to AFP by many investigators. Most workers have agreed on the failure of AFP to appear in normal serum.

Abelev (*1*) and Uriel *et al.* (*3, 4, 11*) carried out further studies on AFP, concluding that the appearance of this substance was an excellent and specific indicator of PHC. α-Fetoprotein was positive in the sera of 50 to 80.7% of patients with hepatoma, according to these investigators. Although other reports (*3, 4, 9*) stated that AFP was also positive in the serum of patients with liver cirrhosis, coexistent hepatoma was not completely ruled out, since the diagnoses were based on the liver biopsy alone.

Endo *et al.* (*6*) reported the measurement of AFP in 815 cases. Among them, 18 cases were diagnosed as positive. They comprised 16 cases of primary hepatoma and two cases of liver cirrhosis. Sixteen cases out of 25 patients with primary hepatoma showed positive AFP (64%).

α-Fetoprotein appears in the serum of a large proportion of patients with hepatocellular carcinoma, but not with cholangiocarcinoma. If both kinds of tumor happen to be mixed and the hepatocellular component is prominent, AFP appears in the serum (*2*). Our case of resected cholangiocarcinoma also showed negative AFP.

2. Correlation between AFP and histological type of hepatoma

In Case 1 with hepatoma of a thin trabecular-type, Edmondson's grade I, AFP was negative. In Cases 2, 3, 4, and 5 with hepatoma of the trabecular-type, Edmondson's grade II, positive AFP was noted in all except Case 5.

The AFP thus appears to be frequently positive in trabecular-type with atypism of Edmondson's grade II group. According to our experience in resected cases, there seems to be some relationship between histological subtype and production of AFP, but further studies are necessary for confirmation. Alpert *et al.* (*3*) stated that well-differentiated tumors tended to be AFP-negative, whereas the poorly differentiated tumors tended to be AFP-positive. Recently, O'Conor *et al.* (*9*) have denied any relation between the degree of tumor cell differentiation and AFP. However, our data, based on a strict analysis of resected specimens, should be quite reliable.

3. Postoperative pattern of AFP

In both Cases 2 and 4, a marked initial fall of AFP after removal of the hepatoma was followed by higher values, giving a similar pattern. In spite of the fact that the general condition of these patients was better and the blood chemistry became almost normal after the operation, it should be noted that the concentration of AFP, which initially decreased postoperatively, gradually increased again. At this stage, no abnormal physical findings, including abdominal masses, were noted and the patients had good appetite.

In Case 3, on the other hand, AFP remained negative over a period of 3 months after hepatectomy. The recurrence of hepatoma was already suspected on the basis of biochemical findings and hepatoscintigram in the stage with negative AFP. In this case, liver cirrhosis was also found.

4. Correlation between size of tumor and AFP

No grossly visible tumor was found in the residual lobe of the liver at the time of operation in any case in the present series. This was ascertained by the operative findings and also by preoperative liver scintiscanning.

In Cases 2 and 4, the values of AFP were approximately parallel to the size of the tumor as found by liver scan, shown in Table I and Fig. 1. The elevation of AFP in these cases preceded the detection of the recurrent tumor after hepatectomy. Determination of AFP thus appears to be of value in detecting a recurrent tumor.

In Case 3, on the other hand, the volume of the tumor and the AFP value were not parallel. α-Fetoprotein values were less than 1 mg/dl from the 12th to 90th postoperative day. It is of great interest that the value of AFP in the serum is variable in patients with hepatoma. Even when the tumor was quite large, the serum value was not necessarily high, as in Case 3. It seems to depend upon differences of productivity in individual hepatoma. The production of AFP in hepatoma has already been proven by the immunofluorescent technique, but such differences in productivity should be analysed from the standpoint of cellular metabolism, especially catabolism. In general, when the generation time of the tumor is rapid, the production of AFP by the tumor is accelerated.

The production of AFP in the tumor is marked until the tumor develops to some extent. When the nutritional situation of the tumor becomes worse and compression or necrosis also takes place, the production of AFP is thought to become lower.

In 3 cases, AFP decreased rapidly upon removal of the tumor, falling to one-half of the preoperative value within 6 days. In another case of unresectable hepatoma, AFP value was decreased by the use of chemotherapy.

These facts suggest a close relationship between AFP value and the size of the tumor. This fits in well with Kithier's view (*7*) that the AFP value in blood increases with the extension of hepatoma. Alpert *et al.* (*3*) reported that the mean weight of tumors from strongly AFP-positive patients was significantly greater than the mean weight of tumors from AFP-negative patients.

5. Clinical importance of AFP

Clinically, the reappearance of AFP in the serum after hepatectomy suggests the recurrence of the tumor. A periodic check of serum for AFP therefore appears to be quite important for the therapeutic schedule. Such elevation of AFP after removal of the tumor would indicate the need for chemotherapy or reoperation, as in Cases 2 and 4. When the productivity of AFP is low after surgery, as in Case 3, scintiscanning is recommended. Accordingly, routine determination of AFP and liver scanning are absolutely necessary to determine the situation of the residual tissue after resection of hepatoma.

Although no statistically significant difference was evident, AFP-negative patients appeared to have a longer survival time, whereas the strongly AFP-positive patients all died within 4 months (*3*). Our two AFP-negative patients were still alive at the conclusion of this study.

Acknowledgments

Many thanks are due to Dr. Yasuo Endo, Department of Internal Medicine, University of Tokyo, for cordial cooperation in the determination of serum AFP values.

REFERENCES

1. Abelev, G. I. Production of embryonal serum α-globulin by hepatomas: Review of experimental and clinical data. *Cancer Res.*, **28**, 1344–1350 (1968).
2. Abelev, G. I., Assecritova, I. V., Kraevsky, N. A., Perova, S. D., and Perevodchikova, N. I. Embryonal serum α-globulin in cancer patients: Diagnostic value. *Int. J. Cancer*, **2**, 551–558 (1967).
3. Alpert, M. E., Hershberg, R., Schur, P. H., and Isselbacher, K. J. Fetoprotein in human hepatoma: Improved detection in serum, and quantitative studies using a new sensitive technique. *Gastroenterology*, **61**, 137–143 (1971).
4. Alpert, M. E., Uriel, J., and de Nechaud, B. Alpha$_1$ fetoglobulin in the diagnosis of human hepatoma. *New Engl. J. Med.*, **278**, 984–986 (1968).
5. Edmondson, H. A. and Steiner, P. E. Primary carcinoma of the liver. *Cancer*, **7**, 462–503 (1954).
6. Endo, Y., Eto, S., Iino, S., Fujiwara, K., Miyake, K., Kanetaka, T., Yamanaka, M., Suzuki, H., Oda, T., Yoshitoshi, Y., Juji, T., Yokochi, T., and Miura, T. Diagnosis of primary hepatic cancer by α_1-fetoglobulin. *Acta Hepatol. Japon.*, **10**, 143–146 (1969).
7. Kithier, K., Houštěk, J., Masopust, J., and Rádl, J. Occurrence of specific fetal protein in a primary liver carcinoma. *Nature*, **212**, 414 (1966).

8. Mancini, G., Carbonara, A. O., and Heremans, J. F. Immunochemical quantitation of antigens by single radial immunodiffusion. *Immunochemistry*, **2**, 235–254 (1965).
9. O'Conor, G. T., Tatarinov, Y. S., Abelev, G. I., and Uriel, J. A collaborative study for the evaluation of a serologic test for primary liver cancer. *Cancer*, **25**, 1091–1098 (1970).
10. Tatarinov, Y. S. Embryospecific α_1-fetoglobulin in a serum of patient with liver cancer. *Vopr. Med. Khim.*, **10**, 90 (1964).
11. Uriel, J., de Nechaud, B., Stanislawski-birencwajg, Masseyeff, M., Leblanc, L., Quenum, C., Loisillier, T., and Graber, P. Antigènes embryonnaires et le cancer du foie chez l'homme: Association de l'α-fetoprotéine sérique avec l'hépatome primaire. *C. R.*, **265**, 75–77 (1967).

RESULTS IN THE TREATMENT OF HEPATOCELLULAR CARCINOMA
With Special Reference to α-Fetoprotein

Yasuo KUROYANAGI

*Department of Surgery, Aichi Cancer Center Hospital**

Seventy-seven patients with hepatocellular carcinoma were seen at the Aichi Cancer Center Hospital from 1964 to 1971. There were 69 males and 8 females. Forty-five of these patients (58%) had carcinoma combined with cirrhosis, the remaining 32 cases (42%) without cirrhosis. Serum α-fetoprotein (AFP) was studied in 44 patients with hepatocellular carcinoma by the single radial immunodiffusion method. The incidence of positive AFP was 70.5% in all. The half-life of AFP was 5.7 days in a hepatectomized patient. Five of the 77 patients underwent left hepatectomy. In one case, AFP disappeared completely after the operation and results continued to be negative for more than 2 years. In another case, AFP decreased abruptly after excision of the tumor, but rose again 1 month later with the appearance of multiple pulmonary metastases. Others have been living for a period of 1 to 5 years at present, except for 1 case of early death after the operation.

Of 22 patients treated with intra-arterial injection of 30 mg of Mitomycin-C into the celiac axis, 3 patients with a fair liver function showed a good response. The remainder, with impaired liver function, showed no response. Radiation therapy combined with intra-arterial injection of 30 mg of Mitomycin-C was beneficial in the treatment of 13 out of 17 patients. Effective total tumor dose varied from 4,000 to 5,000 rads, judged by evaluating the decrease of AFP in sera.

Intra-arterial injection of Mitomycin-C followed by systemic administration of triple anticancer agents (Mitomycin-C, 5-fluorouracil (5-FU), and cytosine arabinoside) in 1 patient was a fairly useful measure, whereas in the systemic administration of Mitomycin-C alone, there was no improvement of subjective and objective symptoms in 3 patients.

In conclusion, repeated measurements of serum AFP provided satisfactory information on the success of surgical excision of the tumor or responsiveness to various types of treatment. However, in patients with negative AFP, follow-up studies should be performed by means of either hepatoscanning or selective angiography because alkaline phosphatase in the serum would not always be reliable in reflecting tumor regression or growth.

The choice of treatments for hepatocellular carcinoma was in the following order: Hepatic resection, radiation combined with intra-

* Kanokoden 81, Tashiro-cho, Chikusa-ku, Nagoya 464, Japan (黒柳弥寿雄).

arterial Mitomycin-C, systemic triple anticancer agents with intra-arterial Mitomycin-C, and single arterial Mitomycin-C.

In spite of recent progress in the understanding and management of primary liver cancer (PLC), the results are far from satisfactory. This is, of course, due mainly to the nature of cancer in general and also to the coexistence of cirrhosis of the liver. Indeed, the resectability of human hepatocellular carcinoma is less than 10%. However with effective excision, a possibility of cure exists when early diagnosis is made.

In recent years two important aids in the diagnosis of hepatocellular carcinoma have been found. The first is the discovery of α-fetoprotein (AFP) in the serum of patients with this disease, which appears to be a specific immunochemical test, and the second is selective arteriography of the liver, which has become, in practice, a method for determining the localization of tumors within the liver. These new diagnostic aids materially advance our assessment and treatment of liver cancer.

In this report, 77 patients with hepatocellular carcinoma encountered at the Aichi Cancer Center Hospital are described. There were 69 males and 8 females. The age distribution by decades from the year 1964 to 1971 is shown in Table I.

TABLE I. Age in Decades (77 Patients)

Age (yrs.)	No. of hepatoma cases
-10	1
10–19	0
20–29	0
30–39	5
40–49	18
50–59	24
60–69	22
70–	7
Total	77

Dec. 1964–Dec. 1971, at the Aichi Cancer Center Hospital.

In our experience, the incidence of positive AFP was 70.5% in 44 cases examined by single radial immunodiffusion, which was about the same as that of other studies of PLC (*6*). The specificity of AFP for hepatocellular carcinoma appears to be very high, regardless of the existence of cirrhosis, and when present, AFP was persistent. Thus, changes of AFP concentrations in the sera of patients have been considered useful for assessing the efficacy of radical operation and the susceptibility of cancer cells to various types of treatment (*2*, *3*).

It has been considered that cirrhosis of the liver may play a role in developing hepatocellular carcinoma as a possible etiologic factor. As early as 1881, Sabourin first pointed out the association of antecedent cirrhosis in about 70% of patients with hepatocellular carcinoma. In our series, 45 of the patients (58%) suffered from hepatocellular carcinoma in combination with cirrhotic liver, and the remaining 32 cases (42%) were noncirrhotic. The close association of hepatocellular carcinoma with severe cirrhosis indicates that surgical intervention is difficult.

Hepatectomy

In fact, surgical procedures involving extensive resection of the liver for hepatocellular carcinoma have only been possible in about 6.5% of 77 patients encountered in our hospital. We had 6 patients on whom left hepatectomy was performed, of which 5 had hepatocellular carcinoma and 1 had primary liposarcoma of the liver. In this resectable group of hepatocellular carcinoma, 4 have remained alive for periods of 14, 27, 57, and 67 months, respectively, and 1 died from hepatic coma immediately after the operation.

Case 1. A 70-year-old male, previously healthy, was admitted complaining of epigastralgia. A mass was palpable in the epigastrium. No ascites or jaundice. Laboratory data were within normal limits except for the erythrocyte sedimentation rate, which was slightly elevated. Celiac arteriograph revealed a mass related to the left lobe of the liver with hypervascularity. The left hepatic artery was dilated, as shown in a photograph of the arteriogram (Photo 1a) and its schematic representation (Photo 1b). A photograph taken at the operation shows a localization of the tumor (Photo 2). α-Fetoprotein was positive. Histology revealed a well differentiated hepatocellular carcinoma without cirrhosis. An excision of the left lobe of the liver, including the tumor, was performed with the disappearance of AFP for a period of several weeks following the operation, suggesting complete removal of the tumor. This patient is still living uneventfully with continuing negative AFP more than 2 years after the operation.

Case 2. A 54-year-old male was admitted, complaining of a tender epigastric mass. Barium meal revealed marked esophageal varices in the lower part of the esophagus. Impaired liver function tests were found. α-Fetoprotein was positive. These findings were considered to indicate a hepatocellular carcinoma

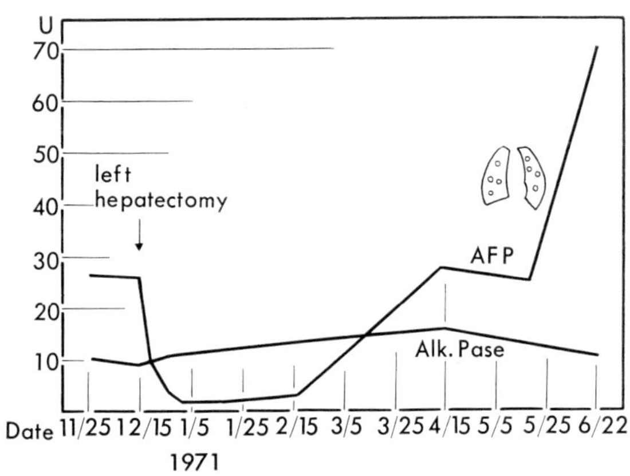

FIG. 1. Levels of serum AFP (arbitrary units/ml) and alkaline phosphatase (King-Armstrong units) in Case 2 following hepatectomy
Alk.Pase: Alkaline phosphatase.

combined with cirrhosis. An extended left hepatectomy was performed. Operative portal venography revealed demonstrable esophageal varices *via* the left gastric vein and nonvisualization of the left portal branch, indicating that the left lobe was involved by the tumor (Photo 3). In this patient the half-life of AFP was 5.7 days.

As shown in Fig. 1, AFP in the serum decreased abruptly after the operation. However, AFP in the serum increased again due to multiple pulmonary metastases 1 month after the operation. Serum alkaline phosphatase remained unchanged. This discrepancy may be a feature of the recurrence of the extrahepatic metastases. The patient is alive, though ill, 1 year after the operation.

Intra-arterial Cancer Chemotherapy

Inoperable hepatocellular carcinoma results in the early death of patients, particularly those with cirrhosis. According to our experience, anticancer chemotherapy administered intra-arterially has been beneficial in some instances. Since malignant neoplasms are mainly supplied with arterial blood, as shown by Mann *et al.* (*4*), the intrahepatic artery route would accordingly seem the best suited for the administration of anticancer agents. Recent progress of selective angiography by Seldinger's percutaneous catheter replacement technique made it possible to inject an anticancer agent into the hepatic artery directly.

It is worthwhile to note the most frequent variations involving the origin of the hepatic artery, and the most common are given below.

(1) The right or entire common hepatic artery originating from the superior mesenteric artery, with no hepatic artery from the celiac axis.

(2) The left hepatic artery arising from the left gastric artery, with the right hepatic coming from the celiac axis.

Attention should be paid to these variations before injection of anticancer agents. Angiographic features of a well-differentiated hepatocellular carcinoma are almost seen as vascular tumors, whereas in anaplastic hepatocellular carcinoma no vascularization is present. These arteriographic findings indicate not only the nature of the tumor, but also the localization of the lesion. These observations may be very important in diagnosing neoplasms of the liver, if AFP is negative.

For intra-arterial anticancer chemotherapy, a short-acting anticancer agent should be used, such as alkylating agents and Mitomycin-C. Mitomycin-C in dosages from 20 to 30 mg was administered into the celiac artery through an Ödman catheter inserted into the femoral artery by Seldinger's method. Of 22 patients treated, 1 had an excellent response and 2 had a good response. The remainder had no response or their condition even worsened. The poor results may be primarily due to an improper selection of patients. Indeed, any symptom relative to extensive parenchymal damage, such as ascites, jaundice, and hemorrhagic tendency would render the patient a poor candidate for any type of treatment.

Case 3. A 64-year-old male was admitted complaining of epigastralgia and weight loss. Hypervascularization was seen in the entire right lobe of the liver in a selective celiac arteriogram. The spleen was not enlarged, suggesting no elevated portal vein pressure (Photo 4). The liver was palpable in 3 finger breadths below the right costal margin. Thirty mg of Mitomycin-C was adminstered *via* the celiac axis. Ten months later, arteriography revealed a shrunken right lobe of the liver with disappearance of the hypervascularization seen before treatment (Photo 5). This patient was the only case that survived for over a year.

Radiation plus Intra-arterial Mitomycin-C Therapy

Regardless of positive or negative AFP, selective celiac arteriography may indicate the form, size, and boundaries of the tumor in determining treatment policies. Vascular proliferation, tumor stain, and A-V shunt formation were considered to be specific features of the arteriogram for hepatocellular carcinoma. These angiographic patterns are quite important in determining the area of the lesions to be irradiated (*1*).

Radiation therapy can be regarded as a hepatectomy, so that the lesion should be limited to certain areas regardless of the anatomic vasculature of the liver. Thus, cancer of the hilum of the liver may also be indicative for radiation therapy.

It is well-known that irradiation of the liver does not detectably impair its function using doses up to 6,000 rads spread over 6 to 8 weeks (*5*). The radiotherapy course can generally be continued to tumor doses of 4,000 or 5,000 rads in total, divided into daily doses of about 200 rads. Attention should be paid to radiation nephritis or colitis. However, so far in our experience these untoward effects have not been serious, as the tumor dose was limited up to 5,000 rads in total.

Of 17 patients with hepatocellular carcinoma given more than 4,000 rads tumor dose with 30 mg of Mitomycin-C intra-arterially, there was marked tumor regression with a remarkable decrease in the hypervascularity of the lesion on repeated angiographies in 13 patients. In regard to AFP-positive cases, 6 out of 9 patients responded well concerning the decrease of AFP in sera. The average survival time was 8.7 months.

Case 4. A 56-year-old male was admitted with a 4-month history of increasing weakness and pain in the right flank. Physical examination on admission revealed the liver to be enlarged, and it had a hard, irregular lower margin. α-Fetoprotein was positive, and alkaline phosphatase was markedly elevated. Celiac arteriography revealed a vascularized lesion involving the major portion of the right lobe of the liver, and the gastroduodenal artery was interrupted at its root. Since the tumor was far too extensive to be resected, the patient was given 30 mg of Mitomycin-C into the celiac axis followed by Lineac radiation therapy with 3,990 rads total tumor dose (Fig. 2). Both AFP and alkaline phosphatase in the sera decreased markedly, with relief of pain and tumor regression. The patient was discharged at once to return to his work for a period of 9 months. However, elevated AFP was found again, suggesting intrahepatic invasion, with an elevated

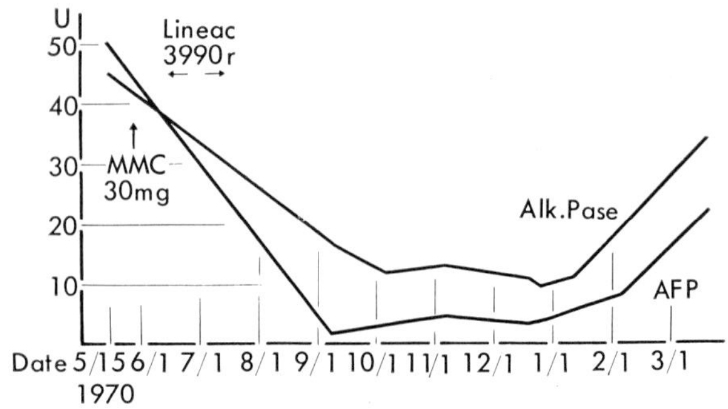

FIG. 2. Levels of serum AFP and alkaline phosphatase in Case 4, after radiation combined with Mitomycin-C therapy
MMC, Mitomycin-C; r, rads.

alkaline phosphatase in the serum. The patient died of severe liver damage due to spreading of the cancer cells within the liver after 11 months' survival.

Case 5. A 46-year-old male, complaining of a mass in the epigastrium, whose liver function tests were within normal limits, suggesting no cirrhosis. Positive AFP was found. Positive Australia antigen was detected by Nishioka's immunoadherance method.* The primary lesion, located in the left lobe of the liver, as confirmed by celiac arteriography, was considered to be nonresectable due to continuous invasion into the medial part of the right lobe. Therefore, 30 mg of Mitomycin-C was injected into the celiac axis through a catheter, followed by

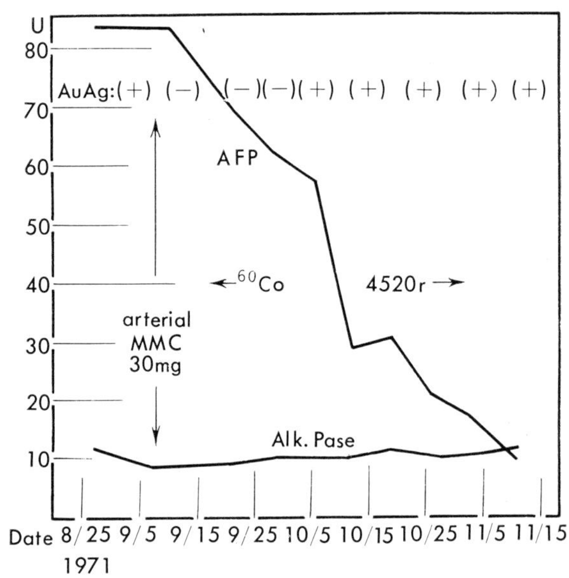

FIG. 3. Levels of serum AFP and alkaline phosphatase in Case 5, after radiation combined with Mitomycin-C therapy
AuAg, Australia antigen; MMC, Mitomycin-C.

* Serum taken from Case 5 was kindly examined for Australia antigen by Dr. K. Nishioka, National Cancer Center Research Institute, Tokyo.

^{60}Co radiation therapy with a total dose of 4,520 rads in 5 weeks. There was remarkable regression of the tumor with a gradual decrease of AFP in the serum during the clinical course of treatment, as shown in Fig. 3. In this case, it is very interesting to note that positive Australia antigen became negative after injection of Mitomycin-C intra-arterially, and this lasted for 1 month. The reason for this remains elusive, but it may be of importance in a discussion on the etiology of hepatocellular carcinoma.

Since inoperable hepatocellular carcinoma was so often radiosensitive after receiving Mitomycin-C, this combination method would improve the result of hepatectomy if performed preoperatively.

Systemic Administration of Anticancer Agents

When hepatic scintiscanning or celiac arteriography reveals widespread dissemination of cancer cells in both lobes of the liver, chemotherapy *via* the systemic venous route is the only way which can be chosen. Despite the number of anticancer agents available for this type of chemotherapy, we prefer to use intravenous injection of Mitomycin-C, 5-fluorouracil (5-FU), and cytosine arabinoside in doses of 0.08, 10, and 0.8 /kg of body weight, respectively, twice a week for a period of up to 5 weeks.

We anticipated that these different drugs might exert some synergic effects on cancer cells, because Mitomycin-C acts as an alkylating agent and is usually fixed to the cells rapidly, whereas 5-FU is metabolized slowly over a prolonged period. Unfortunately we have so far had only 1 suitable case, shown in Fig. 4. Case 6. A 64-year-old male was admitted to the hospital complaining of intermittent fever. Multiple pulmonary metastases were found on routine chest X-ray before detection of the liver tumor. α-Fetoprotein was positive. Blood chemistry showed a cirrhotic pattern. The primary lesion was confirmed, by selective arteriography of the liver, to be occupying the entire right lobe with some invasion into the left lobe. The patient responded well to treatment and survived for

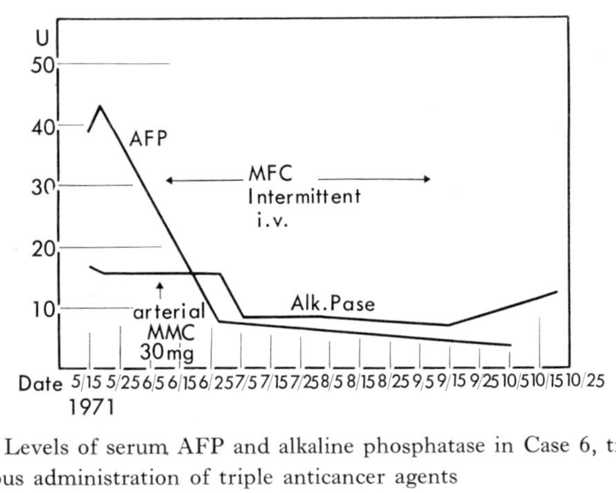

FIG. 4. Levels of serum AFP and alkaline phosphatase in Case 6, treated by intravenous administration of triple anticancer agents
MFC, Mitomycin-C, 5-FU and cytosine arabinoside; MMC, Mitomycin-C.

9 months. In the systemic administration of Mitomycin-C alone, there was no improvement of subjective and objective symptoms in 3 patients. The average survival was 2 months.

DISCUSSION

Since the discovery of AFP, positive AFP in the serum of a patient suspected of harboring a hepatocellular carcinoma appears to be the 1st specific immunochemical test for a specific cancer, in practice. Furthermore, repeated quantitative estimation of AFP in the serum offers the most valuable information regarding the effectiveness of treatment.

Negative AFP does not rule out the presence of a suspected hepatocellular carcinoma. In such a case, selective celiac arteriography can be a useful measure in the diagnosis and planning of proper treatment. An elevated alkaline phosphatase level in the serum may be nonspecific, but it is one of the sensitive indicators for follow-up studies after treatment of patients with negative AFP for hepatocellular carcinoma.

The most favorable hepatocellular carcinoma patients for hepatic resection are those with noncirrhotic liver. One such case is expected to be perfectly curable in our series (Case 1). However, one of our patients with cirrhotic liver showed progressive impairment in liver function tests, after hepatectomy and proximal gastrectomy for preventing hemorrhage from the varices, with resultant poor prognosis. Therefore, the most important consideration in selecting patients for hepatectomy was the extent of the cancer and the status of liver function.

The rather satisfactory results obtained by irradiation combined with intra-arterial Mitomycin-C therapy offer hope of improving the benefits of hepatectomy, if performed before the operation. Less satisfactory results in intra-arterial administration of Mitomycin-C were inevitable in most cases due to improper selection of patients. Therefore, in general, analysis of the results of treatments should be evaluated on the basis of the extent of the cancer and the grade of liver damage.

Acknowledgments

The guidance of Dr. Hajime Imanaga, the Director of Aichi Cancer Center Hospital, is gratefully acknowledged.

REFERENCES

1. Imanaga, H., Kuroyanagi, Y., Kaneko, M., and Kitagawa, T. Radiation combined with Mitomycin-C therapy on hepatocellular carcinoma (in Japanese). *Rinsho Hōshasen* (*Jap. J. Clin. Radiol.*), **16**, 374–380 (1971).
2. Imanaga, H., Kuroyanagi, Y., Kaneko, M., and Yoshida, T. O. Hepatectomy on primary cancer of liver—with special reference to α-fetoprotein (in Japanese). *Jap. Med. J.*, **2400**, 13–16 (1970).
3. Kuroyanagi, Y., Yoshida, T. O., Akaza, T., and Kobayashi, H. Diagnostic significance of serum α-fetoprotein in hepatocellular carcinoma (in Japanese). *Jap. Med. J.*, **2459**, 43–44 (1971).

4. Mann, J. D., Wakim, K. G., and Baggenstoss, A. H. The vasculature of the human liver: A study by injection-cast method. *Proc. Mayo Clin.*, **28**, 227–232 (1953).
5. Phillips, R. F. *In* " Tumors of the Liver," ed. by G.T. Pack and A. H. Islami, Springer-Verlag, Berlin, pp. 272–276 (1970).
6. Portugal, M. L., Azevedo, M. S., and Manso, C. Serum α-fetoprotein and variant alkaline phosphatase in human hepatocellular carcinoma. *Int. J. Cancer*, **6**, 383–387 (1970).

EXPLANATION OF PHOTOS

PHOTO 1a. Case 1, a 70-year-old male with hepatocellular carcinoma
Selective celiac arteriography demonstrates the dilated left hepatic artery with remarkable vascularity in the arterial phase.

PHOTO 1b. A schematic representation of the arteriogram in the same Case 1
LHA, left hepatic artery; RHA, right hepatic artery; SA, splenic artery; GDA, gastroduodenal artery; RGEPA, right gastroepiploic artery.

PHOTO 2. A photo of the mass of the tumor located in the left lobe taken during the operation, in the same Case 1

PHOTO 3. Case 2, an operative portal venogram shows tortuous, dilated, esophageal varices with no opacification of the left branch of the portal vein before operation

PHOTO 4. Case 3, a 64-year-old male with hepatocellular carcinoma
A celiac arteriography revealed demonstrable vascularity of the right hepatic artery in the arterial phase, before treatment.

PHOTO 5. Case 3, the hypervascularity seen previously on the arteriogram disappeared with regression of the tumor 10 months after treatment

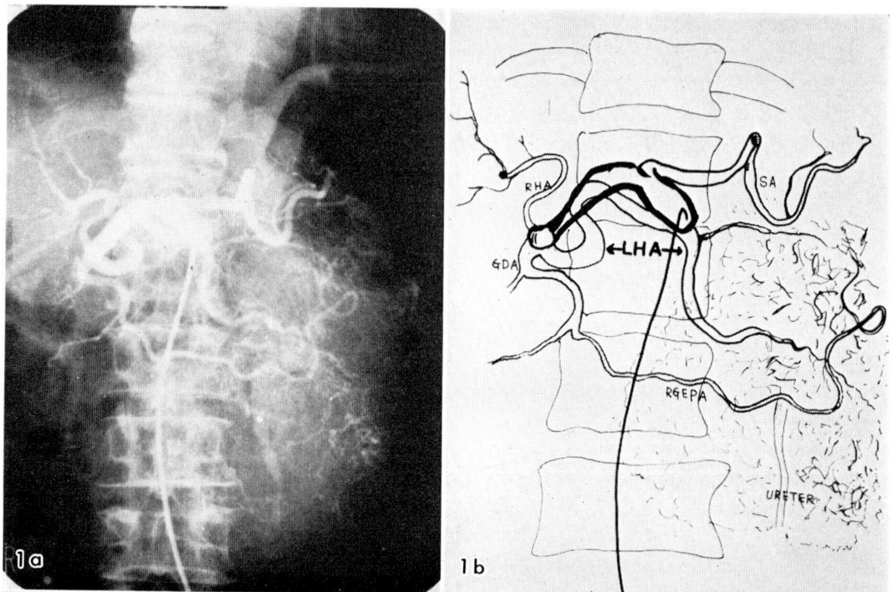
1a
RHA
SA
←LHA→
GDA
RGEPA
URETER
1b

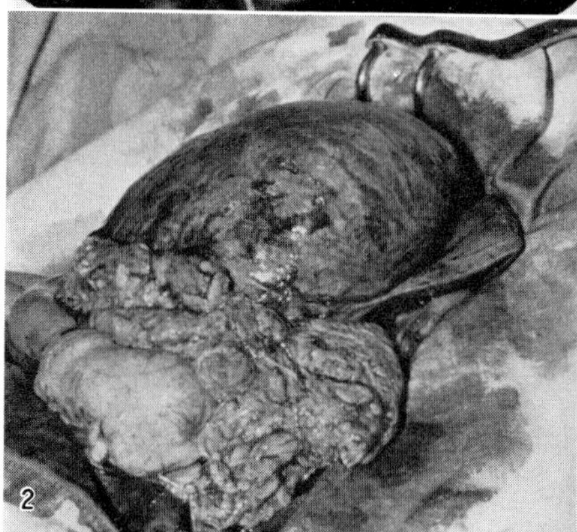
2

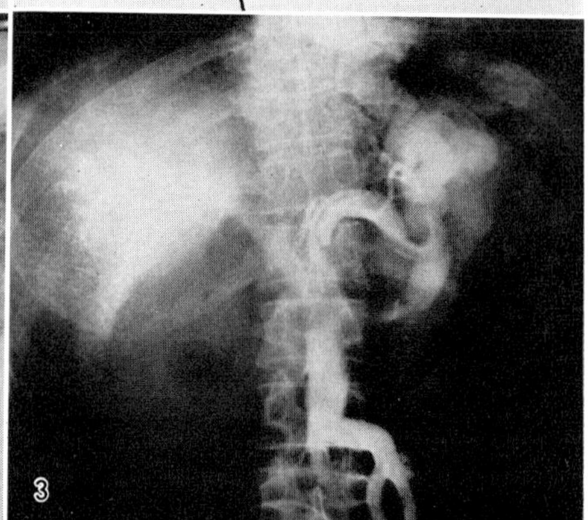
3

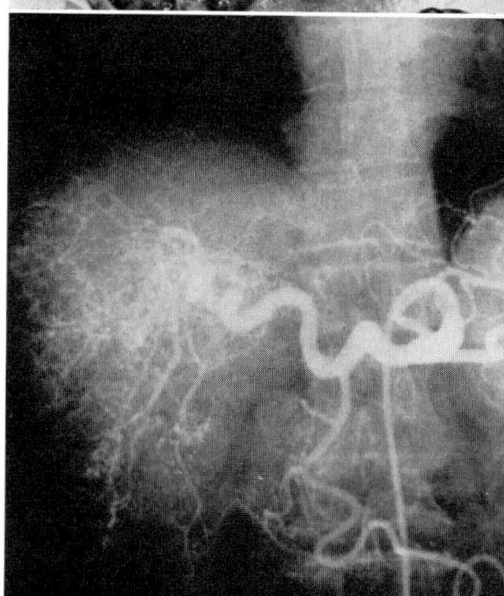
4

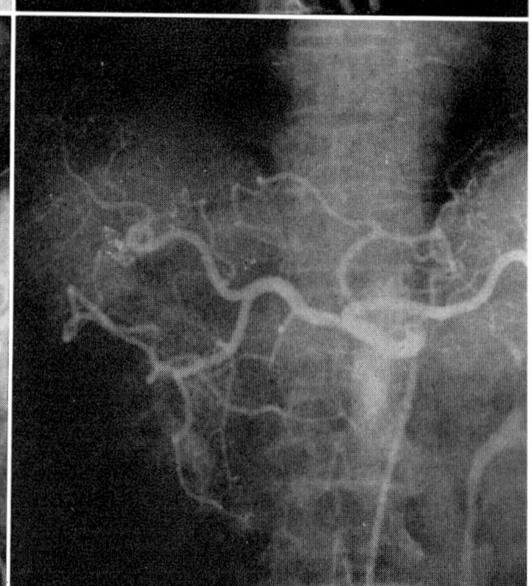
5

FETOPROTEINS AND CHILDREN'S TUMORS

Denise BUFFE

*Laboratoire d'Immunochimie, Institut de Recherches Scientifiques sur le Cancer**

The presence of 4 different fetoproteins (FP) was studied by immunological methods in the sera of children with tumors: α_1-FP, α_2H two β, fetal hemoglobin and βs. Only one has a practical diagnostic significance: It is α_1-FP which is found in 90% of sera from children with hepatoma and 80% of sera from children with teratoma. Under efficient chemotherapy or after surgery this protein disappears; it reappears and its level increases in case of metastasis or recurrency.

The presence of α_1-FP is not absolutely specific of the tumor. One can find it in some hepatopathies of young children, generally infant, but it is transitory and generally in lesser amounts than in tumors. A special point is the presence of α_1-FP in some metabolic diseases, tyrosinemia and Indian cirrhosis.

Though not tumor-specific, the other studied proteins, α_2H and β, could be valuable tools to alert the clinician.

Children's tumors are different from adult tumors in nature: They are embryonic tumors most frequently, and their symptomatology is often very poor and makes diagnosis very difficult before the sudden appearance of the tumor. The prognosis is dreadful because the evolution is very accelerated and the earlier the tumor is detected, the greater is the chance of survival. That is the reason we have been interested in studying embryonic proteins in children's tumors.

Studies on the antigenic structure of tumors comparative to fetal tissue and normal tissue from the same origin have been carried out in our laboratory for several years. The presence of these antigens, or of some of them, has been studied in the serum of children to aid in the diagnosis and prognosis. Some fetal proteins of electrophoretic mobilities α_1, α_2, and β have been studied by different authors (*1–3*, *14*, *15*, *17*, *20–23*) and especially by us (*5–7*, *12*, *13*). They are two proteins with α electrophoretic mobility: α_1-fetoprotein (α_1-FP) and α_2H-globulin (H because hepatic origin) and two β-globulins: Fetal hemoglobin and βs.

All these proteins have been studied by immunological methods: Simple immunoprecipitation in gel according to Ouchterlony's and Mancini's method with monospecific antisera and also, only for α_1-FP and α_2H, by the radio-autographic technique with ^{125}I- or ^{131}I-labeled monospecific antibodies.

The evaluation of embryonic antigens is only semiquantitative by both methods. We use a pool of fetal serum undiluted and after dilution as a reference

* 94800 Villejuif, France.

for α_1-FP and fetal hemoglobin; and for α_2H the reference is a fraction of purified α_2H-globulin (*8*). The antisera are prepared by immunization of rabbits or sheep with fetal sera, fetal hemoglobin, and purified α_2H. Before being used, antisera against α_1-FP are absorbed with pooled human adult plasma, fetal hemoglobin, and α_2H-globulin to make them monospecific for α_1-FP. For the study of βs the antiserum was given us by Takahashi *et al.* (*19*), and reference serum has been obtained from a patient with hepatocarcinoma.

α_1-*Fetoprotein**

α-Fetoprotein (AFP) is a normal embryonic serum globulin which disappears from the serum after birth. It is found in traces until 3 weeks of age. In premature babies it can persist in serum for a longer time, but in healthy infants it was never found after the first month of life by simple immunoprecipitation. The AFP reappears in serum samples from adults with primary hepatocarcinoma, as Abelev *et al.* (*1, 2*), Tatarinov (*18*), and many workers (*3, 17, 20*) from different countries have shown, in about 70% of cases and in some cases of testicular teratoblastoma (*2, 3, 12, 13*).

1. Pathological presence of α_1-*FP in nonneoplastic diseases*

α-Fetoprotein has also been detected in cases of infants with hepatopathies of different etiology. Masopust *et al.* (*15*) has found AFP in the serum of 17 infants, 5 to 6 months old, with hyperbilirubinemia. He explained the synthesis of the protein as a possible prematurity. In 10 cases of icterus and hepatomegaly AFP was present in the serum. These infants of 3 to 4 months of age had been treated in the first week of life with blood or plasma transfusions.

In our practice, we have found AFP in 13 cases of hepatitis out of 114 cases of hepatopathy and in 2 cases of tyrosinosis (*9*) (Table I). Generally the fetoprotein was present in these diseases in lower concentration than in hepatomas and teratomas, and disappeared from the serum during recovery. Masopust has been able to detect fetoprotein in some cases for a period of about 40 to 50 days during the illness. It was the same in 3 of our cases. The other 10 were positive only on one or two samples.

TABLE I. α_1-Fetoprotein in Nonneoplastic Liver Disease in Children 2 Months to 14 Years Old

Number of cases	α_1-FP +	% +	Ref.
143	31[a]	21	(15)
114	15[b]	13	—
42	19[c]	45	(*16*)
28	2[d]	7	(*16*)
9	9	100	(*4*)

[a] All infants. [b] 2 tyrosinosis. [c] Indian childhood cirrhosis. [d] 1 neonatal hepatitis. 1 sibling of a patient with Indian childhood cirrhosis.

* In this article the abbreviation α_1-FP is used instead of AFP.

TABLE II. α_1-Fetoprotein in Cancerous Child Sera

Hepatoblastoma	Malignant teratoma	Other various tumors	Ref.
1/1	5/8	0/126	(*15*)
39/41	27/57	3/369	—

Tyrosinosis cases were different: We observed one of the first cases, a boy, and later his sister. The first positive test was found in the serum of the 3-month-old boy. Many samples were tested, and all were positive until now; the child is 3 years old. The fetoprotein level varied with the diet; when the metabolic perturbations are corrected well enough, the AFP level decreased but it has never been nil. In the girl's case the test had constantly been positive until she died of meningitis. Necropsy did not show hepatoma or teratoma, only a metabolic cirrhosis.

Recently, Belanger *et al.* (*4*) reported 9 cases of hereditary tyrosinemia with α_1-FP in the serum. Noyak *et al.* (*16*) have indicated the presence of AFP in 19 cases out of 42 children with another metabolic disorder, Indian childhood cirrhosis. None of the other metabolic diseases we have tested (galactosemia, fructosemia, Wilson's disease) was positive.

2. *Serum α_1-FP in tumors*

In 1966, Masopust *et al.* (*14*) showed the presence of α_1-FP in sera of children with hepatoblastoma, and ovarian and testis teratoma. He had never found α_1-FP in 72 other cases of malignancies in children, embryonic tumors included. We have confirmed these results (*13*).

Table II summarizes the results of our AFP investigations in children older than one month with various forms of cancer. These results concern the first examination. Table III shows the results of sera obtained from children with various tumors except hepatoma and malignant teratoma.

TABLE III. α_1-Fetoprotein in Sera of Children with Various Tumors Except Hepatoma and Malignant Teratoma

Neuroblastoma	0/11	0/87
Nephroblastoma	0/7	0/89
Lymphoreticulosarcoma	0/44	0/35
Osteosarcoma	0/4	0/27
Embryonal sarcoma	—	0/41
Brain tumor	0/4	0/34
Seminoma	—	3/5
Benign teratoma	—	0/15
Liver tumor		
Hamartome	—	0/5
Angioma		0/3
Various	0/56	0/28
	0/126	0/369
Ref.	(*15*)	(*7, 13*)

The 3 positive tests were from 2 ovarian seminoma and one testis seminoma. Two of these young children had chromosomal abnormalities (Down's syndrome). Only traces of α_1-FP have been found; the radioimmunoprecipitation method was necessary to achieve these positive results. We have no theory to explain this positivity. Until now, the cases of seminoma have always been negative. We have begun a systematic study to investigate if α_1-FP is related to tumor or chromosomal abnormalities.

In the hepatoma group, 38 sera were positive out of 41 by simple immunodiffusion techniques, and one was positive only with the autoradiographic test. The two negative tests concern one hepatoblastoma and one carcinoma of the hepatic cell cords. All these patients were tested in the acute phase, before the surgery or on the day of operation.

Figures 1 and 2 illustrate the changes in serum level of α_1-FP in children with hepatoma after surgery.

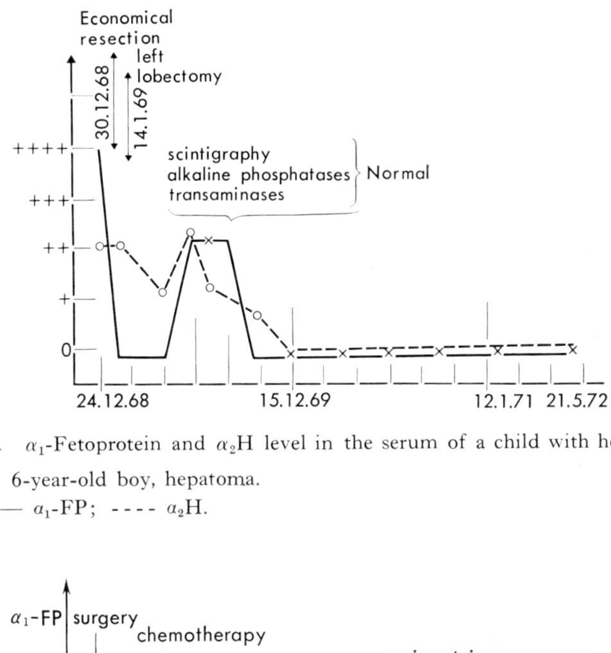

FIG. 1. α_1-Fetoprotein and α_2H level in the serum of a child with hepatoma Pa... 6-year-old boy, hepatoma.
——— α_1-FP; ---- α_2H.

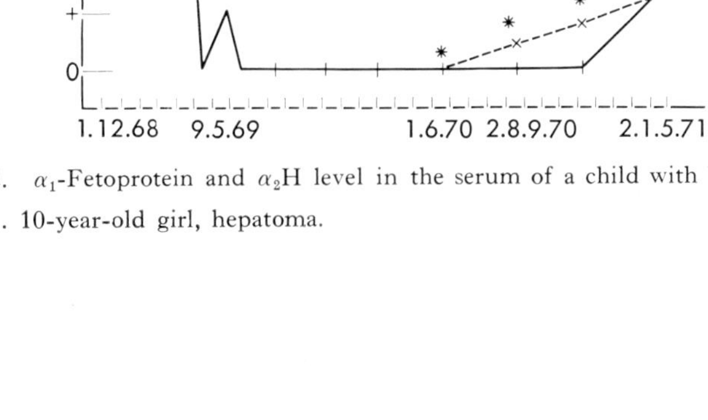

FIG. 2. α_1-Fetoprotein and α_2H level in the serum of a child with hepatoma Ba... 10-year-old girl, hepatoma.

In case Pa, a 6-year-old boy (Fig. 1), the surgeon, who was sure of having to deal with a benign tumor (hamartoma), in spite of a positive α_1-FP test before the operation, made a resection of the tumor pedicule. The pathologist then corroborated the diagnosis of hepatoma. Then in another operation, a left hepatic lobectomy was performed. The α_1-FP had disappeared from the serum between the two operations. Five months later and in 3 different and successive blood samples, the α_1-FP has been detected again at a low level.

All the clinical investigations have given normal results (scintillography, alkaline phosphatase, transaminase), and there was no sign of metastasis. Without any treatment α_1-FP became negative again after a few weeks. This child received no chemotherapy at any time during the disease. The α_1-FP occurrence on the 5th month after surgery might have been due to a spontaneous abortive recurrence or to the end of regeneration. This boy is still in good health after 3 years, and all samples are negative except one in September 1970 which was weakly positive only with labeled antibody. Perhaps it was another abortive recurrence.

In case Ba, a 10-year-old girl (Fig. 2), the first sample was positive before left lobectomy (*1*, *12*) and, 4 months later, the second sample contained even more α_1-FP. The α_1-FP level decreased and disappeared after chemotherapy. During 18 months, all samples were negative except one weakly positive by the autoradiographic method, and the young girl was apparently in good health. In September 1970 and January 1971, two samples were negative by simple immunoprecipitation and positive with labeled antibodies, the second more positive than the first. At this time there was no clinical evidence of recurrence. In May 1971 an already inoperable epigastric tumor was detected and AFP was present in the serum with simple immunodiffusion technique.

This case shows how valuable the determination of AFP on repeated blood samples taken during treatment is to evaluate therapy effect and detect recurrences, and how important the use of more and more sensitive methods is to follow the evolution and to detect residual disease.

TABLE IV. Serum α_1-FP in 57 Cases of Teratoma

	No. of cases	+	−	% +
In active phase	37	27	10	72
In therapeutic remission	20	0	20	0

In the malignant teratoma group (Tables IV and V) we have detected α_1-FP in the sera of 27 patients out of 37 with tumors *in situ* or just after surgery. Among the negative cases (20 in therapeutic remission without evidence of recurrence or metastasis and 10 in active disease), 8 became positive during the evolution when a recurrence occurred (Table VI). Four remained negative:

In one case a 9-year-old girl with ovarian embryonic carcinoma was operated on 1 month before the first test. This girl had no recurrence for 30 months and was always in good health. In the three other negative cases the test has constantly been negative in spite of a bad evolution. From the 18 other negative

TABLE V. Serum α_1-FP in Teratoma According to Localization

	No. of cases	In active phase		In therapeutic remission	
		+	−	+	−
Ovarian	20	9	1	0	10
Testis	10	5	1	0	4
Mediastinal	4	2	2	0	0
Retro peritoneal	6	4	1	0	1
Sacro-coccygeal	16	7	4	0	5
Other	1	0	1		
Total	57	27	10	0	20
		37			

TABLE VI. Evolution of Serum α_1-FP in 57 Cases of Teratoma

57 → 27⊕ = 48%

57 → 30⊖ →

20 in complete remission:
- 1 always ⊖ with a good evolution for 3 years
- 6 with a recurrence → 5⊕
- 13 only 1 or 2 tests. No additional information

10 in active phase:
- 2 always ⊖ in spite of worse evolution
- 3⊕ during evolution
- 5 only 1 sample. No information

tests, we received only one sample, and we do not know the ulterior evolution.

Figures 3 and 4 show the evolutive diagram of two cases of ovarian teratoma.

Case Pr (Fig. 3) was a 15-year-old-girl with ammenorrhea; 1 month later, ascites was present. Cytology of the ascitic fluid showed clusters of malignant cells. The α_1-FP was found in her serum at the end of February 1968. The patient received a first course of chemotherapy: Actinomycin, cyclophosphamide, and methotrexate. Under therapy the test became negative, while the ascites

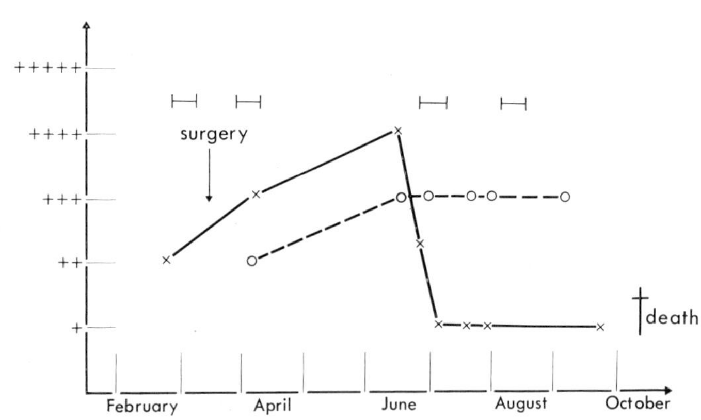

FIG. 3. α_1-FP and α_2H level in the serum of a child with teratoma
Pr... 15-year-old girl, ovarian teratoma.
——— α_1-FP; ---- α_2H; ⊢⊣ chemotherapy (actinomycin, cyclophosphamide, methrotrexate)

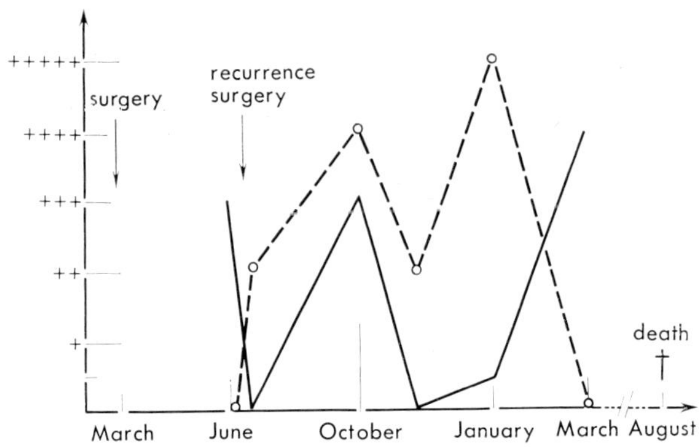

FIG. 4. α_1-Fetoprotein and α_2H level in the serum of a child with teratoma G. A.... 9-year-old girl, ovarian teratoma.
——— α_1-FP; ---- α_2H.

regressed as well as the volume of the tumor, hence allowing an excision, but there were peritoneal parietal metastases which could not be removed. At the end of June, α_1-FP was again present at the time of a recurrence and decreased after a second round of chemotherapy. One month later two serum samples were again positive in spite of another course of chemotherapy, and the girl died in October. Histological examination showed multiple necrotic area.

Case G. A., a 9-year-old girl with ovarian teratoma (Fig. 4), was operated on March 1970. Three months later, there was a recurrence, and the first test done at this time was positive in spite of chemotherapy. A second operation was made and a voluminous tumor was removed; 15 days later α_1-FP had disappeared from the serum. Several courses of chemotherapy and radiotherapy were done but did not prevent a worse evolution with AFP alternately positive and negative. Then the AFP level increased in the serum in spite of chemotherapy and radiotherapy, and the girl died in August 1971.

3. α_1-Fetoprotein presence in surgical cancerous organs

We have never detected α_1-FP in soluble extracts of the different tumors studied, except in extracts of hepatomas and some teratomas. Two aqueous extracts of hepatoma have been tested. α_1-Fetoprotein was detected by immunoelectrophoresis. In 2 cases of hepatomas, we were able to study by immunofluorescence the α_1-FP localization in cells. Only a few clusters of malignant cells were fluorescent with labeled antibodies. A cytoplasmic fluorescence was observed. Normal hepatocytes were not positive, only very dedifferentiated cells were labeled.

Five cases of teratoma have been studied for their content of α_1-FP. In case Pr, the tumor supernatant contained α_1-FP in a concentration at least 12 times higher than in the serum for the same total amount of protein.

In another case, Be, the tumor was removed following chemotherapy, and the α_1-FP had disappeared from the serum before the operation. No traces of α_1-FP were found in the tumor.

In case G. A., the operated voluminous tumor showed many necrotic areas with no recognizable structures, perhaps due to the chemotherapy. In its soluble extracts we did not find a higher amount of α_1-FP than in the patient's serum.

In another case of sacro-coccygeal teratoma, at the time of the operation, the serum did not contain any detectable α_1-FP but the sacro-coccygeal cyst contained a mucoid liquor with a high α_1-FP level. By immunofluorescence, all epithelial cells of the wall of the cyst were labeled. This was a secreting pseudo clump of cells contained α_1-FP in their cytoplasm.

We have also found α_1-FP in tumoral cells from pleural liquid in a case of abdominal teratoma with pulmonary metastasis.

In conclusion, the detection of α_1-FP has first of all a diagnostic value. The frequency of positivity is very high: 92% of hepatomas and 72% of active malignant teratomas. Such a fidelity gives remarkable diagnostic arguments.

(1) To confirm malignancy: α_1-FP is negative in liver metastasis and in liver benign tumors, in benign teratomas with an adult differentiation, and in operated patients with complete remission.

(2) To aid in a quick differential diagnosis between hepatoma, neuroblastoma, and nephroblastoma when the site of the tumor is in the right hypochondrium and between a genital or abdominal tumor if a liver cancer and a hereditary tyrosinemia have been excluded.

(3) The repetition of the test is very important in case of hepatopathy. The quick decrease of α_1-FP level is an argument for benign hepatopathy.

α_2H-Globulin

α_2H-globulin is a macroglobulin with iron in its molecule. It shows an immunological identity with ferritin. This globulin has never been found in the serum of normal adults and children of more than 2 months of age. α_2H-globulin is found in fetal and adult liver (*8*). In the serum of patients with tumors we have found α_2H very frequently, *i.e.*, in 50% of adults and in 80% of children (*56*).

The presence of α_2H in serum is not related to the localization, the volume, or the histological characters of the tumor, as shown by the results of the first examination in Tables VII and VIII. The α_2H-globulin level is not very quickly modified by operation or chemotherapy. It decreases slowly and disappears if the evolution is good, but in cases of recurrence or metastasis it reappears or its level increases about 2 months before the clinical detection of recurrence.

In case Pa (hepatoma, Fig. 1), α_2H-globulin decreased slowly, and its level was not detectable by our techniques: Simple immunodiffusion or radioimmunodiffusion in the 9th sample on December 1969. Now all samples are negative.

In case Pr (ovarian teratoma, Fig. 3), while α_1-FP decreased and became nil with surgery and chemotherapy, the α_2H amount increased and remained high until the α_1-FP reappearance and the girl's death.

In another case of ovarian teratoma in which we had never detected α_1-FP, we have observed an increase of α_2H-globulin in a sample of serum taken 1 month before the clinical recurrence had been detected.

TABLE VII. α_2H-Globulin in Serum of Children 2 Months to 16 Years Old

	No. of cases	+	−	% +
With tumor	453	362	91	80
Healthy or with benign disease	177	16	161	9

TABLE VIII. α_2H-Globulin in Serum of Children with Tumors

	No. of cases	α_2H +	α_2H −	% +
Hepatoma	41	37	4	90
Teratoma	43	21	22	48
Neuroblastoma	87	67	20	77
Nephroblastoma	88	77	11	87.5
Lymphoreticulosarcoma	35	30	5	85.7
Osteosarcoma	27	20	7	74
Embryonic sarcoma	41	33	8	80
Brain tumor	34	29	5	80
Various	56	45	11	80
Total	452	359	93	79%

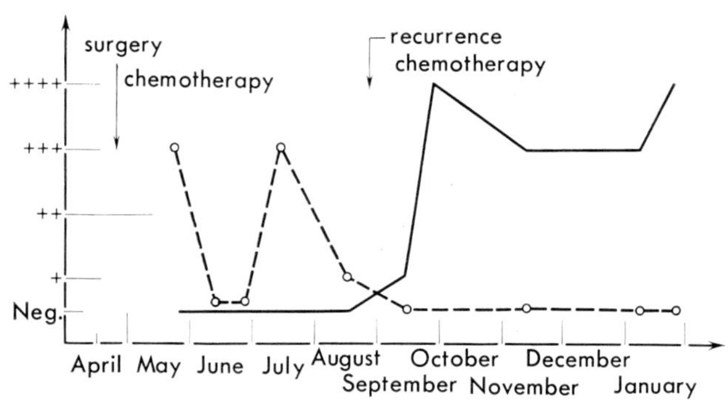

FIG. 5. α_1-Fetoprotein and α_2H level in the serum of a child with teratoma K... 2-year-old girl, ovarian teratoma.
——— α_1-FP; - - - - α_2H.

The same observation was made in another case of ovarian teratoma (K, Fig. 5); the α_2H level increased 2 months before the reappearance of α_1-FP in the serum and the clinical detection of the recurrence.

We have very often observed in the cases with high levels of α_1-FP a decrease of α_2H-globulin. We have no definite explanation for this phenomenon but perhaps α_2H and α_1-FP are synthesized by the same cell in a different state of retro differentiation. This hypothesis may be taken into consideration in hepatomas and teratomas. In fact, we have found α_1-FP and α_2H-globulin by the immunofluorescence technique in the same undifferentiated cell in a few cases of hepatoma. But it does not hold true for all the tumors and especially for tumors without α_1-FP.

We have detected α_2H-globulin by radioimmunodiffusion in all extracts of tumors tested and especially in liver metastasis in peritumoral areas, and by immunofluorescent techniques α_2H has been found in reticuloendothelial cells.

Is α_2H-globulin a stimulating factor for cell division, or a growth factor? Or does it act immunologically by blocking leucocyte reactions ? It is possible that it acts by both mechanisms, as some preliminary results suggest. This protein exists in normal liver. By what mechanism it goes through the cellular membrane into the serum, we do not know. Whatever the mechanism, one fact remains: α_2H detection in serum is a valuable evolutivity test.

Two β-FP Found in Many Children with Tumors

Fetal hemoglobin has been detected by simple immunoprecipitation in 77% of children 2 months to 6 years old. All cases of hepatoma were positive. In 1967, Takahashi *et al.* (*19*) reported the presence of a new serum protein βs in hepatoma extracts, in sera of patients with primary hepatoma, and in cord and fetal sera. In 1970, these authors (*23*) found βs also in other malignancies and in a small number of cases with nonneoplastic liver diseases.

We have tested sera of children with different tumors by Ouchterlony's method with an antiserum given to us by Takahashi and we have found βs in 60% of tested cases. When the test was done in the evolutive phase of the disease we have noted it in 85% of the cases and in 100% of tested hepatoma and teratomas. These results are not surprising because in our experiments βs showed an immunological identity with C-reactive protein.

CONCLUSIONS

Out of the 4 fetoproteins studied in children with tumors, only one has a practical diagnostic significance: α_1-FP, in hepatoma and teratoma cases in spite of its presence in some hepatopathies of childhood.

Though not tumor-specific, α_2H-globulin can help also for diagnosis and prognosis. When this protein is detected in sera in case of α_1-FP nonproducing tumors, clinicians must search for a malignant process. The fact that α_2H practically always precedes the reappearance of α_1-FP in the serum is a valuable tool to alert clinicians.

The clinical value of the two β-proteins is not yet proved and needs further investigation. The high percentage of positivity in children is perhaps related to age, the synthesis of these proteins being not yet completely repressed. It is necessary to repeat and to multiply controls with different sera from children in good health or with nonneoplastic diseases. In our preliminary experiments βs is not a fetoprotein, though it was found in fetal serum in the second part of pregnancy, it is the C-reactive protein which is known to be present in pregnant women's sera and in newborn sera. The results of these tests together with the increase of haptoglobin and ceruloplasmin, though they are nonspecific, can give a useful index to appreciate the efficiency of the therapy and to permit more precociously a diagnosis of a generalization of recurrency.

The presence of α_1-FP in metabolic diseases and especially in congenital tyrosinemia seems to us very important. In fact, a physiological tyrosinemia is known in premature and in newborn children less than 2 weeks old, *i.e.*, when the presence of α_1-FP in the serum is also a physiological phenomenon.

These remarks open up a new field in the research on cellular differentiation. They suggest that α_1-FP is related to the molecular events of cell differentiation and is a sort of marker of embryonic cells.

A better knowledge of the different steps of cellular metabolism and of factors acting on them could help in understanding the malignant transformation.

Added in Proof

All the results we reported here concern clinical observations done before March 1972. Now we have got 2 other cases of tyrosinosis with α_1-FP which have been published elsewhere (*Biomedicin*, No. 19 (1973)).

REFERENCES

1. Abelev, G. I., Assecritoval, I. V., Kraevsky, N. A., Perova, S. D., and Perevodchikova, N. I. Embryonal serum α-globulin in cancer patients. Diagnostic value. *Int. J. Cancer*, **2**, 551–558 (1967).
2. Abelev, G. I. α-Fetoprotein in ontogenesis and its association with malignant tumors. *Adv. Cancer Res.*, **14**, 295–558 (1971).
3. Alpert, M. E., Uriel, J., and de Nechaud, B. α_1-Fetoglobulin in the diagnosis of human hepatoma. *New Engl. J. Med.*, **278**, 984–986 (1958).
4. Belanger, L., Belanger, M., and Larochelle, J. Une cirrhose infantile associée à la néoproduction d'α-foetoprotéine. Perspectives nouvelles dans la tyrosinémie héréditaire. *Nouv. Presse Med.*, **1**, 1503–1504 (1972).
5. Buffe, D., Rimbaut, C., and Burtin, P. Présence d'une protéine d'origine tissulaire, l'α_2H-globuline, dans le sérum de sujets atteints d'affections malignes. *Int. J. Cancer*, **3**, 850–856 (1968).
6. Buffe, D., Rimbaut, C., Lemerle, J., Schweisguth, O., and Burtin, P. Présence d'une ferroprotéine d'origine tissulaire, l'α_2H-globuline dans le sérum des enfants porteurs de tumeur. *Int. J. Cancer*, **5**, 85–87 (1970).
7. Buffe, D., Rimbaut, C., and Burtin, P. Recherche de l'α_1-foetoprotéine et de l'α_2H-globuline dans le sérum d'enfants porteurs d'hépatome et de tératome. Intérêt diagnostic et pronostic. Congr. Biochem. Clinical, Praha, Sept. 1971.
8. Buffe, D., Rimbaut, C., Fuccaro, C., and Burtin, P. Isolement et caractérisation d'une ferroprotéine tissulaire l'α_2H-globuline. *Annu. Inst. Pasteur*, **123**, 129–142 (1972).
9. Dommergues, J. P., Odievre, M., Buffe, D., and Nocton, F. Synthèse prolongée d'α_1FP chez 2 frères atteints de tyrosinose congénitale. *Arch. Pédiatr.*, **29** (1972).
10. Ishak, K. G. and Glunz, P. R. Hepatoblastoma and hepatocarcinoma in infancy and childhood. *Cancer*, **20**, 396–422 (1967).
11. Kithier, K., Houstek, J., Masopust, J., and Radl, J. Occurrence of specific foetal protein in primary liver carcinoma. *Nature*, **212**, 414 (1966).
12. Mawas, C., Kohen, M., Lemerle, J., Buffe, D., Schweisguth, O., and Burtin, P. Serum α_1-foetoprotein (fetuin) in children with malignant ovarian or testicular teratomas. Preliminary results. *Int. J. Cancer*, **4**, 76–79 (1969).

13. Mawas, C., Buffe, D., Schweisguth, O., and Burtin, P. α_1-Fetoprotein and children's cancer. *Rev. Eur. Clin. Biol.*, **16**, 430–435 (1971).
14. Masopust, J., Kithier, J., Fuchs, V., Kotál, L., and Rádl, J. Fetoprotein: A specific α_1-globulin of human fetuses. Its ontogenesis and importance for pathology. *In* "Intra Uterine Dangers to the Fetus," ed. by J. Horsky and Z. K. Stembera, Proc. Symp. Prague, October 11–14, 1966, Exc. Med. Found., Amsterdam, pp. 30–35 (1967).
15. Masopust, J., Kithier, J., Rádl, J., Koutecky, J., and Kotál, L. Occurrence of fetoprotein in patients with neoplasms and nonneoplastic diseases. *Int. J. Cancer*, **3**, 364–373 (1968).
16. Nayak, N. C., Chawla, V., Malaviya, A. N., and Chandra, R. K. α-Fetoprotein in Indian childhood cirrhosis. *Lancet*, **1**, 68 (1972).
17. O'Conor, G. T., Tatarinov, Yu. S., Abelev, G. I., and Uriel, J. A collaborative study for the evaluation of a serologic test for primary liver cancer. *Cancer*, **25**, 1091–1098 (1970).
18. Tatarinov, Yu, S. Content of embryospecific α-globulin in blood serum of human foetus, newborn and adult man in primary cancer of liver. *Vopr. Med. Khim.*, **11**, 20–24 (1965).
19. Takahashi, A., Yachi, A., Anzai, T., and Wada, T. Presence of a unique serum protein in sera obtained from patients with neoplastic diseases and in embryonic and neonatal sera. *Clin. Chim. Acta*, **17**, 5–12 (1967).
20. Uriel, J., de Nechaud, B., Stanislawski-birencwajg, M., Masseyeff, R., Leblanc, L., Quenum, C., Loisillier, F., and Grabar, P. Antigènes embryonnaires et cancer du foie chez l'homme. Association de l' α_1-foetoprotéine sérique avec l'hépatome primaire. *C. R.*, **265**, 75–78 (1967).
21. Uriel, J. Transitory liver antigens and primary hepatoma in man and rat. *Pathol. Biol.*, **17**, 877–884 (1969).
22. Uriel, J. and de Nechaud, B. La recherche d'α_1-foetoprotéine en pathologie humaine. Etat actuel de la question. *Annu. Inst. Pasteur*, **122**, 829–839 (1972).
23. Wada, T., Anzai, T., Yachi, A., Kawaharada, M., Ikebe, M., and Takahashi, A. Diagnostic significance of two fetal proteins αF and βs in hepatoma and other neoplastic diseases. *Protides Biol. Fluids*, **18**, 221–225 (1970).

EMBRYONAL CARCINOMA AND α-FETOPROTEIN
With Special Reference to Hepatoblastoma

Hiroshi HASEGAWA,*1 Tatsu MUKOJIMA,*2 Nobu HATTORI,*2 Ryozo SANO,*3 and Teruyuki HIROTA*3

*Department of Surgery,**1 *Department of Clinical Laboratory,**2 *and Department of Clinical Pathology,**3 *National Cancer Research Institute*

The problem of α-fetoprotein (AFP) with regard to embryonal carcinomas, in children's hepatocellular tumors in particular, appears unique: The serum AFP titer in hepatoblastoma is markedly high in comparison with the titer observed in adult hepatoma and other neoplastic diseases. This paper refers to the particular properties of these tumors with special reference to the clinical course, AFP titer, and histopathological features.

Six cases of children's hepatocellular tumor were positive in AFP, all with very high titers. In 3 cases of hepatectomy, the postoperative diminution curves of AFP titer were drawn, and the half-life of AFP in the sera was calculated. A case with a half-life of 6.79 days and another of 5.35 days died due to recurrence of the tumor, and a case with a half-life of 3.69 days is now surviving 2 years after radical hepatectomy. In the latter case, cannulation infusion chemotherapy administered intra-arterially was effective: The regression of the tumor paralleled the diminution of AFP titer. After a radical resection of the tumor in the 2nd operation, the AFP titer became zero. With regard to the histopathological findings, one case with an extraordinarily high titer of AFP demonstrated the features of hepatocarcinoma of an adult type, and the remaining 5 cases showed features of fetal, embryonal, or mixed types of hepatoblastoma.

Two cases of sacrococcygeal teratoma presented positive findings in AFP survey. The AFP titer was checked in one of the cases throughout its course.

Four cases of testicular and other embryonal carcinomas were examined. In half of them, the AFP survey gave negative results, but no definitive histopathological difference was suggested among the AFP-negative and AFP-positive cases. Twelve cases of common neoplastic diseases in infancy and childhood were also examined and all presented negative findings.

The clinical and histopathological problems concerning α-fetoprotein (AFP) in infancy and childhood appear unique: The serum AFP titer in hepatoma in

*1,*2,*3 Tsukiji 5-1-1, Chuo-ku, Tokyo 104, Japan (長谷川　博, 向島　達, 服部　信, 佐野量造, 広田映五).

TABLE I. α-Fetoprotein Titer and Liver Cell Carcinoma in Children

Case No.	Sex	Age	Operation and treatment	AFP
1	Female	$2^{3}/_{12}$	R. hepatectomy Postop. radiation	++ 1,050→62
2	Male	$7^{8}/_{12}$	Cannulation infusion chemotherapy (5-FU)[a]	+++ 16,000
3	Male	$1^{5}/_{12}$	Extend. L. hepatectomy Postop. radiation	+++ 14,900
4	Female	$1^{10}/_{12}$	Extend. R. hepatectomy Postop. death	++ 1,276
5	Male	$^{5}/_{12}$	Cannulation infusion chemotherapy (VCR)[b] L. hepatectomy	++ 3,220→0
6	Male	$1^{4}/_{12}$	Extend. L. hepatectomy Cannulation infusion chemotherapy (VCR)[b]	++ 1,850→24→5,650

[a] 5-FU=5-fluorouracil. [b] VCR=vincristine.

children is markedly high in comparison with the values observed in adult hepatoma and other neoplastic diseases. The cause of such differences is not known as yet, but the biological character or the relative amount of the AFP-producing cells may be responsible. The present paper intends to treat these problems with reference to the clinical course, laboratory findings, and histopathological features of embryonal carcinomas obtained in our experience.

As shown in Tables I and II, 6 cases of hepatoblastoma and 4 cases of other embryonal neoplasmas were analyzed. All of the total of 10 cases were positive in AFP examination. However, there were 2 other cases of embryonal carcinoma in adults in which AFP was negative. Twelve cases of common neoplastic diseases in infancy and childhood were also examined. α-Fetoprotein surveys by our single radial immunodiffusion method (*6*) presented negative findings in all.

Case presentation will be made for 3 groups: Hepatoblastoma, sacrococcygeal teratoma, and testicular and other malignancy.

Hepatoblastoma

Six patients under 7 years old were subjected to surgery and 3 children receiving hepatectomy were submitted to repeated examination of serum AFP

TABLE II. α-Fetoprotein Titer in Malignant Sacrococcygeal Teratoma and Testicular Malignancy

Case No.	Sex	Age	Diagnosis and treatment	AFP
7	Male	$3^{10}/_{12}$	Sacrococcygeal teratoma Partial resect., chemoth., and radiation	222→28→265
8	Female	$1^{9}/_{12}$	Sacrococcygeal teratoma treated in other hospital	61
9	Male	$^{6}/_{12}$	Testicular embryonal ca. Orchiectomy, radiation, and chemoth.	78
10	Male	45	Teratoca., (seminoma and embry. ca.) Orchiectomy, radiation, and chemoth.	285→525

postoperatively in order to obtain the diminution curves of the titer. The operations performed on these 6 cases were: Right hepatectomy in 2 cases, left hepatectomy in 3 cases, and exploratory laparotomy in 1 case.

Case presentation will be made with reference to the changes in the serum AFP titer in relation to the clinical and histopathological findings in these 6 patients.

Case 1: A 2-year-3-month-old girl. A huge mass was palpated on the upper right quadrant of the abdomen. In the preoperative examination, no distant metastasis was found and radical right hepatectomy was performed along Cantlie's line. The huge tumor, occupying the whole right lobe, seemed to be covered by a pseudocapsule, but several very small nodules were observed on the outside of the pseudocapsule near Cantlie's line, demonstrating the spread of the tumor to the remaining left lobe. After the operation, radiation therapy was performed on the stump of the remnant liver in addition. However, in the 6th month after surgery, the girl died suddenly because of intraperitoneal hemorrhage due to the rupture of the recurrent liver tumor, and autopsy was performed in another hospital.

The AFP level in sera had not been measured during her life since the appropriate laboratory technique was not established at the time of the operation. The measurement was, therefore, made on blood samples which were taken repeatedly after surgery and stored in a deep-freezer for more than a year. The postoperative AFP diminution curve in the stored sera is shown in Fig. 1. The calculated half-life of AFP in the patient's circulating blood was 5.35 days, which was later judged as too prolonged in comparison with the half-life of Case 5 with whom a permanent cure is expected.

Histopathological diagnosis on the surgical specimen was hepatoblastoma of a fetal type, and its histological pattern was trabecular in most of the tumor

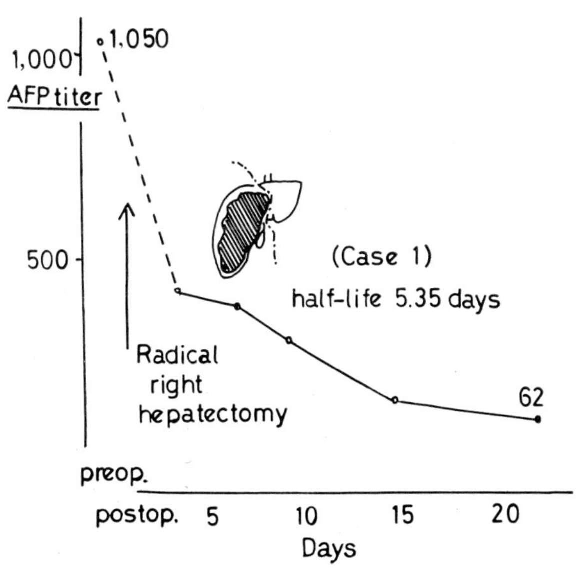

FIG. 1. Diminution curve of AFP titer in Case 1

with embryonal cell pattern observed only in a few areas (Photo 1).

Case 2: A 7-year-8-month-old boy. This patient was subjected to exploratory laparotomy in another hospital 2 months before our examination, and clinically diagnosed as Wilms' tumor with extensive liver metastases. On his admission to our hospital, no distant metastasis was identified but hepatoblastoma was suspected. On surgical exploration, the liver tumor was found occupying the whole of the liver. Since there was no extrahepatic spread of the tumor, biopsy and hepatic intra-arterial cannulation through the right gastroepiploic artery were performed. After surgery, a continuous infusion of chemotherapeutic agent was combined with radiotherapy. But a total dose of 3,950 mg of 5-fluorouracil (5-FU) with radiation was not at all effective, and the tumor enlarged gradually. On autopsy, the tumor occupied the whole liver and weighed 2,930 g, which was about one-seventh of the body weight at the time of death (22 kg).

α-Fetoprotein was checked in this patient on 2 occasions: On the 15th day and on the 65th day, or 10 days before death, after the beginning of the cannulation infusion chemotherapy with 5-FU. In the earlier blood sample, the AFP level was 8,500 units, and in the later sample, it was 16,000 units. This was the highest titer of fetoproteinemia ever obtained in our laboratory.

A histological examination was performed on the biopsy and autopsy specimens. The tumor consisted of hepatocarcinoma cells of an adult type (Photo 2). The cells were large in size, the cytoplasm contained abundant vacuoles, and the nuclei showed marked atypia. No definite findings suggesting embryonal liver cells were found. In the autopsy specimen, massive necrosis and degeneration of the tumor cells were found. The reason for the extraordinarily high titer of AFP is unknown, but it may be attributed to the huge tumor mass, which was relatively large compared to the body weight of the patient, leaving only a scanty residual mass of normal liver that was engaged in the metabolism of protein.

Case 3: A 1-year-5-month-old boy. This patient was subjected to partial hepatectomy on 2 occasions in another hospital. Both resections of the tumor located on the left lobe were incomplete, according to the report from the surgeon. During medical treatment and observation in our hospital, the serum cholesterol level was proved to have elevated, and a 3rd surgery was therefore decided on by our team. Macroscopically, the 3rd intervention successfully resected the tumor completely: Left hepatectomy was performed along Cantlie's line shifted markedly to the right. However, 5 months later, the boy died because of lung metastases, and recurrence in the remnant right lobe of the liver. The total mass of the tumor at the time of autopsy was not as large as in Case 2, and the titer of AFP in sera examined before death was nearly as high. It was 14,900 units.

The histopathological diagnosis was hepatoblastoma with two patterns: In some areas, trabecular patterns consisting of cells with basophilic cytoplasm, and in other areas small foci of tumor cells with abundant clear cytoplasm on Hematoxylin-Eosin staining. In this case, the high value of AFP may be related to the biological character of the tumor cells.

Case 4: This case was admitted to another hospital, but extended right hepatectomy was performed by one of the authors, and AFP and histological ex-

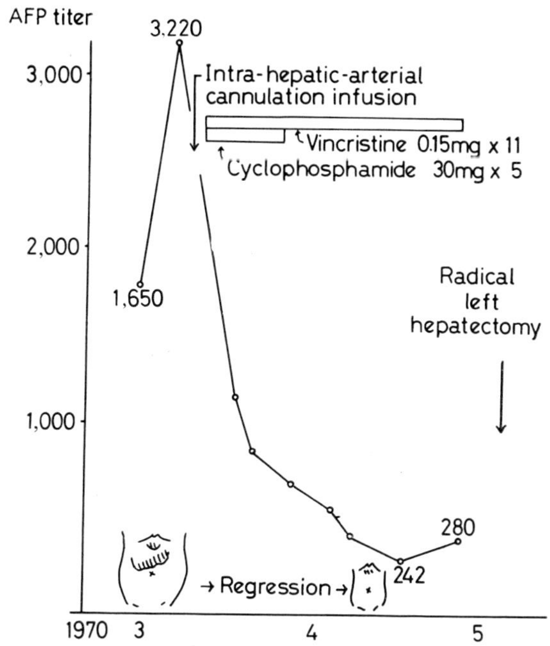

FIG. 2. Diminution curve of AFP titer in Case 5 (effect of intra-arterial cannulation infusion)

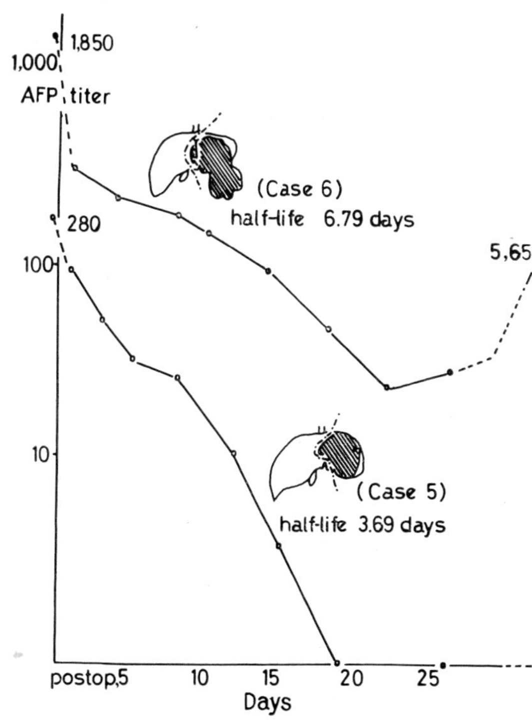

FIG. 3. Diminution curve of AFP titer after hepatectomy in Cases 5 and 6

aminations were made in our hospital. In spite of the success of the operation, the girl died on the day after the operation of an unknown cause. The histopathological diagnosis was hepatoblastoma of mixed fetal- and embryonal-type cells. The titer of AFP before the operation was moderately high (1,276 units).

Case 5: A 5-month-old boy. A large mass was found in the center of the liver on palpation and on a hepatoscintigram. Because the tumor seemed inoperable, the first operation was performed for the purposes of biopsy and cannulation infusion chemotherapy. A fine Teflon tube was introduced through the right gastroepiploic artery, and was fixed so that the tip of the tube was kept just in the proper hepatic artery. The chemotherapy was started on the day of the operation under the following schedule: Vincristine 0.5 mg/m^2 and cyclophosphamide 100 mg/m^2, each 3 times a week. On the 5th day after the operation, regression of the tumor was noticed and in 1 month, the upper abdominal tumor had almost disappeared. In total, Vincristine was administered intra-arterially 11 times at 0.15 mg per dose, and cyclophosphamide 5 times at 30 mg per dose. It was quite interesting that the titer of AFP in the sera decreased sharply from 3,220 to 242 units coincident with the regression of the tumor. On the 2nd laparotomy, the tumor was completely removed. The diminution curve of AFP is demonstrated in Figs. 2 and 3. After complete removal of the tumor, AFP disappeared with a half-life of 3.69 days: The disappearance is shown on a semilogarithmic scale in Fig. 3.

The histopathological finding was a mixed type of hepatoblastoma. The majority of epithelial cells consisted of fetal and embryonal types, the rest were mesenchymal components made up of uncalcified osteoid tissue and small foci with fibroblastic proliferation (Photo 3). This is the first case in our experience which responded dramatically to chemotherapy, and the third case surviving more than 2 years after surgery for hepatoblastoma in the children we have operated upon.

Case 6: A 1-year-4-month-old boy. On a hepatoscintigram and on palpation, a large mass was found in the left lobe of the liver. On laparotomy, neither extrahepatic invasion nor spreading to the right side of Cantlie's line was found, and radical, extended, left hepatectomy was performed. The titer of AFP, however, did not decrease as rapidly as in Case 5. The calculated half-life of AFP in the sera was 6.79 days (Fig. 3). At the end of the 1st month after the operation, the titer did not go down to zero, and began to increase again with recurrence of the upper abdominal tumor. A 2nd operation performed 2 months after the 1st elucidated that the remnant right lobe was completely occupied with the spread of the tumor. Intra-arterial cannulation infusion chemotherapy using a fine Teflon tube was therefore performed, and Vincristine and cyclophosphamide were administered repeatedly. The therapy was not at all effective and the patient died 4 months after the hepatectomy.

The histological diagnosis was hepatoblastoma, but the tissue contained a great deal of mesenchymal components—osteoid tissue was found throughout the specimen, and in some areas fibroblastic proliferation was also found. The epithelial component consisted of fetal-type cells with clear cytoplasm and a few cells of an embryonal type (Photo 4). This pattern seems to explain the ineffectiveness of the anticancer drugs and the relatively low titer of AFP throughout the patient's clinical course.

Sacrococcygeal Teratoma

Two cases of sacrococcygeal teratoma with malignant changes were examined for AFP, and both were found to be positive, but weaker than hepatoma. The results are as follows:

Case 7: A 3-year-10-month-old boy. Three months before his visit to our hospital, his mother noticed a disturbance in defecation and in another hospital, an incision to the swelling of the coccygeal region was performed under the diagnosis of inflammation. On admission to our hospital, defecation and micturition were completely halted by a tumor occupying the whole pelvic space. An emergency operation was performed to make a colostomy. On opening the peritoneum, an intrapelvic mass was verified, which extended up to the bifurcation of the common iliac artery.

One week later, partial resection of the sacrococcygeal and intrapelvic mass was performed by sacral approach, but the majority of the mass was too soft to enucleate or remove. Following the partial resection, a systemic intravenous administration of chemotherapeutic agents was made: Vincristine 1.5 mg/m^2 and cyclophosphamide 300 mg/m^2 per week. The lower abdominal mass and edema of the legs and scrotum had decreased in size by the end of the week after the initiation of chemotherapy, and disappeared by the end of 1 month after chemotherapy. At that time, the AFP titer in the blood had also decreased from the initial value of 222 units to 28 units, as shown in Fig. 4. Thereafter, how-

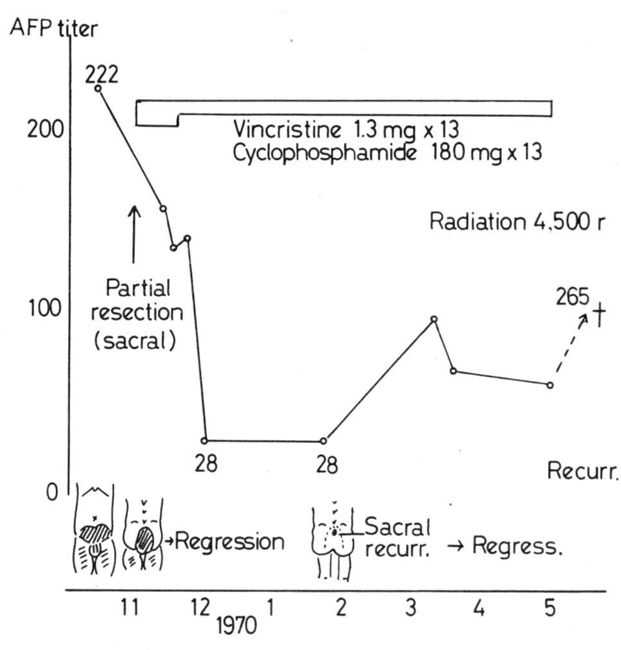

FIG. 4. Change of AFP titer in relation to treatment and recurrence

ever, AFP titer increased preceding recurrence, and then decreased with the regression of the tumor by radiation therapy and chemotherapy. At the time of death, the titer was rather higher than the value obtained before treatment. The histopathological diagnosis was sacrococcygeal teratoma with a malignant change, *i.e.*, embryonal carcinoma. No definite histological finding resembling embryonal liver cells was obtained in surgical or autopsy specimens.

Case 8: A 1-year-9-month-old girl. Malignant sacrococcygeal teratoma was diagnosed on the patient's first visit to our hospital, and AFP examination was found to be positive, as with the preceding case. She was operated upon in another hospital and histopathological findings were proved to be quite the same as in Case 7.

Teratocarcinoma of the Testis and Other Miscellaneous Malignancies

Case 9: A 6-month-old boy. On the 5th month after birth the mother of the patient noticed a swelling of the testis. Orchiectomy was performed on this case in the 1st hospital where he was examined. The AFP level was examined a year after this, when he was admitted to our hospital for the treatment of multiple recurrence of the teratocarcinoma. The titer was 78 units, and histopathological diagnosis was teratocarcinoma of the testis.

Case 10: A 45-year-old male. This was a case of multiple recurrence after orchiectomy. About 2 weeks before death, the AFP titer was 525 units, and histopathological diagnosis on an autopsy specimen was teratocarcinoma of the testis.

Two other cases of embryonal carcinoma in adults were examined. The AFP was negative, and no histological difference was suggested between the negative and positive cases. Twelve other cases of miscellaneous common neoplastic diseases in infancy and childhood were surveyed for AFP. They were all negative (leukemia 3, Wilms' tumor 3, neuroblastoma 2, 1 case each of rhabdomyosarcoma, brain tumor, anaplastic carcinoma, and dysgerminoma).

DISCUSSION

Since the discovery of the relationship between AFP and cancer by Tatarinov (*7*) in 1965, many clinical papers (*1–8*) have been presented concerning the diagnosis and specificity of the AFP test in adult hepatoma. However, by 1968, Houstek *et al.* (*3*) had proved the presence of the protein in a child's hepatoma, and in 1971 a definitive paper (*5*) was presented by the group in Villejuif, France, on AFP and children's cancer. According to the group in Villejuif, 23 cases of hepatoma, 27 cases of malignant teratoma, and 150 other miscellaneous tumors of infants and children were examined by the immunological method of Mancini and the excellent results shown below were obtained:

Hepatoma, 21/23 positive (histological evidence in 21)
Malignant teratoma, 15/27 positive (other 12 cases were negative, but they are cured or complete remission cases.)

Wilms' tumor	0/43
Neuroblastoma	0/42
Osteosarcoma	0/19
Embryonal sarcoma	0/17
Lymphoma	0/17
Brain tumor	0/7
Others	0/5

They also reported the diminution of AFP in the postoperative course. In Case B of their report, the preoperatively positive data became zero on the 18th day after the operation, with a half-life of 9 days. From the impression obtained from Cases 1, 5, and 6 in our hospital, the half-life that they report in Case B is too long, so that a permanent cure cannot be expected. Since there was a recurrence in Case B, as they reported in the same paper, we believe that our view that " the postoperative half-life of AFP in the sera must be less than 4 days " will be strongly supported in the future. However, they report an interesting case that suggests an abortive recurrence, or a possible exception to the postoperative relationship between the tumor and AFP: In Case P of their report, AFP became zero after a left hepatectomy and 3 consecutive examinations performed during the following 5 months revealed negative results. Nevertheless, the AFP finding became weakly positive thereafter on 2 successive occasions, and, quite curiously, it became zero again without any treatment. Since Case P is reported to have been living for more than 8 months without any sign of recurrence, such an abortive recurrence, if this is correct, may offer some interesting solutions to problems related to the immunotherapy of AFP-positive neoplasms.

Further improvement of survey techniques may elucidate the relationship between the presence or absence of AFP and histologically verified embryonal carcinoma. Our single radial immunodiffusion method (*6*) is, as reported elsewhere by Mukojima and Hattori, an excellent method for detection and the evaluation of AFP titer. However, radioimmunoassay, presented in this issue of Monograph by others, has increased the sensitivity several hundredfold, and is presenting some difficulties because the detection is too sensitive.

Histopathological findings have, at least at present, no definite relation to the presence or the level of AFP in the sera, but in the near future, the coordination of histochemical and electron microscopic studies may reveal a direct relationship.

In any case, the reversal of cellular function of some neoplasms towards the embryonal state, as discovered in isoenzyme research and in the paraendocrine syndrome, has been verified by recent advances in medicine and biology. Thus, further study of AFP in embryonic neoplasm may link cancerology and embryology.

Acknowledgment

This study was partly funded by the Children's Cancer Association of Japan.

REFERENCES

1. Alpert, M. E. and Seeler, R. A. α-Fetoprotein in embryonal hepatoblastoma. *J. Pediatr.*, **77**, 1058–1060 (1970).
2. Alpert, M. E., Uriel, J., and de Nechaud, B. α-Fetoglobulin in the diagnosis of human hepatoma. *New Engl. J. Med.*, **278**, 984–986 (1968).
3. Houštěk, J., Masopust, J., Kithier, J., and Rádl, J. Hepatocellular carcinoma in association with specific fetal α-globulin, fetoprotein. *J. Pediatr.*, **72**, 186–193 (1968).
4. Masopust, J., Kithier, K., Rádl, J., Koutecky, J., and Kotál, L. Occurrence of fetoprotein in patients with neoplasms and non-neoplastic diseases. *Int. J. Cancer*, **3**, 364–373 (1968).
5. Mawas, C., Buffe, D., Schweisguth, O., and Burtin, P. α-Fetoprotein and children's cancer. *Rev. Eur. Etude Clin. Biol.*, **16**, 430–435 (1971).
6. Mukojima, T., Shimodaira, K., Hattori, S., Hasegawa, H., and Kitaoka, H. The diagnosis of primary cancer of the liver by α-Fetoglobulin; with special reference to the single radial diffusion method (in Japanese). *Kanzo* (*Liver*), **11**, 325–333, (1970).
7. Tatarinov, Yu. S. Content of embryo-specific α-globulin in blood serum of human fetus, new-born and adult man with primary cancer of liver. *Vopr. Med Khimi.*, **11** (2), 20–24 (1965) (cited from M. E. Alpert *et al. New Engl. J. Med.*, **278**, 984–986 (1969)).
8. Uriel, J., de Nechaud, B., Stanislawski-birencwajg, M., Masseyeff, R., Leblanc, L., Quenum, C., Loisillier, F., and Grabar, P. Antigènes embryonaires et cancer du foie chez l'homme. Association de l'α-fétoprotéine sérique avec l'hépatome primaire. *C. R.*, **265**, 75–78 (1967).

EXPLANATION OF PHOTOS

PHOTO 1. Hepatoblastoma (fetal type)

The structure resembles the liver cell plate, and the cells are relatively small without marked nuclear atypia.

PHOTO 2. Hepatocarcinoma (adult type)

Cancer nestle formations are seen in various size. The tumor cells are irregular and large in size with abundant cytoplasm and hyperchromatic nuclei.

PHOTO 3. Hepatoblastoma (mixed type)

The majority of the tumor cells are epithelial components of fetal and embryonal type. Osteoid tissue is seen on the left side.

PHOTO 4. Hepatoblastoma (mixed type)

A generous mixture of pure epithelial components and mesenchymal derivation can be observed.

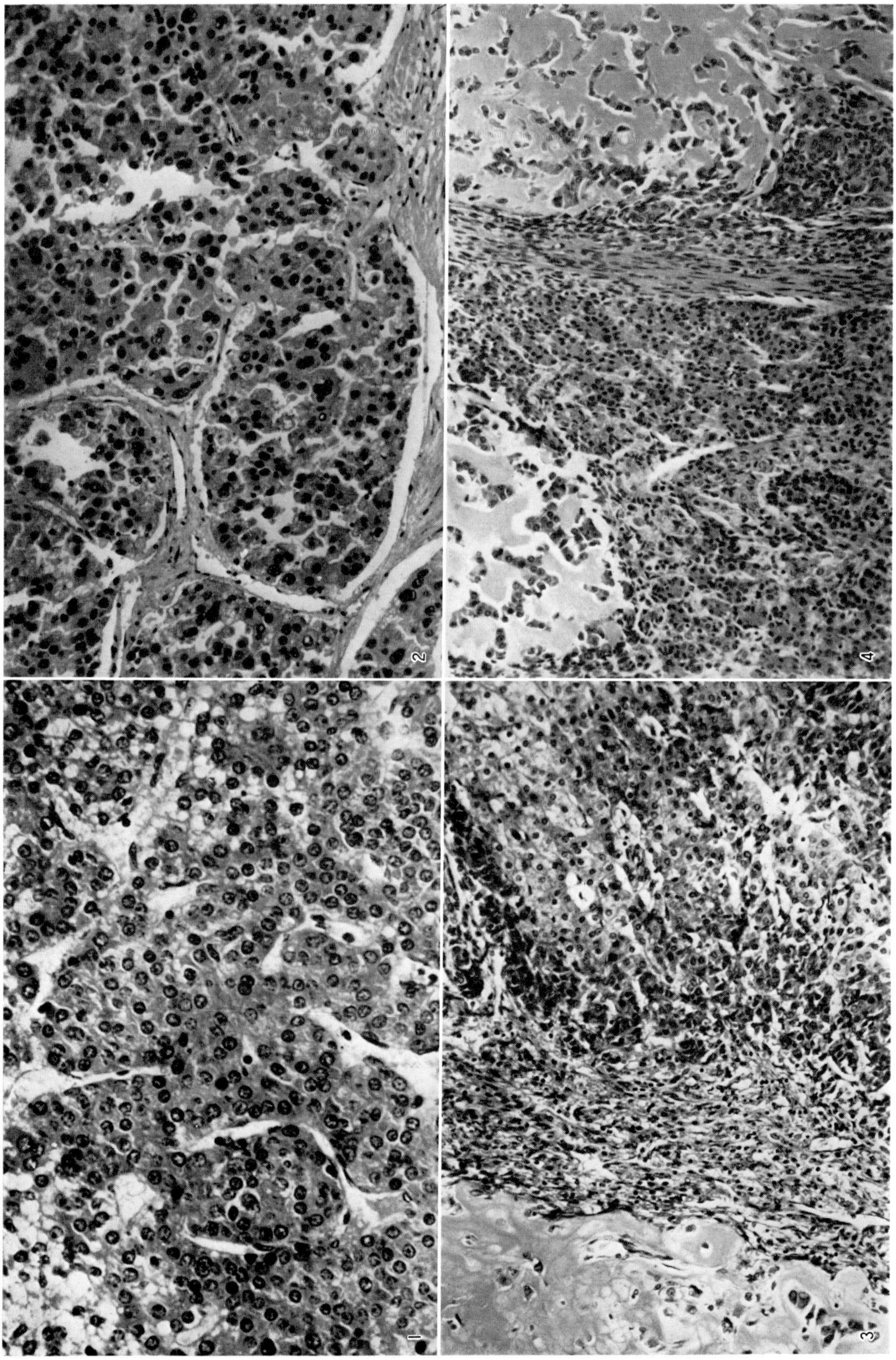

GANN Monograph on Cancer Research 14, 1973

EMBRYONAL CARCINOMA AND α-FETOPROTEIN

Yoshiaki TSUCHIDA, Keiko OHMI, and Yasuo ENDO
*Departments of Pediatric Surgery, Pediatrics and Internal Medicine, Faculty of Medicine, University of Tokyo**

Reactions for α-fetoprotein (AFP) were studied in children admitted to the Department of Pediatric Surgery and the Department of Pediatrics of the University of Tokyo Hospital. α-Fetoprotein appeared in 2 types of tumors only; in hepatocellular carcinomas (2 cases) and in embryonal carcinomas (2 testicular and 1 presacral). Sequential evaluations in these instances revealed that the production rate of AFP closely parallels the total amount and viability of the malignant tumor tissue. Reactions were negative in neuroblastoma, Wilms' tumor, hepatic neuroblastoma, rhabdomyosarcoma, and benign teratoma. Therefore, it appears that AFP tests are valuable in the differential diagnosis of malignant tumors and in follow-up of these patients.

The pertinent literature was reviewed with special regard to the relationship between embryonal carcinoma and AFP. It is a unanimous conclusion that AFP is synthesized by embryonal carcinomas, not only of the testis, but also of various other sites. However, it remains to be determined how and why the tumor cells of embryonal carcinoma produce AFP. It is noteworthy that implantable testicular teratocarcinoma of mice also produce AFP.

In 1964, Tatarinov (*14*) first detected α-fetoprotein (AFP) in the sera of patients with primary hepatoma. Since then, a great number of similar observations have been made and its detection in serum is now considered diagnostic of hepatocellular carcinoma.

Recently, AFP has also been found in the serum of some children with the so-called teratocarcinoma or embryonal carcinoma. Since other malignant tumors in the pediatric age group such as neuroblastoma, Wilms' tumor, rhabdomyosarcoma, *etc.*, apparently never produce AFP (Table I), this particular relationship has attracted the attention of many clinicians and investigators.

In 1967, Abelev and his associates (*2*) reported that AFP appears not only in hepatic tumors, but also in testicular tumors. They further mentioned that AFP was positive in 13 of 32 cases with testicular teratoblastoma and the rate of positivity was higher in those with the features of embryonal carcinoma (*1*). Unfortunately, the ages of the patients were not recorded.

Masopust and his colleagues (*10*) stated, in their extensive analysis of 732 cases in 1968, that AFP appears in 2 types of tumors only; in hepatocellular carcinoma and in malignant undifferentiated teratoma. They detected AFP in

* Hongo 7-3-1, Bunkyo-ku, Tokyo 113, Japan (土田嘉昭, 近江恵子, 遠藤康夫).

TABLE I. Occurrence of AFP in Children Suffering from Neoplasms

Diagnosis	Masopust *et al.* (*10*)		Present series	
	No. of cases	AFP-positive	No. of cases	AFP-positive
Neuroblastoma	11	0	3	0
Ganglioneurinoma	3	0	—	—
Nephroblastoma	7	0	1	0
Mediastinal teratoma	—	—	1	0
Ovarian teratoma	5	2	—	—
Testicular teratoma	2	2	2	2
Presacral teratoma	1	1	1	1
Dysgerminoma	1	0	—	—
Rhabdomyosarcoma	—	—	1	0
Leukemia	44	0	—	—
Hepatocellular carcinoma	1	1	2	2

patients with ovarian, testicular, and presacral teratoblastomas. Reports by these 2 groups (*1*, *10*) and by other investigators (*3*, *4*, *7*, *8*, *11*, *12*, *16*) thereafter are summarized in Table II. The number of cases of ovarian, retroperitoneal, and presacral teratomas is smaller than those of testicular tumors, but the rate of AFP positivity in the former group appears to be higher than that in testicular teratocarcinomas. In any event, these results show that teratocarcinomas or embryonal carcinomas, not only of the testis, but also of various other sites have the potential to produce AFP.

TABLE II. Occurrence of AFP in Malignant Teratomas

Authors	No. of cases	AFP-positive	Histologic type
A. Testicular teratoma			
Abelev (*1*)	24	12	Teratoblastoma
Masopust *et al.* (*10*)	2	2	Embryonal carcinoma
Hull *et al.* (*8*)	40	10	Embryonal cell carcinoma
Mawas *et al.* (*11*)	21	15	Teratocarcinoma
Smith (*13*)	7	2	Embryonal cell carcinoma
Bourgeaux *et al.* (*4*)	2	2	Embryonal tumor
Present series	2	2	Embryonal carcinoma
B. Ovarian teratoma			
Masopust *et al.* (*10*)	5	2	Malignant teratoma
Ushijima (*16*)	1	1	Embryonal carcinoma
C. Retroperitoneal teratoma			
Hull *et al.* (*8*)	4	4	Teratocarcinoma
Akasaka *et al.* (*3*)	1	1	Malignant teratoma
D. Presacral teratoma			
Masopust *et al.* (*10*)	1	1	Malignant teratoblastoma
Hasegawa (*7*)	1	1	Embryonal carcinoma
Present series	1	1	Embryonal carcinoma

Pathology of Embryonal Carcinoma

It seems that there still exists some confusion regarding the terminology of malignant teratomas. Dillard and his associates (*6*) divided all teratomas into 3 groups; mature, immature, and malignant. The immature teratoma is one in which the focal areas show incomplete maturation. This is, in our experience, clinically not malignant (*12*). Malignant teratomas are those tumors composed predominantly of malignant tissue which shows infiltration and metastases. Most malignant teratomas in our series were embryonal carcinomas, which have a characteristic structural pattern of cellular anaplastic adenocarcinoma. The prognosis was fatal in the majority of cases.

Chretien and his co-workers (*5*) found that malignant sacrococcygeal teratomas in their 21 consecutive patients were all embryonal adenocarcinomas. The prognosis was fatal in all. Associated teratoid elements were present in 7 of the 21 cases (*5*). Our 3 cases with positive reaction for AFP belong to " embryonal adenocarcinoma " (Photo 1), according to the terminology of Chretien *et al.* (*5*). It would appear that " embryonal adenocarcinoma " may also be known as " malignant teratoma," " teratocarcinoma," " teratoblastoma," " teratoblastoma with the features of embryonal carcinoma," or simply " embryonal carcinoma."

Among our 13 cases of embryonal carcinoma, a few had focal areas appearing typical of " endodermal sinus tumor " (*15*), but were classified as " embryonal carcinoma " in this report.

AFP in Individual Cases

From the viewpoint of controlling tumor growth with AFP evaluation in the course of therapy, it may be of interest to review the individual case histories of 3 of our patients. Every patient was studied by the Ouchterlony method, but semiquantitative assay was also used in some instances.

Case 1: Y. O., 2½-year-old male. When the patient was 19 months old, the mother noticed an enlargement of the left testis. Left orchiectomy was performed at the age of 27 months and a huge left retroperitoneal metastasis was detected at the age of 30 months, with positive reaction for AFP. After removal of the huge tumor, serum AFP disappeared. Three months later it reappeared with left subphrenic metastasis. The patient subsequently died of cachexia. The final diagnosis was embryonal carcinoma of the left testis with retroperitoneal metastasis.

Case 2: S. K., 23-month-old male. At the age of 17 months, right orchiectomy was performed for testicular embryonal carcinoma. Six months later, a huge metastatic tumor was noted in the right retroperitoneal area, with positive reaction for AFP. After radiation treatment and chemotherapy with Actinomycin-D, the metastatic tumor regressed in size and the reaction for AFP became negative. The necrotic mass was excised. Paralysis due to vertebral metastasis was followed by wound disruption and intestinal fistula, and the patient died of malnutrition.

TABLE III. Infants and Children with Positive Reaction for AFP Admitted to the University of Tokyo Hospital

Case No.	Age (yr. mo.)	Sex	Clinical diagnosis	Histologic type	Remarks
1. Y.O.	2, 6	Male	Metastatic testicular tumor	Embryonal carcinoma	
2. S.K.	1, 11	Male	Metastatic testicular tumor	Embryonal carcinoma	
3. C.T.	1, 1	Female	Intrapelvic presacral tumor	Embryonal carcinoma	
4. Y.K.	3, 5	Male	Hepatic tumor with jaundice	Hepatocarcinoma (adult type)	Initially negative
5. H.K.	2, 6	Male	Virilizing hepatic tumor	Hepatoblastoma	

Case 3: C. T., 13-month-old female. Urinary retention and lower extremity weakness were noted at the age of 13 months. Rectal examination revealed a large mass in the intrapelvic presacral space, and the reaction for AFP was positive. Colostomy and biopsy of the tumor were performed and the diagnosis of embryonal carcinoma was confirmed histologically. After radiation and chemotherapy, serum AFP disappeared, but reappeared 3 months later with widespread metastases. The patient died of cachexia at the age of 19 months. The final diagnosis was embryonal carcinoma of the presacral region with widespread metastases.

At this Department of Pediatric Surgery, reaction for AFP was studied in other children with malignant tumors. Positive reaction was shown in 2 cases, namely hepatocarcinoma (adult type) due to biliary cirrhosis and virilizing hepatoblastoma (Table III). Reaction was negative in neuroblastoma, Wilms' tumor, hepatic neuroblastoma, rhabdomyosarcoma, and benign teratoma (Table I).

Clinical Applications of AFP Tests

As was shown in our 3 cases of embryonal carcinoma, AFP in the serum parallels tumor growth. It was positive when the patient was first seen with a huge tumor, but turned negative after removal of the tumor or after reduction in size following tissue necrosis. Tissue necrosis was histologically confirmed in 2 of our cases (Cases 2 and 3).

A parallel relation between tumor growth and positivity of AFP was also demonstrated in a 3-year-old child with hepatocarcinoma. He underwent exploratory laparotomy for suspected protracted infantile hepatitis and hepatocarcinoma with a negative reaction for AFP was incidentally detected, though AFP later appeared in the serum with the growth of the tumor.

To our way of thinking, AFP may also be valuable in follow-up of neonates with benign teratoma, particularly sacrococcygeal teratoma. If the surgeon is not completely confident of total removal of the tumor, the patient should be followed for years with AFP tests, because embryonal carcinoma sometimes arises from the residual tissue of sacrococcygeal teratoma (*5*).

Mawas and his colleagues (*11*) reported that the AFP test was positive in 15 (65%) of 21 children with teratocarcinoma, whereas the rate was 15–23% in adults (*11*). They also noted that the incidence of positive tests in hepatocellular carcinoma is higher in children (90%) than in adults (70%). It seems that the results considerably encourage clinical application of AFP test in the field of pediatric oncology.

Components Synthesizing AFP in Embryonal Carcinoma

It is of interest to discuss which component of embryonal carcinoma produces AFP. Possible explanations previously offered are (i) synthesis by particular tumor cells destined to become embryonic liver cells or (ii) an effect of the tumor cells on the host liver, causing a resumption of AFP synthesis. From our observations it would appear that the activities of tumor cells having a typical glandular pattern (Fig. 1), the predominant component of embryonal carcinoma, closely parallel the production rate of AFP. Therefore, it is also plausible that all these tumor cells produce AFP themselves. Kahan and Levine (*9*) found that implantable testicular teratocarcinoma cells of mice synthesize AFP, not only *in vivo* but also *in vitro*. This is an important finding, which tends to confirm specific AFP production by malignant teratomas. It must be taken into account that a teratoma is a peculiar tumor, embryologically akin to fetus, which normally synthesizes AFP.

Possible Applications in Pathology

The authors particularly expect that AFP tests will be of assistance in the distinct pathological classification of malignant teratomas, specifically with regard to differentiation among immature teratoma, teratocarcinoma, embryonal carcinoma, and endodermal sinus tumor (*15*).

Acknowledgments

We are indebted to Dr. Y. Urano, Department of Pathology, University of Tokyo, for his advice and also to Dr. S. Saito and Prof. M. Ishida, Department of Surgery, University of Tokyo, for their assistance in, and permission for, the preparation of this report.

This study was supported by a Grants-in-Aid for Scientific Research from the Ministry of Education and from the Ministry of Health and Welfare, Japan.

REFERENCES

1. Abelev, G. I. Production of embryonal serum α-globulin by hepatomas: Review of experimental and clinical data. *Cancer Res.*, **28**, 1344–1350 (1968).
2. Abelev, G. I., Assecritova, I., Kraevsky, N., Perova, S., and Perevodchikova, N. Embryonal serum α-globulin in cancer patients: Diagnostic value. *Int. J. Cancer*, **2**, 551–558 (1967).
3. Akasaka, T. Two cases of retroperitoneal teratoma. Oral presentation before

the 8th Annual Meeting of the Japanese Society of Pediatric Surgeons, Osaka, Japan, June, 1971.

4. Bourgeaux, C., Martin, F., Cabanne, P., Aupecle, P., and Guerrin, J. Value of α-fetoprotein in the diagnosis and postoperative survey of testicular embryonal tumors. *Presse Med.*, **79**, 1589–1590 (1971).
5. Chretien, P. B., Milam, J. D., Foote, F. W., and Miller, T. R. Embryonal adenocarcinomas (a type of malignant teratoma) of the sacrococcygeal region. *Cancer*, **26**, 522–535 (1970).
6. Dillard, B. M., Mayer, J. H., McAlister, W. H., McGavrin, M., and Strominger, D. B. Sacrococcygeal teratoma in children. *J. Pediatr. Surg.*, **5**, 53–59 (1970).
7. Hasegawa, H. α-Fetoglobulin in malignant tumors in children. Oral presentation before the 7th Annual Meeting of the Japanese Society of Pediatric Surgeons, Sendai, Japan, May, 1969.
8. Hull, E. W., Miertel, C. G., and Carbone, P. P. Serum α-fetoprotein in cancer patients. *Clin. Res.*, **17**, 403 (1969).
9. Kahan, B. and Levine, L. The occurrence of a serum fetal α-1-protein in developing mice and murine hepatomas and teratomas. *Cancer Res.*, **31**, 930–936 (1971).
10. Masopust, J., Kithier, K., Rádl, J., Koutecky, J., and Kotál, L. Occurrence of fetoprotein in patients with neoplasms and non-neoplastic diseases. *Int. J. Cancer*, **3**, 364–373 (1968).
11. Mawas, C., Buffe, D., and Burtin, P. Influence of age on α-fetoprotein incidence. *Lancet*, **1**, 1292 (1970).
12. Saito, S., Sato, T., Tsuchida, Y., and Ishida, M. Clinico-pathological study of abdominal teratomas in children. Oral presentation before the 8th Annual Meeting of the Japanese Society of Pediatric Surgeons, Osaka, Japan, June, 1971.
13. Smith, J. B. α-Fetoprotein: Occurrence in certain malignant diseases and review of clinical applications. *Med. Clin. N. Am.*, **54**, 797–803 (1970).
14. Tatarinov, J. Detection of embryospecific α-globulin in the blood sera of patient with primary liver tumor. *Vopr. Med. Khim.*, **10**, 90–91 (1964).
15. Teilum, G. "Special Tumors of Ovary and Testis: Comparative Pathology and Histological Identification," Munksgaard, Copenhagen, pp. 31–372 (1971).
16. Ushijima, H. Clinico-pathological study of ovarian tumors in children. Oral presentation before the 8th Annual Meeting of the Japanese Society of Pediatric Surgeons, Osaka, Japan, June, 1971.

EXPLANATION OF PHOTO

PHOTO 1. Photomicrograph of embryonal carcinoma

The predominant histologic pattern is that of a cellular anaplastic adenocarcinoma. Characteristic glandular pattern with papillary features is seen in all cases. Associated teratomatous elements are present in some cases. Hematoxylin-Eosin staining.

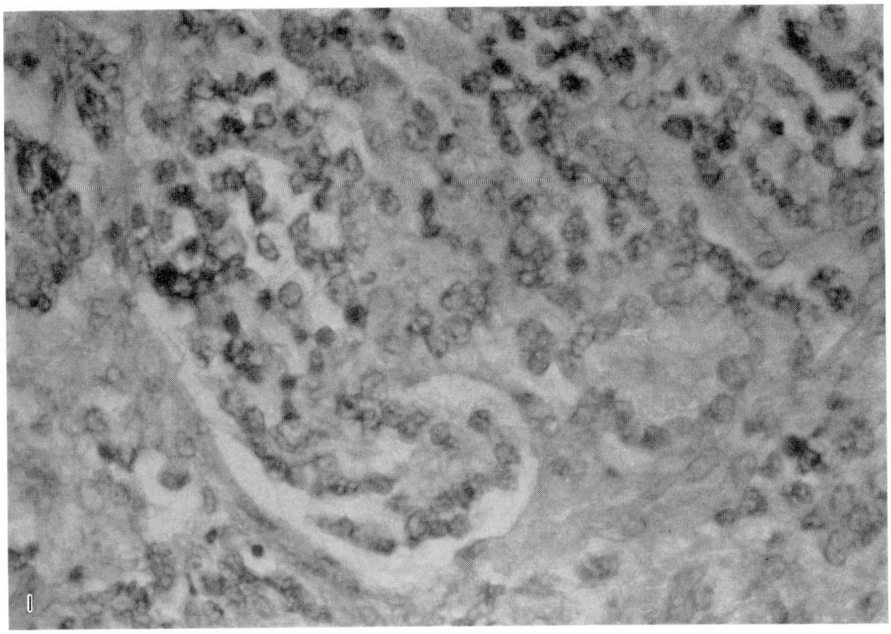

GANN Monograph on Cancer Research 14, 1973

SERUM α-FETOPROTEIN-POSITIVE STOMACH CANCER

Sadahiko AKAI and Kiyoshi KATO
*Prefectural Cancer Center, Niigata Hospital**

α-Fetoprotein (AFP) is, on occasion, seen in the serum of patients with carcinoma of the digestive tract but without primary liver cancer, especially carcinoma of the stomach. Many of these patients have metastases to the liver. The incidence of AFP among patients with cancer of the stomach is much lower than in those with hepatoma, and even in the AFP-positive cases its level is relatively low. The immunological properties of AFP in these cases, however, seem to be identical with those of AFP found in fetuses and hepatomas.

α-Fetoprotein is not present in the serum of healthy adults. Although this protein has sometimes been encountered in some pathological conditions, such as teratoblastoma and embryonal carcinoma of the testis and the ovary, it has been thought to be almost specific to hepatocellular carcinoma (hepatoma). In Japan, it is positive in approximately 80% of patients with hepatoma. Clinically, therefore, detection of AFP is indispensable in establishing a diagnosis of hepatoma.

Recently, as α-fetoprotein (AFP) has been investigated in a greater number of patients and as it has become more easily detectable technically, more AFP-positive cases, though still only a few in number, have been found among disorders other than hepatoma, such as hepatitis, hepatic cirrhosis, metastatic cancer of the liver, and in pregnancy. These cases are often called "false positives."

The diagnostic merit of AFP in relation to hepatoma is reduced if there are a considerable number of "false positive" cases. Moreover, the presence of AFP in patients with metastatic cancer of the liver indicates that AFP may be synthesized in cancer cells of epithelial origin other than hepatic cells.

An inquiry was sent in June, 1972, to major institutions where extensive investigations of AFP have been carried out in an attempt to collect AFP-positive cancer cases, excluding hepatoma, and testicular and ovarian neoplasms. Tables I and II summarize the answers from 44 institutions and a report from the National Cancer Center, Tokyo (*2*). A total of 57 cases of carcinoma with positive AFP were reported. Autopsies were done in 29 cases, the presence of hepatoma being excluded in these cases. Forty-eight of these 57 cases were cancers of the stomach. Of these 48 cases, all except 12 with gastric cancer had hepatic metastases.

* Kawagishi-cho 2, Niigata 951, Japan (赤井貞彦, 加藤　清).

TABLE I. AFP-positive Cancers

Institution	No. of cases
1. Hokkaido Univ. Hospital	2
2. Sapporo Med. College Hospital	0
3. Tokyo Univ. Hospital	2
4. Nihon Univ. Hospital	0
5. Tokyo Med. and Dental Univ. Hospital	1
6. Jikei Univ. Hospital	1
7. Central Hospital, Japanese National Railways	1
8. Cancer Institute Hospital, Tokyo	0
9. Japan Red Cross Central Hospital	0
10. National Cancer Center Hospital, Tokyo	13
11. Chiba Univ. Hospital	0
12. Niigata Univ. Hospital	3
13. Prefectural Cancer Center, Niigata Hospital	3
14. Nagaoka Red Cross Hospital	5
15. Toyama City Hospital	0
16. Nagoya City Univ. Hospital	1
17. Aichi Cancer Center Hospital	1
18. Gifu Univ. Hospital	1
19. Kyoto Univ. Hospital	0
20. Kyoto Hospital of Japan Monopoly Corporation	0
21. Osaka Univ. Hospital	1
22. Hospital, Center for Adult Diseases, Osaka	2
23. Nara Med. Univ. Hospital	3
24. Wakayama Med. Univ. Hospital	1
25. Kobe Univ. Hospital	7
26. Okayama Univ. Hospital	2
27. Prefectural Kagawa Central Hospital	1
28. Yamaguchi Univ. Hospital	3
29. Kurume Univ. Hospital	1
30. Nagasaki Univ. Hospital	2
Total	57

TABLE II. AFP-positive Cancers Other than Hepatoma

Initial lesion	No. of cases	Liver metastases		
		+	−	?
Stomach	48	35 (21)	12 (2)	1 (1)
Pancreas	3	2 (2)	0	1 (?)
Duodenum	2	1 (1)	1 (0)	0
Gallbladder	2	1 (1)	1 (1)	0
Unknown	2	2 (0)	0	0
Total	57	41 (25)	14 (3)	2 (1)

Number of autopsied cases is shown in parentheses.

Cancer of the Stomach Combined with Hepatoma

Double cancers, *i.e.*, cancer of the stomach combined with hepatoma, are rare. The following case, however, illustrates the possibility that the use of AFP in diagnosing hepatoma may be complicated by the presence of double cancers.

M. S., 43 yrs., female: With a principle complaint of epigastralgia, the patient underwent examinations of the gastrointestinal tract including fluoroscopy and gastroscopy. With a diagnosis of cancer of the pylorus, the patient underwent subtotal gastrectomy. There were two Borrmann II-type cancers in the antrum. Histological examination revealed one of them to be adenocarcinoma papillotubulare and the other carcinoma simplex. There were no palpable masses in the liver at surgery. Serum AFP measured preoperatively was 1.1 mg/dl, and it was thought then that this was an AFP-positive cancer of the stomach. A mass was felt in the right upper quadrant 230 days postoperatively and AFP at this time was 17.5 mg/dl. On laparotomy a tumor, 14×13×10 cm, in the right hepatic lobe was removed. There were no signs of recurrence of the cancer of the stomach in the peritoneal cavity. Histology of the hepatic tumor showed a hepatocellular carcinoma of a trabecular type. Serum AFP increased gradually to reach a level of 94.0 mg/dl and the patient died 505 days after the 1st operation (Fig. 1). Autopsy showed a large hepatoma, supposedly an intrahepatic metastasis, but there was no recurrence of the cancer of the stomach.

Ten cases of combined cancers of the stomach and the liver have been reported to date in Japan (*1*). This fact, together with the case described above, indicates that in cases of a hepatic mass with positive AFP, either hepatoma or hepatic metastasis of an AFP-positive cancer of the stomach must be suspected, and in cases of cancer of the stomach with positive AFP the possible simultaneous presence of hepatoma must be borne in mind.

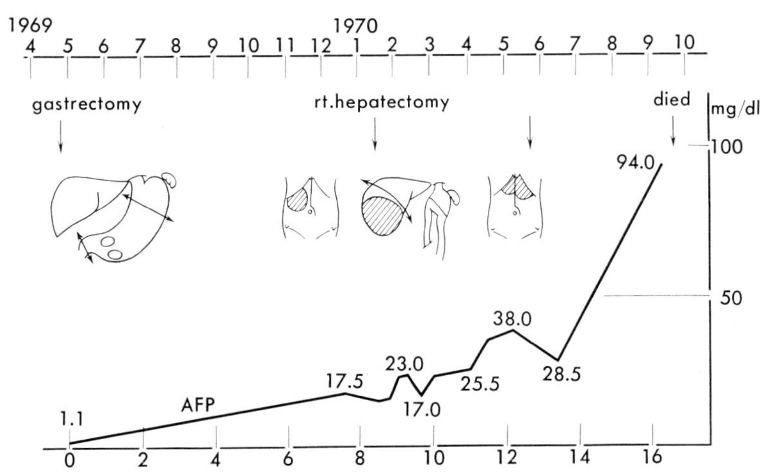

FIG. 1. Case M. S., with cancer of the stomach and hepatoma
Serum AFP level gradually rose with the size of the hepatoma. M. S., 43-year-old female.

TABLE III. Gross Anatomical Appearance of AFP-positive Gastric Cancer

Classification		No. of cases
Early cancer		1
Borrmann type	I	1
	II	17
	III	20
	IV	4
Unknown		5
Total		48

Pathology of AFP-positive Cancer of the Stomach

On gross anatomical examination, the majority of these 48 AFP-positive cases had cancer of the stomach of Borrmann II and III types, *i.e.*, ulcerating types (Table III). Histologically well-differentiated cancers outnumbered poorly differentiated ones (Table IV). These features are suggestive of frequent metastases to the liver. There were, however, no morphological characteristics specific to AFP-positive cancer of the stomach. There were metastatic tumors in the liver in 35 of 48 cases. In the other cases, either regional lymph node involvement or intraperitoneal implantation was found, but there were no hepatic metastases. An autopsy was done in 2 of these 12 cases. In the other, a subtotal gastrectomy, though of palliative nature, was carried out. Serum AFP measured preoperatively in the latter case, by radioimmunoassay, was 74.0 ng/ml, declining to 14.6 ng/ml after the operation. Thus, hepatic metastases are likely to be present in cases of AFP-positive cancer of the stomach, though this is not absolutely the case.

TABLE IV. Histological Types of AFP-positive Cancer

Well-differentiated	35
Poorly differentiated	3
Unknown	19
Total	57

Level of AFP in AFP-positive Cancer of the Stomach

Quantification of serum AFP was carried out in 45 of the 48 cases, as shown in Fig. 2. It is generally lower than in patients with hepatoma, but there was a value as high as 400 mg/dl.

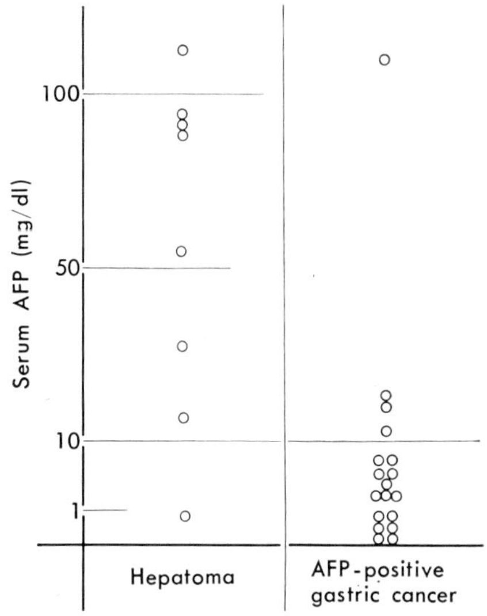

FIG. 2. Serum AFP levels of hepatoma and AFP-positive gastric cancer

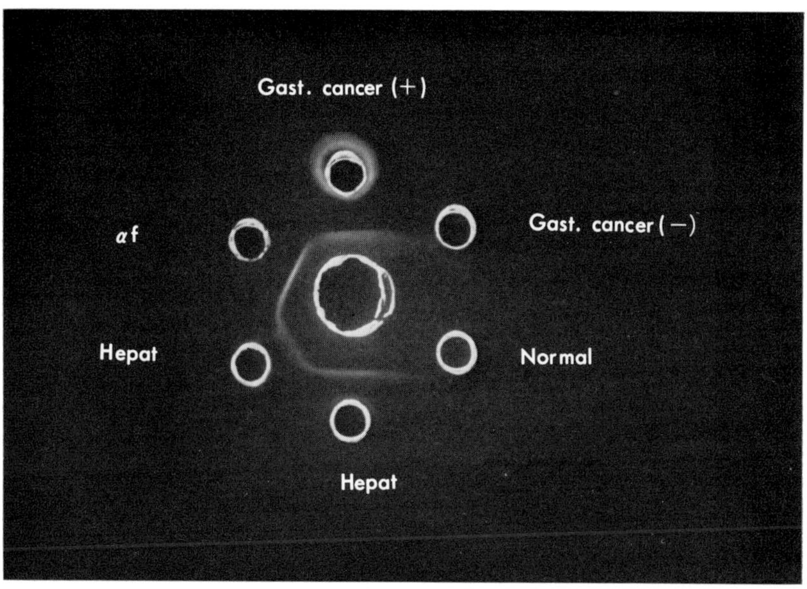

FIG. 3. Immunologic studies of AFP by the double diffusion method

Fetal AFP (αf), hepatoma sera (Hepat) and AFP-positive gastric cancer serum (Gast. cancer (+)) cross-react completely when a horse antiserum against fetal AFP is allowed to diffuse from the center well. This suggests substantial or complete immunologic identity. Neither normal adult serum (normal) nor AFP-negative gastric cancer serum (Gast. cancer (−)) react with the antiserum.

Immunological Properties of Serum AFP of Fetus, Hepatoma, and AFP-positive Gastric Cancer

The precipitin line of serum of AFP-positive cancer of the stomach fuses with the lines of hepatoma and fetal AFP to form a continuous line (Fig. 3). AFP of cancer of the stomach, therefore, seems to have an antigenicity identical with that of hepatoma AFP and purified fetal AFP (*3*). The biochemical properties may be assumed to be also identical. It is, therefore, not justified to designate AFP-positive cancers other than hepatoma as " false positive."

Incidence of Positive AFP in Cases of Cancer of the Stomach

In the Niigata Cancer Center Hospital, AFP has been investigated in 231 cases of cancer of the stomach by means of double immunodiffusion, immunoelectrosyneresis, and radioimmunoassay. It was positive in 3 cases (1.3%). Many of these patients were, however, in advanced or terminal stages of the disease. Investigations on a larger scale, using a more sensitive method of detection such as radioimmunoassay, seem necessary to settle the matter.

REFERENCES

1. Akai, S., Kato, K., Shimada, K., Tobita, Y., Tsunoda, H., Iwabuchi, S., Yoshida, K., and Tashiro, S. Significance of measurements of α-fetoprotein in the surgery of hepatic cancer (in Japanese). *Gan-no-Rinsho* (*Cancer Clinic*), **18**, 59–66 (1972).
2. Kitaoka, H., Hattori, N., and Mukojima, T. α_1-Fetoprotein and metastatic liver cancer with special reference to gastric cancer (in Japanese). *Igaku-no-Ayumi* (*The Stride of Medicine*), **79**, 129–130 (1971).
3. Nishi, S. Isolation and characterization of a human fetal α-globulin from the sera of fetuses and a hepatoma patient. *Cancer Res.*, **30**, 2507–2513 (1970).

SOME OTHER ANTIGENS AND HEPATOMAS

IMMUNOCHEMICAL STUDIES ON ANTIGENIC COMPONENTS COMMON TO CARCINOMA AND FETUS, AND THEIR DIAGNOSTIC SIGNIFICANCE

With Special Reference to the Connection with α-Fetoprotein

Takeo WADA, Tetsuro ANZAI, and Akira YACHI
*Department of Internal Medicine, Sapporo Medical College**

Three different fetal serum proteins, α-fetoprotein (AFP), α_2H, and βs, were detected by immunoprecipitation in agar gel plates, and their incidence in the sera of patients with primary hepatoma and other malignant diseases, and the sera of patients with liver diseases was compared. In hepatoma patients, the incidence of AFP was 75% and that of α_2H 66%, while the incidence of βs was 47%. None of the serum samples of patients with malignant diseases other than primary hepatoma contained AFP, whereas α_2H and βs were detected in some of these serum samples. Both α_2H and βs were also found in some serum samples from patients with liver diseases other than primary hepatoma. None of the normal control sera contained any of these fetal protein components. Comparison of the incidence of AFP and βs in 43 serum samples from patients with primary hepatoma revealed that simultaneous tests aiming at the detection of either of these may improve diagnostic sensitivity up to 92%.

Comparison of histological findings in AFP-producing and βs-producing hepatoma cases suggested that the degree of differentiation of AFP-producing hepatoma was lower than that of βs-producing hepatoma. Serum levels of orosomucoid, α_1-antitrypsin, and haptoglobin in βs-producing hepatoma cases were generally higher than the levels in sera containing AFP but not βs, suggesting a relatively reduced ability of the liver in AFP-producing hepatoma cases to synthesize and release these normal serum proteins, as compared with βs-producing hepatoma cases.

From the results of experimental *in vitro* synthesis of AFP by tissue slices, it was found that, in fetuses, not only the liver but also a wide variety of organs and tissues participate in the biosynthesis of AFP. The same experimental procedures demonstrated the synthesis of AFP by hepatoma tissue.

α-Fetoprotein and Other Serum Proteins Common to Hepatoma Patients and Fetuses

It is well known that fetal sera contain protein components that are different from adult human serum proteins (*2, 5, 6*). Detection of fetal serum proteins in

* Minami-1-jo, Nishi-17-chome, Chuo-ku, Sapporo 060, Japan (和田武雄, 安斎哲郎, 谷内 昭).

the sera of cancer hosts was initiated by Abelev *et al.* (*1*), who studied the serum proteins of hepatoma-bearing mice. Tatarinov (*11*) was the pioneer of similar studies on human fetal proteins appearing in the sera of patients with primary hepatoma. The fetal serum protein reported in these studies has been termed α-fetoprotein (AFP), and a number of studies have since been carried out on this subject. In this country also, studies in this field have flourished, yielding a number of new observations.

The present authors have been concerned with studies on serum protein components that are common to cancer and fetal tissues, not only AFP but also other components such as the so-called carcinoembryonic antigen (CEA, Gold and Freedman (*8*)), and isolation of these protein components has been attempted. In the present paper, some of the findings obtained during studies on hepatoma-specific serum protein components will be described. In 1967, Takahashi *et al.* (*10*) reported a new fetal serum protein, βs, in the sera of hepatoma patients, and a series of studies on this component have been reported from this laboratory. On the other hand, Burtin *et al.* (*4*) described another fetal serum protein, α_2H, and later reported the presence of this protein in the sera of patients with hepatoma and other malignant diseases (*3*). Results obtained by comparing these 3 components, AFP, βs, and α_2H, will now be presented.

The physicochemical properties of these 3 components apparently differ from each other. As can be seen in the immunoelectrophoretic patterns shown in Fig. 1, they have different electrophoretic mobilities, and Fig. 2 shows that the ion exchange chromatographic patterns of sera of patients with hepatoma and of umbilical cord sera yield elution diagrams of the 3 components which are different from each other.

Results obtained by employing specific antisera for detection of the components in clinical materials, as well as some of the results obtained by basic studies, are described below.

Comparison between the Incidences of AFP, α_2H, and βs in the Sera of Patients with Various Malignant Diseases

Detection of the 3 fetal serum protein components, AFP, α_2H, and βs, was carried out by double diffusion precipitation in agar gel plates. Serum samples obtained from patients with primary hepatoma and various other malignant diseases, as well as normal control sera, were subjected to the tests and the incidences of the 3 components were compared. As can be seen in Table I, AFP was detected in 32 of 43 cases (75%) with primary hepatoma and α_2H was detected

TABLE I. Incidences of AFP, α_2H, and βs

Diagnosis	AFP	α_2H	βs
Primary hepatoma	32/43 (75%)	25/38 (66%)	21/45 (47%)
Malignant diseases other than primary hepatoma	0/27	8/27 (30%)	18/148 (12.2%)
Non-neoplastic liver diseases	0/22	3/17 (18%)	3/27 (11%)
Healthy adult	0/40	0/40	0/61

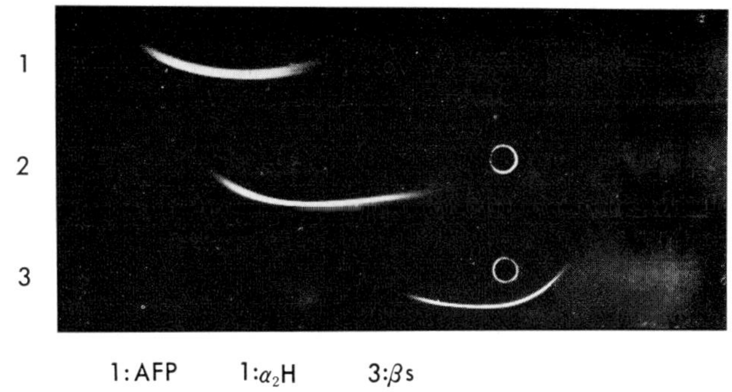

FIG. 1. Comparison of immunoelectrophoretic precipitin lines of AFP, α_2H, and βs

Anode to the left.

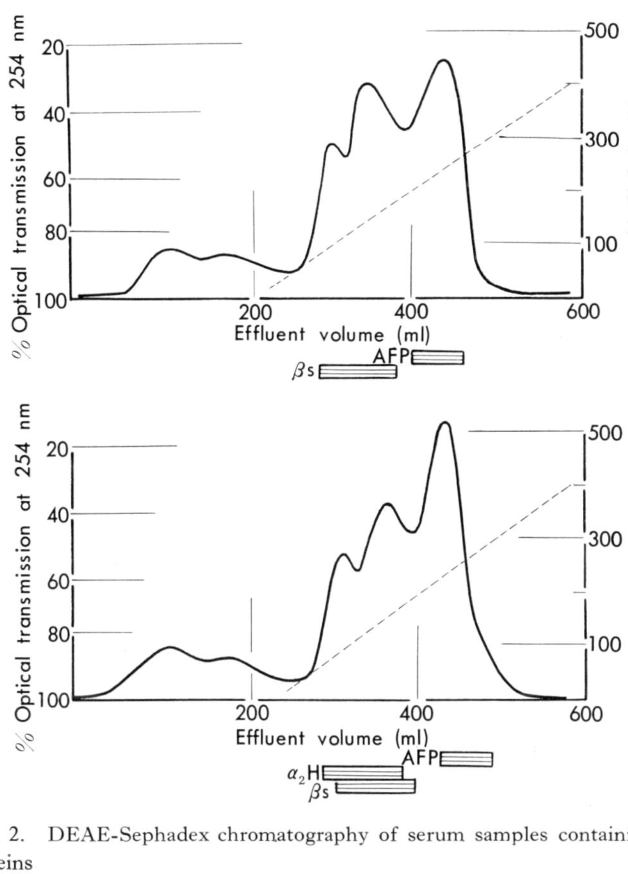

FIG. 2. DEAE-Sephadex chromatography of serum samples containing fetal proteins

Upper figure: Serum of a patient with primary hepatoma, containing AFP and βs. Hepatoma serum 10 ml, DEAE-Sephadex A-50, 2.5×40 cm, 0.1 M Tris-HCl buffer, pH 8.0, flow rate 35 ml/hr, gradient elution system. Bottom figure: Umbilical cord serum containing AFP, α_2H, and βs. Fetal proteins in the effluent fractions were detected immunochemically. Umbilical cord serum 10 ml, DEAE-Sephadex A-50, 2.5×40 cm, 0.1 M Tris-HCl buffer, pH 8.0, flow rate 35 ml/hr, gradient elution system.

in 25 of 38 cases (66%) with primary hepatoma, while the incidence of βs in hepatoma was 21 out of 45 cases (47%), the incidence of AFP being the highest of the 3 in hepatoma sera. Serum samples from patients with malignant neoplastic diseases other than primary hepatoma, as well as normal control sera, were all AFP-negative, so that the hepatoma specificity of AFP was the highest of the 3 fetal proteins tested. On the other hand, α_2H was detected in 8 of 27 sera from patients with malignant diseases other than primary hepatoma, and in 3 of 17 sera from patients with liver diseases other than primary hepatoma, whereas the incidence of βs in the sera of patients with malignant diseases other than primary hepatoma was 18 out of 148 cases, and the incidence in sera of patients with liver diseases other than primary hepatoma was 3 out of 27 cases. None of the normal control sera, however, contained any of these 3 fetal serum protein components.

TABLE II. Incidence of AFP and βs in Various Malignant Diseases

Clinical diagnosis	No. of cases	AFP-positive	βs-positive (%)
Hepatocellular carcinoma	49	37 (75.5%)	21 (47.7)
Cholangiocarcinoma	1	0	1 (100.0)
Carcinoma of stomach	62	0	10 (16.1)
Carcinoma of colon	5	0	2 (40.0)
Carcinoma of rectum	8	0	1 (12.5)
Carcinoma of pancreas and biliary system	9	0	1 (11.1)
Carcinoma of lung	22	0	3 (13.6)
Acute myelogen. leukemia	15	0	4 (26.6)
Chronic myelogen. leukemia	12	0	1 (8.3)
Multiple myeloma	26	0	3 (11.6)
Malignant lymphoma	16	0	3 (18.7)
Total	225	37	50 (22.2)

The incidences of AFP and βs in the sera of patients with various malignant diseases other than primary hepatoma are shown in Table II. As stated above, none of the serum samples tested contained AFP, whereas βs was detectable in a relatively wide range of malignant neoplastic diseases, as previously reported, together with results of basic studies on this protein (*12*, *13*). Thus, the above results indicate that, regarding specificity to primary hepatoma, AFP is the most specific. On the other hand, both α_2H and βs, although the specificity as such

TABLE III. Comparison of the Incidences of AFP and βs in 43 Cases of Primary Hepatoma

AFP	βs	No. of cases (%)
+	−	19 (44.2%)
+	+	16 (37.2%)
−	+	4 (9.3%)
−	−	4 (9.3%)
35 (81.4%)	20 (46.5%)	43

is less than that of AFP, are at least not detectable in normal control sera, but are also found in some of the serum samples from patients having disease processes in the liver, or having malignant neoplastic diseases in the body not necessarily limited to the liver. Recent progress in methods for detection of AFP has permitted increased sensitivity by application of the radioimmunoassay system, and this enhanced sensitivity may lead to the recognition of AFP, hitherto considered to be a strictly hepatoma-specific protein, as merely a product of nonspecific reactions. If this is the case, it might be possible that the differences in the incidences of the 3 fetal proteins may reflect differences in the antibody titers of the specific antisera used, and differences in the concentrations of these proteins in the serum samples.

Serum samples from 43 patients with primary hepatoma were investigated for the presence of AFP and βs. As shown in Table III, 16 of the 43 sera (37%) contained both proteins, and 19 sera (44%) contained AFP but not βs, whereas 4 sera (9%) contained βs but not AFP. In the remaining 4 sera (9%), neither AFP nor βs was detected. It is therefore concluded that, although it appears that the diagnostic sensitivity of AFP is 81% at the most, which is still higher than the value of 47% in the case of βs, simultaneous tests aiming at detection of either of these may enhance the diagnostic sensitivity up to 39 out of 43, or 92%.

For the purpose of immunochemical diagnosis of primary hepatoma, although it is important to enhance the sensitivity by introducing more sensitive detection methods for AFP, another point of importance is to supplement these with the detection of βs, which is chemically and biologically different from AFP.

It is also presumed that the discrepancies between cases, as stated above, may derive from the different biological properties of cells which produce these serum proteins. In relation to this, results obtained by fluorescent antibody demonstrations of different rates of serum protein production in tissues of the same cases have previously been reported (*12*). Additional evidence is now presented in a case of primary hepatoma whose clinical course was followed for a relatively long period of time. In the initial stage, βs alone was detected in the patient's serum, but after 15 months, AFP became detectable for the first time. Comparison of histological findings regarding the liver tissues, one obtained surgically during the initial stage and the other obtained at autopsy, revealed that trabecular arrangements and glandular structures of hepatoma cells in the former tissue were relatively better preserved than in the tissue in the AFP-producing stage obtained at autopsy, and bile production was also demonstrated in the initial stage. The autopsy material, representing the AFP-producing terminal stage, was characterized by more marked changes.

Collation with findings in other cases studied from the pathohistological standpoint has led us to deduce that AFP-producing hepatoma may be accompanied by a relatively lower degree of differentiation than that of βs-producing hepatoma.

Relation between the Incidences of AFP and βs, and the Concentrations of Several Other Serum Protein Components

In the preceding section, the speculation has been presented that the difference between the incidence of AFP and that of βs might be related to the differences in the nature and grades of differentiation of AFP-producing and βs-producing hepatoma cells. In connection with this, the concentrations of orosomucoid, α_1-antitrypsin, and haptoglobin, known to increase in the sera of tumor hosts, were studied and the correlation between these values and the presence or absence of AFP and βs was investigated. As can be seen in Fig. 3, the levels of orosomucoid and α_1-antitrypsin in βs-positive sera were generally higher than the levels in sera containing AFP but not βs. As shown in Fig. 4, determination of the seromucoid fraction, which includes both of these protein components, resulted in an even more clear-cut demonstration of the above tendency. Haptoglobin levels in sera containing AFP but not βs were also lower than the levels in βs-positive sera, although precise evaluation of the results is complicated by the fact that the normal range of serum haptoglobin levels differs according to genetic types.

The above results lead us to assume a possible correlation between the ability of the liver to synthesize these normal serum proteins and the ability of hepatoma cells to synthesize either AFP or βs. From such a viewpoint, we may postulate a relatively reduced ability of the liver in AFP-producing hepatoma cases to syn-

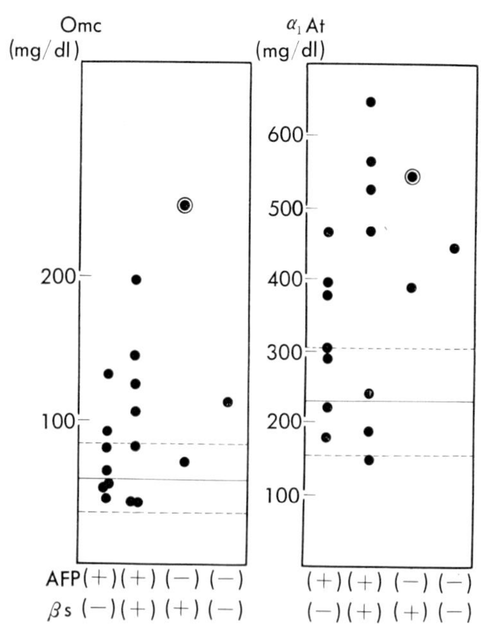

FIG. 3. Comparison of serum levels of orosomucoid (Omc) and α_1-antitrypsin (α_1At) between AFP-producing and βs-producing hepatoma cases
◉ cholangiocarcinoma.

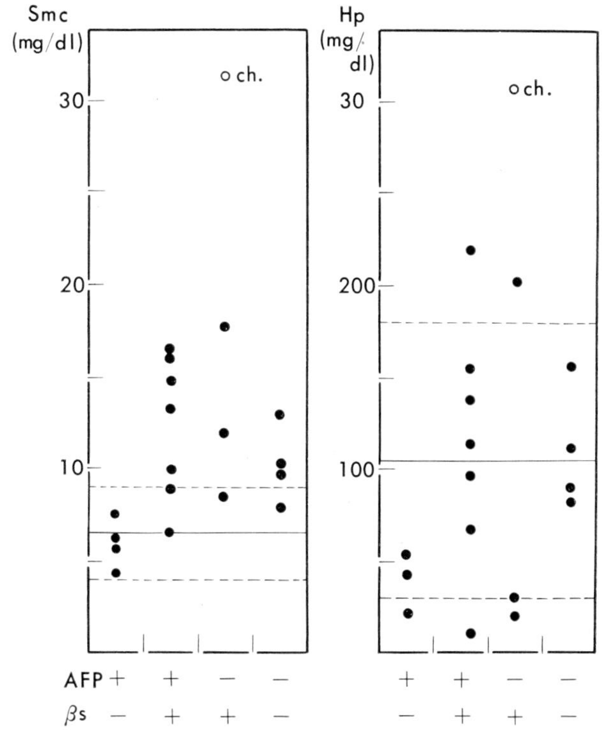

FIG. 4. Comparison of serum levels of seromucoid (Smc) and haptoglobin (Hp) between AFP-producing and βs-producing hepatoma cases
The mark " ch." indicates cholangiocarcinoma.

thesize and release these normal serum protein components as compared to its ability in βs-producing hepatoma cases. In other words, the deduction is warranted that not only the degree of differentiation of hepatoma tissue, but also the functional states of the liver as a whole, may be related in some way or other to the above observation.

Experiment in in vitro *Synthesis of AFP*

Hochwald *et al.* (*9*) and Williams *et al.* (*14*) demonstrated *in vitro* protein synthesis by tissue slices after incubation in a culture medium containing ^{14}C-isoleucine and ^{14}C-lysine, followed by detection of the synthesized protein using radioautoimmunoelectrophoresis. This method was used to demonstrate the synthesis of AFP by fetal tissues and carcinoma tissues. As shown in Fig. 5, materials which showed a reaction on radioautoimmunoelectrophoresis after incubation were the liver, thymus, stomach, and colon of a 6-month-old fetus obtained legally by a tocological operation. Tissue material of a metastasis to the lung from primary hepatoma also produced ^{14}C-labeled AFP, although the precipitin line was faint since the blood level of AFP in this case was rather low, and also since the material was taken by autopsy carried out after a certain lapse of time after the patient's death. No radioactive precipitin line reacting with the

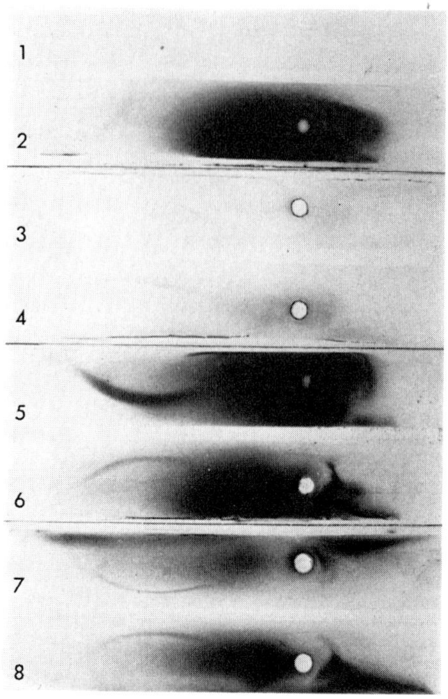

FIG. 5. Radioautoimmunoelectrophoretic demonstration of *in vitro* synthesis of AFP by tissue slices

Anode to the left, 1, control serum; 2, normal adult liver; 3, primary hepatoma, primary site; 4, primary hepatoma, metastasis to the lung; 5, fetal liver; 6, fetal thymus; 7, fetal stomach mucosa; 8, fetal colon mucosa.

anti-AFP serum was detected in the radioautograms of the incubation media of adult liver and of normal control serum. It was therefore concluded that, in fetuses, not only the liver but also other organs participate in the production of AFP.

Demonstration of AFP synthesis by fetal liver has already been reported by Abelev *et al.* (*1*) and by Gitlin and Boesman (*7*). The present results demonstrate *in vitro* biosynthesis of AFP by hepatoma tissue, and by a relatively wide variety of fetal organs and tissues in addition to the fetal liver.

CONCLUSIONS

In relation to studies in our laboratory on antigenic components that are common to carcinoma and fetus, some results on AFP, as well as on βs and α_2H, have been described.

The significance of simultaneous detection of AFP and βs in the diagnosis of hepatoma has been stressed, and the relation between the presence or absence of AFP and βs, and the function of the liver in the synthesis of normal serum proteins was discussed. It was also reported that, from the results of *in vitro* synthesis of AFP by tissues, the biosynthesis of AFP in fetuses was demonstrated not only by the liver but also by a wide variety of other organs and tissues. The same experimental procedures were also used to demonstrate the biosynthesis of AFP by hepatoma tissue.

Acknowledgments

This study was supported by a Grant-in-Aid for Scientific Research from the Ministry of Health and Welfare, a Grant-in-Aid for Special Scientific Research on Cancer from the Ministry of Education, and a grant from Chiyoda Life Insurance Co., Research Foundation.

REFERENCES

1. Abelev, G. I., Perova, I., Khramkova, N. I., Postnikova, Z. A., and Irlin, I. S. Production of embryonal α-globulin by transplantable mouse hepatomas. *Transplantation*, **1**, 174–180 (1963).
2. Bergstrand, C. G. and Czar, B. Paper electrophoresis study of human fetal serum protein with demonstration of a new protein fraction. *Scand. J. Clin. Lab. Invest.*, **9**, 277–286 (1957).
3. Buffe, D., Rimbaut, C., and Burtin, P. Présence d'un protéine d'origine tissulaire, l'α_2H-globuline, dans le sérum de sujets atteints d'affections malignes. *Int. J. Cancer*, **3**, 850–856 (1968).
4. Burtin, P., von Kleist, S., and Buffe, D. Étude sur les antigènes foetaux humaines. I. Étude immunoélectrophorétique des antigènes du sérum foetal humaine absents du sérum adulte. *Bull. Soc. Chim. Biol.*, **49**, 1389–1398 (1967).
5. de Muralt, G. and Roulet, D. L. A. Étude immunologique des protéines sériques foetales humaines. *Helv. Pediatr. Acta*, **16**, 517–533 (1961).
6. Galdo, A., Casado, J. P., and Talavera, R. Démonstration dans le sérum du foetus humain d'une nouvelle fraction protéique du moyen de l'électrophorèse sur papier. *Arch. Fr. Pédiatr.*, **16**, 954–962 (1959).
7. Gitlin, D. and Boesman, M. Sites of serum α-fetoprotein synthesis in the human and in the rat. *J. Clin. Invest.*, **46**, 1010–1016 (1967).
8. Gold, P. and Freedman, S. O. Demonstration of tumor specific antigens in human colonic carcinoma by immunological tolerance and absorption techniques. *J. Exp. Med.*, **121**, 439–462 (1965).
9. Hochwald, G. M., Thorbecke, G. J., and Asofsky, R. Sites of formation of immune globulins and of a component of C'_3. I. A new technique for the demonstration of the synthesis of individual serum proteins by tissues *in vitro*. *J. Exp. Med.*, **114**, 459–470 (1961).
10. Takahashi, A., Yachi, A., Anzai, T., and Wada, T. Presence of a unique serum protein in sera obtained from patients with neoplastic diseases and in embryonic and neonatal sera. *Clin. Chim. Acta*, **17**, 5–12 (1967).
11. Tatarinov, Y. S. Content of embryo-specific α-globulin in fetal and neonatal sera and sera from adult humans with primary carcinoma of the liver. *Fed. Proc.*, **25**, 344–346 (1966).
12. Wada, T., Anzai, T., Yachi, A., Takahashi, A., and Sakamoto, S. Incidences of three different fetal proteins in sera of patients with primary hepatoma. *Protides Biol. Fluids*, **18**, 221–226(1970).
13. Wada, T., Yachi, A., Anzai, T., Kawaharada, M., Ikebe, M., and Takahashi, A.

Diagnostic significance of two fetal proteins, AFP and βs, in hepatoma and other neoplastic diseases. *J. Clin. Oncol.*, **2**, 1–8 (1972).

14. Williams, R. C., Jr., Asofsky, R., and Thorbecke, G. J. Plasma protein formation *in vitro* by tissues from mice infected with staphylococci. *J. Exp. Med.*, **118**, 315–326 (1963).

AUSTRALIA ANTIGEN AND HEPATOCELLULAR CARCINOMA

Kusuya NISHIOKA,[*1] Takeshi HIRAYAMA,[*1] Teruaki SEKINE,[*1]
Kazuo OKOCHI,[*2] Makoto MAYUMI,[*2] Sung Juei-LOW,[*3]
Liu Chen-HUI,[*3] and Lin Tong-MIN[*3]

National Cancer Center Research Institute,[*1] *Blood Transfusion Service, Tokyo University Hospital,*[*2] *and National Taiwan University*[*3]

In collaboration with universities, research institutes, and hospitals in Japan, Formosa, and Manila, 354 sera of hepatocellular cancer patients including appropriate control groups, were obtained. It was found that 37.3%, 54.8%, and 70% of the sera from Japan, Formosa, and Manila, respectively, showed positive Australia (Au) antigen as detected by the immune adherence hemagglutination test, which is known as one of the most sensitive techniques for the detection of antigen. This showed a significantly high aggregation of Au antigen in hepatocellular cancer patients as compared with control groups. The antigen was demonstrated in a persistent form. The positive rate of antibody against Au antigen in hepatocellular cancer patients was much less than in control groups, and no antibody could be demonstrated by passive hemagglutination in the sera of hepatocellular cancer patients with positive Au antigen.

Impaired immunological states in hepatocellular cancer and/or the existence of a permissive factor allowing chronicity of Au antigen were discussed with regard to family and age factors in primary exposure.

A relationship between α-fetoprotein (AFP) and Au antigenemia in primary hepatocellular cancer (PHC) was demonstrated.

In Uganda (*20*), Senegal (*13*), and Spain (*18*), higher positive rates of Australia (Au) antigen were found in hepatocellular cancer patients than in the normal population, but this relation was not found in hepatocellular cancer patients in the U.S.A. and East Asia before we undertook a survey, and it has generally been considered that Au antigen has little or no relationship with hepatocellular cancer in East Asia (*12*, *14*, *15*, *17*) and the U.S.A. (*13*, *17*, *21*).

We have established an immune adherence hemagglutination (IAHA) method as one of the most sensitive methods for immune reaction (*9*) at the

[*1] Tsukiji 5-1-1, Chuo-ku, Tokyo 104, Japan (西岡久寿弥, 平山　雄, 関根暉彬).
[*2] Hongo 7-3-1, Bunkyo-ku, Tokyo 113, Japan (大河内一雄, 真弓　忠).
[*3] Jen-ai Road, Taipei, Taiwan (宋瑞楼, 劉禎輝, 林東明).

National Cancer Center, Tokyo. This has been applied to the detection of Au antigen on a large scale since 1971 (*8*). It gave 1,000-fold greater sensitivity than the agar gel diffusion and was 100-fold more sensitive than the complement fixation tests. As a result, a much higher frequency of Au antigen was found in hepatocellular cancer patients in Singapore, Taiwan, Japan, and Manila. Immunological problems concerning this finding will be described below.

Positive Rate of Au Antigen in the Sera of Hepatocellular Cancer Patients as Detected by IAHA

Through collaboration with Drs. T. Mukojima and N. Hattori (National Cancer Center, Tokyo), Dr. M. Ishii (Kobe University), Drs. T. Miyaji and M. Sakurai (Osaka University), Drs. H. Hirai and S. Nishi (Hokkaido University), Dr. C. Hirayama (Kyushu University), Drs. Y. Kuroyanagi and T. Yoshida (Aichi Cancer Center), Drs. J. L. Sung, C. H. Liu, and L. T. Lin (National Taiwan University), and Dr. G. F. Basa (Philippine Cancer Society), a large number of sera of hepatocellular cancer patients, including appropriate control groups, were obtained.

The Au antigen-positive rates in the sera of the cancer patients are shown in Table I. High Au antigen-positivity was observed in hepatocellular cancer patients, and in Japanese hepatocellular cancer patients, 97 out of 260 sera (37.3%) gave positive Au antigen by IAHA. This is significantly higher than in groups with metastatic liver cancer, gastric cancer, breast cancer, other cancer, and healthy persons in the National Cancer Center, Tokyo, and may be compared with 113 out of 4,387 (2.6%) for healthy blood donors. In Table II, results by

TABLE I. Positive Rate of Au Antigen in the Sera of Hepatocellular Carcinoma Patients as Detected by IAHA

Patients with hepatocellular carcinoma			Comparison groups		
	No. studied	Au-positive No. (%)		No. studied	Au-positive No. (%)
(NCC)	80	33 (41.3)	Metastatic liver cancer (NCC)	68	1 (1.5)
(KOU)	64	22 (34.3)	Gastric cancer (NCC)	83	3 (3.6)
(ACC)	5	3 (60.0)	Breast cancer (NCC) (ACC)	46	0 (0)
(HOU)	81	26 (32.1)	Other cancer (NCC)	52	2 (3.8)
(KYU)	30	13 (43.3)	Healthy control (NCC)	376	5 (1.3)
Total in Japan	260	97 (37.3)	Blood donors	4,378	113 (2.6)
Total in Taipei	84	46 (54.8)	Blood donors	278	34 (12.2)
			Other cancer	347	47 (13.5)
Total in Manila	10	7 (70.0)			
Total in Singapore[a]	113	38 (33.6)	Blood donors	1,516	117 (7.8)
			Other cancer	204	12 (5.8)

NCC: National Cancer Center, Tokyo. KOU: Kobe University. ACC: Aichi Cancer Center. HOU: Hokkaido University. KYU: Kyushu University. [a] Ref. (*16*)

TABLE II. Comparison of Positive Rate of Au Antigen in the Sera of Hepatocellular Carcinoma Patients as Detected by IAHA and Other Methods

Area	Method	Hepatocellular carcinoma		Control groups	
		No. tested	Au antigen-positive No. (%)	No. tested	Au antigen-positive No. (%)
Singapore	EOD (*15*)	114	3 (2.6)	1,653[a] 108[b]	69 (9.2) 1 (0.9)
	IAHA (*16*)	113	38 (33.6)	1,516[a] 204[b]	117 (7.8) 12 (5.8)
Japan	ID (*12*)	19	1 (5.3)	5,246[a]	54 (1.0)
	IAHA	260	97 (37.3)	4,387[a] 249[b]	113 (2.6) 6 (2.4)
Philippines	EOD	10	1 (10.0)		
	IAHA	10	7 (70.0)		

EOD: Electro-osmodiffusion. ID: Immunodiffusion.
[a] Healthy blood donors. [b] Other cancer patients.

the IAHA method are compared with results by other, less sensitive methods which failed to demonstrate higher Au antigen-positivity in the sera of hepatocellular cancer patients.

Features of Au Antigen Detected in the Sera of Hepatocellular Cancer Patients

One of the main features of the prevalence of Au antigen in the sera of hepatocellular cancer patients is that the amount of Au antigen in most cases is not high enough to be detected by other, less sensitive methods. As shown in Fig. 1, the

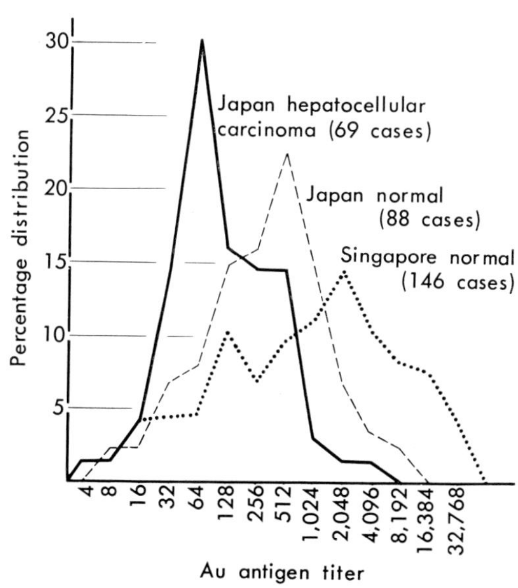

FIG. 1. Distribution by Au antigen titer measured by IAHA

frequency distribution curve of Au antigen titer in serum as determined by IAHA in the blood donor group and that in the hepatocellular cancer patients showed different patterns. The peak in hepatocellular cancer patients is 64, while the peaks of the blood donor groups in Japan and in Singapore are 512 and 2048, respectively. Antigen titer was expressed as the highest serum dilution giving positive IAHA. In general, sera with a titer less than 128 could not be detected by other, less sensitive methods. This could account for the results reported until now, that the frequency of Au antigen in hepatocellular cancer patients in East Asia did not show a significantly higher frequency than control groups, presumably due to the fact that a significantly greater number of hepatocellular cancer patients have Au antigen, but in levels so low as to be detectable only by sensitive methods such as IAHA. The second feature is that Au antigen was detected in a persistent form in all sera of hepatocellular cancer patients tested. We reexamined 17 sera of hepatocellular cancer patients from the National Cancer Center Hospital, Tokyo. These samples were bled from each patient at intervals of at least 1 month and showed persistence of Au antigen, except in 2 cases of infantile hepatocellular cancer who received blood transfusions in the course of surgical operations and showed positive Au antigen transiently.

Impairment of Immune Response to Au Antigen in Hepatocellular Cancer Patients

The passive hemagglutination technique for the detection of antibody against Au antigen was established by Imai *et al.* (*3*) and was applied for measurement of Au antibody in sera. In healthy controls, 69 out of 376 (18.4%) and in other cancer, 33 out of 229 cases (14.4%) showed positive Au antibody, as detected by the phytohem-agglutination (PHA) technique. In contrast, only 6 out of 80 cases of hepatocellular cancer (7.5%) showed positive Au antibody and Au antibody could not be demonstrated in the sera of hepatocellular cancer patients with positive Au antigen.

As PHA is highly sensitive, these results suggest that the levels of anti-Au antibody in hepatocellular cancer patients were much lower than in control groups, indicating a possibility of specific impairment of an immunological state or immunological tolerance to Au antigen. There may be factors allowing Au antigen to be persistently positive in the sera of hepatocellular cancer patients. The so-called " immunological tolerance " to Au antigen could be considered as a background mechanism allowing persistent Au antigen in hepatocellular cancer, as observed in oncogenic RNA viruses in experimental animals.

Family and Age Factors

As for factors allowing immunological tolerance in infection by Au antigen, two main host factors were observed in our collaborative studies in Japan. The first is the family as a host determinant and the second is the age of primary exposure of the host to Au antigen.

Concerning the first problem, Ohbayashi *et al.* (*10*) first described familial clustering of Au antigenemia, chronic liver disease, and hepatocellular cancer in Japan. Similar clustering was preliminarily reported later in Chile (*19*) and the U.S.A. (*2*).

According to Ohbayashi, the familial clustering of chronic liver diseases and hepatocellular cancer is not rare in Japan. Since 1971, Ohbayashi, Okochi, and Mayumi have carried out the IAHA test for Au antigen in sera from 54 individuals of families with multiple occurrence of chronic liver disease and hepatocellular cancer.

Summarizing the results of Au antigen and anti-Au antibody tests, 19 (91%) out of 21 male and female siblings were positive for Au antigen, and 20 (83%) of the 24 offspring of the female siblings were also positive. On the other hand none of the 8 offspring of the male siblings were positive for Au antigen, except for 1, in whose mother anti-Au was detected.

To compare the pattern of a normal family, Kaji (*5*) studied members of 33 of Au antigen-positive families in Nichinan and 8 in Iriomote, and a very high positive rate of Au antigen was obtained. These cases of familiar aggregation of Au antigen indicate a high rate of exposure to a viral agent in the family. In those cases, not associated with clustering of chronic liver diseases, the transmission is not limited to the maternal line, but some other mode of spread among the family is strongly indicated.

To elucidate the mode of spread through the maternal line, and to determine the time of primary exposure to Au antigen, Okada (*11*) observed that the time of infection through the maternal line is not intrauterine, but rather the time of delivery. He found 44 Au antigen-positive cases out of 1,439 at the initial stages of pregnancy. Of these, 21 cases were followed up for the presence of Au antigen in the blood of the mother and children during the course of pregnancy and after birth. Au antigen disappeared from 14 cases and none of these children were positive for Au antigen. Seven cases showed persistance of Au antigen even after birth. Australia antigen could not be found in either cord blood or in blood younger than 4 months old. At the age of 4 or 5 months, 3 children born from mothers who were Au antigen-positive at birth showed the presence of Au antigen in the blood. The other 4 cases were younger than 4 months old at this time and follow-up studies are now being continued.

These observations suggest that, in high risk families, Au antigen or an Au antigen-related infective agent was transmitted from mother to child, and was also responsible for the development of persistent Au antigenemia, chronic hepatitis, cirrhosis of the liver, and eventual hepatocellular cancer.

These familiar clusterings of Au antigen associated with hepatocellular cancer and chronic liver diseases strongly indicate that the transmission of the infective agent occurred at the neonatal or infant stage, leading to a chronic carrier state associated with these liver diseases. Immunological tolerance could be induced by primary exposure to the infective agent, as observed in many cases of oncogenic viruses of experimental animals.

Comparison of Au Antigen with Oncogenic RNA and DNA Viruses

Based on these new observations in Japan, comparison of Au antigen with typical oncogenic DNA and RNA viruses was proposed. This would be useful

TABLE III. Comparison of Oncogenic DNA, RNA Viruses, and ICRON with Regard to Host Response

Viruses	Oncogenic DNA virus	Oncogenic RNA virus	ICRON
Primary exposure in adult	Solid immunity	Solid immunity	Solid immunity
Primary exposure in newborn	Tumor after maturity	Tumor after maturity	Cryptogenic disorders tumor?
Presence of host component in particle	—	+	+
Persistency in circulation	—	+	+
Tolerance	—	+	+

for the next step towards understanding of carcinogenesis by ICRON (*1*), a new biological unit particle represented by Au antigen. This is briefly summarized in Table III. An essential feature common to these 3 groups is the effect of the time of primary exposure of the host to infective agent. When primary exposure occurred in adults, all 3 resulted in solid immunity and a tumor was not induced in the host. For Au antigen, this includes most cases of antibody production after Au antigen-positive blood transfusion in the adult. However, in the newborn, tumors developed after maturity in both oncogenic RNA and DNA viruses.

For Au antigen or ICRON, this will result in cryptogenic hepatic disorders or persistent Au antigenemia without antibody formation or tolerance, as observed in most cases of oncogenic RNA viruses. It is well known that primary exposure to the virus in the newborn results in persistence of the virion in circulating blood and impairment of the specific immune reaction (tolerance). Therefore, it is understandable that the persistence of Au antigen in circulation and suppressed immune response to Au antigen, as observed in hepatocellular cancer patients, could be induced by primary exposure at the newborn stage through the maternal line, and such phenomena could be considered as plausible prerequisite factors for the persistence of Au antigen with regard to immunological host response.

Relationship between AFP and Au Antigen in the Sera of Hepatocellular Cancer Patients

The relationship between the prevalence of Au antigen as detected by IAHA in the sera of hepatocellular cancer patients and AFP, which was measured using the single radial immunodiffusion method by Ishii (*4*), Mukojima, and Nishi, is shown in Table IV. It was found that 74 out of 169 AFP-positive hepatocellular cancer cases showed the presence of Au antigen in sera, considerably higher than the 7 out of 40 cases of AFP-negative hepatocellular cancer, showing significance at the 1% level by the χ^2 test.

Except for 2 transient Au-positive cases which turned negative 1 month after blood transfusion, sera from 9 infantile hepatocellular cancers and 5 embryonal carcinoma which contained a large amount of AFP gave negative IAHA for Au antigen.

TABLE IV. Relation of AFP and Au Antigen in Sera

	No. studied	No. positive	(%)
AFP+Hepatocellular carcinoma total	169	74	(43.8)
(KOU)	59	22	(37.3)
(NCC)	54	30	(55.6)
(HOU)	56	22	(39.2)
AFP−Hepatocellular carcinoma total	40	7	(17.5)
(KOU)	5	0	(0)
(NCC)	26	3	(11.5)
(HOU)	19	4	(21.1)
AFP+Infantile hepatocellular carcinoma	11	(2)	
AFP+Embryonal carcinoma	5	0	

( ): Transient positive.

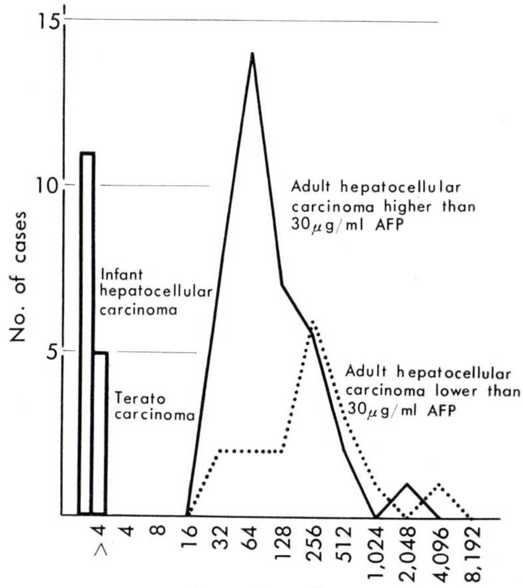

FIG. 2. Australia antigen titer in different disease groups

As shown in Fig. 2, when the amount of Au antigen was plotted according to the Au antigen titer determined by IAHA, it was found that adult hepatocellular cancer cases with a larger amount of AFP, more than 30 μg/ml, were found in cases with less Au antigen titer in the sera, showing a peak at 64. Cases with less AFP (less than 30 μg/ml) showed a distribution pattern with a peak at an Au antigen titer of 256. As mentioned above, no persistence of Au antigen was found in infantile liver cancer and teratocarcinoma with a large amount of AFP in the sera.

According to the above observations, the relative risk in Au antigen-positive persons for various cancers was calculated as compared with Au antigen-negative cases. The relative risk in Au antigen-positive cases as compared with Au antigen-negative is 1.1 for metastatic liver cancer, 2.7 for gastric cancer, and 1.9 for other cancer, which does not indicate a very significant elevation. On the other hand, the risk in Au antigen-positive persons was extremely high (89.0 times higher) for AFP-positive hepatocellular cancer as compared with Au-negative persons in Japan. The value for AFP-negative hepatocellular cancer was 9.6.

The association of AFP and Au antigen in the sera of PHC patients indicates a possibility for improved chances of detecting clinically unapparent forms of hepatocellular cancer in adults in the early stage by combined measurements of AFP and Au antigen in persons in endemic areas for hepatocellular cancer, such as Japan and other East Asian areas.

Acknowledgments

Collaborations of Mrs. H. Yamashita and F. Tsuda for detection of Au antigen and antibody and Miss. H. Kato for preparation of the manuscript are gratefully acknowledged. This study was supported by research grants from the Ministry of Health and Welfare and from the Ministry of Education, Japan.

REFERENCES

1. Blumberg, B. S., Millman, I., Sutunick, A. I., and London, W. T. The nature of Australia antigen and its relation to antigen-antibody complex formation. *J. Exp. Med.*, **134**, 320–329 (1971).
2. Denison, E. K., Peters, R. L., and Reynolds, T. B. Familial hepatoma with hepatitis-associated antigen. *Annu. Internal Med.*, **74**, 391–394 (1971).
3. Imai, M. Takahashi, T., Mayumi, M., and Okochi, K. Detection of antibody to Australia antigen by passive hemagglutination (in Japanese). *Igaku-no-Ayumi* (*The Stride of Medicine*), **78**, 759 (1971).
4. Ishii, M. " Proceedings of Regional Meeting on Australia Antigen and Hepatocellular Carcinoma," National Cancer Center Research Institute, Tokyo, December 7, 1971.
5. Kaji, M. " Proceedings of Regional Meeting on Australia Antigen and Hepatocellular Carcinoma," National Cancer Center Research Institute, Tokyo, December 7, 1971.
6. Kendall, M. G. and Buckland, W. R. "A Dictionary of Statistical Terms," (3rd Ed.), Oliver & Boyd, Edinburgh, p. 128 (1971).
7. Mayumi, M., Okochi, K., and Nishioka, K. Australia antigen in hepatoma. Hepatitis Scientific Memoranda, December 1971.
8. Mayumi, M., Okochi, K., and Nishioka, K. Detection of Australia antigen by means of immuno-adherence hemagglutination test. *Vox Sang.*, **20**, 178–181 (1971).
9. Nishioka, K. Complement and tumor immunology. *Adv. Cancer Res.*, **14**, 231–293 (1971).
10. Ohbayashi, A, Mayumi, M., and Okochi, K. Australia antigen in familial cirrhosis. *Lancet*, **1**, 244 (1971).
11. Okada, K. " Proceedings of Regional Meeting on Australia Antigen and Hepatocellular Carcinoma," National Cancer Center Research Institute, Tokyo, December 7, 1971.
12. Okochi, K. and Murakami, S. Observations on Australia antigen in Japanese. *Vox Sang.*, **15**, 374–385 (1968).

13. Prince, A. M., Leblanc, L., Krohn, K., Masseyeff, R., and Alpert, M. E. SH antigen and chronic liver disease. *Lancet*, **2**, 717–718 (1970).
14. Shih, P. L., Chang, C. K., and Sung, J. L. Personal communication.
15. Simons, M. J., Yu, M., Chew, B. K., Tan, A. Y. O., Yap, E. H., Seah, C. S., Fung W. P., and Shanmugaratnam, K. Australia antigen in Singapore Chinese patients with hepatocellular carcinoma. *Lancet*, **1**, 1149–1151 (1971).
16. Simons, M. J., Yap, E. H., Yu, M., and Shanmugaratnam, K. Australia antigen in Singapore, Chinese patients with hepatocellular carcinoma and comparison group. *Int. J. Cancer*, **10**, 320–325 (1972).
17. Smith, J. B. and Blumberg, B. S. Viral hepatitis, postnecrotic cirrhosis and hepatocellular carcinoma. *Lancet*, **2**, 953 (1969).
18. Teres, J., Guardia, J., Brugubra, M., and Rodes, J. Hepatitis-associated antigen and hepatocellular carcinoma. *Lancet*, **2**, 215 (1971).
19. Velasco, M., Sorensen, R., Carmona, A., Daiber, A., and Katz, R. Australia antigen and primary carcinoma of the liver. *Gastroenterology*, **60**, 729 (1971).
20. Vogel, C. C., Anthony, P. P., Mody, N. J., and Barker, L. F. Hepatitis-associated antigen in Ugandan patients with hepatocellular carcinoma. *Lancet*, **2**, 621–624 (1970).
21. Wright, R., McCollum, R. W., and Klatskin, G. Australia antigen in acute and chronic liver disease. *Lancet*, **2**, 117–121 (1969).

PATHOLOGY OF HUMAN HEPATOMAS AND AFP

ASSOCIATION OF HEPATOCELLULAR CARCINOMA WITH CIRRHOSIS AMONG AUTOPSY CASES IN JAPAN (1958–1967)

Toru MIYAJI

*Department of Pathology, Osaka University Medical School**

The registered 136,475 autopsy cases during the 10 years from 1958 to 1967 in Japan were statistically analyzed with special reference to hepatoma and liver cirrhosis. The results are summarized as follows:

(1) The incidence of hepatoma has been fairly high (2.7% in males and 1.1% in females).

(2) The incidence of cirrhotic changes excluding fibrosis was also comparatively high (7.4% in males and 4.3% in females).

(3) The majority of cirrhosis victims in Japan have multilobular thin septal patterns, which were called B type cirrhosis of Nagoya-Miyake or the posthepatitic type of Gall, in which cirrhosis not otherwise specified could also be included.

(4) When it is limited to these types of cirrhosis, the association with hepatoma was found to be 58.7% in males and 41.4% in females, and the association of hepatoma with cirrhosis was found to be 33.9% in males and 19.0% in females.

Since Berman (*1*), Japan has been noted as a country of high incidence of primary liver carcinoma. As a matter of fact, Segi *et al.* (*6*) and his associates have repeatedly described the same effect based on worldwide mortality statistics. Autopsy cases at the University of Tokyo have also revealed the same findings (*4, 7*). The author and his associates (*3*) have also studied 36,380 autopsy cases carried out at 46 medical schools and 22 hospitals from 1946 to 1955 and found 639 hepatomas, 29 cholangiomas, and 8 mixed types.

Since 1958, Annual of the Pathological Autopsy Cases in Japan has been published as a registry, and it covers more than 95% of the pathological autopsies in Japan each year. The author has studied the incidence of hepatoma and cholangioma, and their association with cirrhotic change based on the registry.

From 10 volumes of the Annual published by the Japanese Pathological Society each year, each registered case was recorded on an IBM-type card following a disease code comprising 1,036 pathological findings. The cards were counted with a mark system selector (Tanac).

As shown in Table I, among 136,475 autopsy cases, there were 61,869 malignancies, including space-occupying lesions in the cranial cavity, pheochromocytomas and islet cell tumors, although the latter two types of tumors were very

* 33 Joan-cho, Kita-ku, Osaka 530, Japan (宮地　徹).

TABLE I. Autopsy Cases in Japan (1958–1967)

Year	Total autopsy cases				Malignancies		
	Male	Female	Unknown	Total	Male	Female	Total
1958	5,193	3,178	150	8,521	2,121	1,414	3,535
1959	5,282	3,574	180	9,036	2,307	1,647	3,954
1960	5,939	3,786	202	9,927	2,729	1,613	4,342
1961	4,476	4,476	205	11,281	3,001	2,087	5,088
1962	6,600	5,064	215	12,599	3,183	2,224	5,407
1963	7,320	5,569	195	14,179	3,987	2,585	6,572
1964	8,415	5,832	245	14,993	4,188	2,715	6,903
1965	11,710	5,240	170	17,120	4,858	2,995	7,853
1966	10,658	7,157	47	17,862	5,177	3,336	8,513
1967	12,472	8,386	99	20,957	5,901	3,801	9,702
Total	82,505	52,262	1,708	136,475	37,452	24,417	61,869

Medical examiner's cases and sex unknown with malignancies are excluded.

infrequent. In the Annual, cirrhosis was customarily divided into the following types; namely, A type, which corresponded to postnecrotic, B type posthepatitic and nutritional type of Gall's classification (*2*) as mentioned by Mori (*5*). A′ type cirrhosis was considered to be one showing histological features of transitional nature between A and B types, and B′ type between B type and fibrosis. Cirrhosis NOS (not otherwise specified) represented those in which no specific type

TABLE II. Association of Hepatoma

Liver	Sex	Total	Fibrosis	Types of cirrhotic: A type cirrh.	A′ type cirrh.	B type cirrh.	Cirrh. NOS
With hepatoma	Male	2,268	22	101	9	537	795
	Female	549	9	15	6	87	140
Without hepatoma	Male	5,173	667	616	37	1,134	1,466
	Female	2,313	332	290	15	403	562

TABLE III. Age Distribution of

	Total	NB	0–1	2–	5–	10–	15–	20–	25–	30–	35–	40–
Male	1,134	0	0	0	5	10	8	7	17	40	66	101
Female	404	0	5	2	3	2	2	6	6	12	22	26

B type cirrhosis corresponds to nutritional and posthepatitic cirrhosis of Gall. NB refers to

TABLE IV. Age Distribution of

	Total	NB	0–1	2–	5–	10–	15–	20–	25–	30–	35–	40–
Male	1,434	3	18	2	3	10	17	25	26	59	81	117
Female	558	1	7	3	7	8	11	11	13	9	20	49

NB refers to newborn.

was mentioned. Fatty, biliary, cardiac, hemochromatic cirrhosis, schistosomiasis including fibrosis and cirrhosis, Wilson's disease, and Budd-Chiari syndrome were also listed.

Various cirrhotic changes with and without heptoma are shown in Table II. Hepatomas are found among cirrhotic changes in 22.8% of males and 10.5% of females, and cirrhotic changes were found among hepatomas in 67.2% of males and 49.4% of females. However, when just cirrhosis NOS and B type (posthepatitic and nutritional) cirrhosis are combined, hepatoma was found in 51.2% of males and 23.5% of females. On the other hand, these cirrhotic lesions among hepatoma cases were found in 58.7% of males and 41.3% of females. Cirrhosis associated with hepatoma was found 35.2% in males and 19.9% in females for NOS type, and 32.1% in males and 17.8% in females for B type (posthepatitic and nutritional of Gall), with no statistically significant difference between them. Due to the difference in number, however, hepatoma asscoiated with cirrhosis NOS were 35.1% in males and 25.5% in females, and those associated with B type cirrhosis were 23.7% and 15.9%, respectively. In addition to this, the age incidences of both cirrhosis and hepatoma were similar with the peak at the 5th decade in both males and females (Tables III, IV, and V). It was assumed that the majority of cirrhosis NOS could be included in B type cirrhosis.

Compared with hepatoma, cholangioma did not have much to do with cirrhotic changes as shown in Table VI, particularly in view of the frequency of cirrhotic changes including fibrosis among all autopsy cases, 8.2% in males and

with Cirrhotic Changes (1958–1967)

changes of the liver							
B′ type cirrh.	Fatty cirrh.	Biliary cirrh.	Cardiac cirrh.	Hemochromatosis	Budd-Chiari syndrome	Wilson's disease	Schistosomiasis fibr. and cirrh.
23	0	9	4	4	8	7	5
5	0	3	3	0	1	1	1
100	56	575	252	60	18	44	124
34	21	402	148	15	8	38	42

Autopsied B Type Cirrhosis (1958–1967)

45–	50–	55–	60–	65–	70–	75–	80–	85–	90–	95–	Age unknown
158	188	162	151	89	64	38	17	3	1	0	9
25	65	56	59	45	25	18	8	3	0	0	3

newborn.

Autopsied Cirrhosis NOS (1958–1967)

45–	50–	55–	60–	65–	70–	75–	80–	85–	90–	95–	Age unknown
141	185	205	196	168	89	62	15	4	1	0	11
59	60	70	83	60	49	25	9	3	1	0	1

TABLE V. Age Distribution of

Sex	Total	NB	0–1	2–	5–	10–	15–	20–	25–	30–	35–	40–
Male	2,268	2	22	13	7	11	19	17	39	62	117	175
Female	549	1	13	3	4	5	7	8	15	15	23	40

NB refers to newborn.

TABLE VI. Association of Cholangioma

Sex	Total	Fibrosis	A type cirrh.	A′ type cirrh.	B type cirrh.
Male	432	7	5	0	18
Female	236	3	4	0	4

TABLE VII. Age Distribution of

Sex	Total	NB	0–1	2–	5–	10–	15–	20–	25–	30–	35–	40–
Male	432	0	1	0	0	0	1	2	4	13	14	19
Female	237	0	0	0	0	0	1	1	1	5	5	10

NB refers to newborn.

5.0% in females. The age incidence of cholangioma was also similar to hepatoma with the peak at the 5th decade (Table VII).

The incidence of cirrhotic changes of the liver excluding fibrosis among all autopsy cases (7.4% in males and 4.3% in females) was fairly high in Japan compared with that found in the literature and cases examined by the author abroad. In addition, the incidence of hepatoma was much higher than could be found in any other countries, and the relationship between hepatoma and cirrhotic changes was more pronounced. In spite of extensive study in regard to the etiological factor or factors of hepatoma and cirrhosis in Japan, it was not quite clear what kinds of agents were really causative, although some work emphasized the potentiality of viral hepatitis as a possible precursor of cirrhosis through chronic hepatitis and fibrosis of the liver.

From a clinical point of view, it is very important to note that cirrhosis in Japan was so closely associated with hepatoma that clinicians should always be alert to the possible development of hepatoma on the basis of cirrhosis. Its early diagnosis is so important that extensive study on fetoprotein is expected to bring a new facet and powerful clue along this line.

REFERENCES

1. Berman, C. *In* " Primary Carcinoma of the Liver. A Study in Incidence, Clinical Manifestations, Pathology and Aetiology," ed. by H. K. Lewis, London, pp. 5–18 (1951).
2. Gall, E. A. Posthepatitic, postnecrotic, and nutritional cirrhosis. A pathologic analysis. *Am. J. Pathol.*, **36**, 241–271 (1960).
3. Miyaji, T. Primary liver carcinoma in Japan, particularly on the association with cirrhosis. *Trans. Soc. Pathol. Japon.*, **54**, 23–38 (1965).

Autopsied Hepatoma (1958–1967)

45–	50–	55–	60–	65–	70–	75–	80–	85–	90–	95–	Age unknown
284	373	384	323	238	111	50	9	4	1	1	8
58	76	95	60	78	25	17	4	0	0	0	3

with Cirrhotic Changes (1958–1967)

Cirrh. NOS	B′ type cirrh.	Fatty cirrh.	Biliary cirrh.	Cardiac cirrh.
29	1	0	35	0
8	0	0	13	1

Autopsied Cholangioma (1958–1967)

45–	50–	55–	60–	65–	70–	75–	80–	85–	90–	95–	Age unknown
35	47	79	66	68	53	22	5	1	0	0	2
16	35	29	44	40	26	16	5	0	0	0	3

4. Miyake, M. Primary hepatic cancer and liver cirrhosis in Japan. *Acta Unio Int. Contra Cancrun*, **17**, 892–897 (1961).
5. Mori, W. Cirrhosis and primary cancer of the liver. Comparative study in Tokyo and Cincinnati. *Cancer*, **20**, 627–631 (1967).
6. Segi, M., Kurihara, M., and Matsuyama, T. "Cancer Mortality for Selected Sites in 24 Countries," No. 5 (1964–1965). Department of Public Health, Tohoku University School of Medicine, Sendai, Japan; Doll, R., Muir, C., and Waterhouse, J. "Cancer Incidence in Five Continents (UICC Monograph)," Springer-Verlag (1966 and 1970).
7. Shikata, T. Studies on the relationship between hepatic cancer and liver cirrhosis. Rescrutinization of the causal relationship between malignant hepatoma and liver cirrhosis in human necropsy cases. *Acta Pathol. Japon.*, **9**, 267–311 (1959).

GANN Monograph on Cancer Research 14, 1973

α-FETOPROTEIN AND THE MORPHOLOGY OF HEPATOMA IN MAN

Masami SAKURAI and Toru MIYAJI
*Department of Pathology, Osaka University Medical School**

The relation between α-fetoprotein (AFP) in serum and morphology of the tumor was studied in 78 cases with hepatoma. The AFP-positive indicates positive results by the ordinary micro-Ouchterlony technique, having a sensitivity above 1 mg/dl of serum concentration. Morphological differentiation of the hepatoma was analyzed by Edmondson's grading.

It was found that 52 (67%) of 78 hepatoma cases were AFP-positive. The peak incidence of AFP-positive results was found in Grade III, poorly differentiated hepatoma comprising 26 (76%) of 34 cases. Grade II, moderately differentiated, and Grade IV, undifferentiated, hepatoma showed lower AFP-positive incidences, about 60% each.

A functional differentiation of hepatoma as "bile-positive" was particularly emphasized. Among 34 bile-positive hepatoma cases, AFP was positive in 27 cases (79%). However, among 44 bile-negative hepatoma cases, AFP-positive decreased to 25 (57%). Among 52 AFP-positive hepatoma, bile was positive in 27 cases (52%), but among 26 AFP-negative cases, bile was positive only in 7 (27%). Furthermore, an immunofluorescent study showed many more AFP-positive hepatoma cells in bile-positive areas than in bile-negative areas of the same case.

Quantitative determination of serum AFP was done in 28 cases. Grade II and III hepatoma revealed much higher AFP values in bile-positive cases than in bile-negative ones, and the highest AFP value was found in bile-positive Grade III hepatoma, reaching 76.2 mg/dl as a mean value of 6 cases. Differences in biological behavior between AFP-positive and AFP-negative hepatoma will be discussed. Finally, it can be said that AFP is positive almost without exception when a hepatoma is poorly differentiated Grade III cytohistologically and is associated with bile-positive results microscopically in the hepatoma.

A large series of studies concerning the relation between serum α-fetoprotein (AFP) and the morphology of the hepatoma in man was reported by Purves *et al.* (*10*) from Johannesburg, South Africa. They found some correlation in that the highest average value of serum AFP occurred in cases with poorly differentiated hepatoma, followed by well-differentiated ones, and the lowest average value

* 33 Joan-cho, Kita-ku, Osaka 530, Japan (桜井幹巳, 宮地　徹).

was found in cases with anaplastic hepatoma. Abelev (*1*) summarized the literature concerning AFP in ontogenesis and its association with malignant tumors. One of the points of interest regarding human hepatoma and AFP is an apparent difference in the incidence of AFP-positive results among different races (*4*, *5*) and different ages of patients (*2*, *7*). These differences may well correspond to morphological differences, but this has not yet been proved. As has been well documented in Miyaji's work (see page 179), hepatoma in Japan has a very high association with cirrhosis and the majority of cases occur over the age of 40.

The present paper reports the analysis of hepatoma as many cases as possible collected throughout Japan* to examine any correlation between AFP-positive results and the morphology of the hepatoma.

Anti-human AFP horse serum was supplied by The Green Cross Corporation (Osaka). Serum AFP was tested by the micro-Ouchterlony immunodiffusion method (*9*) with a sensitivity above 1 mg/dl. Quantitative determination was done in some cases by the single radial immunodiffusion method (*6*) and the radioimmunoassay method (*8*).

For morphological studies, several sections from grossly different areas were taken from each case, stained by ordinary Hematoxylin-Eosin, and examined under a light microscope.

α-Fetoprotein and Cytohistological Grading of Hepatoma

It is well known that the morphology of hepatoma shows a considerable variety in different areas, even in the same liver. Grossly green, yellow, red, or white hepatoma in a single case is not exceptional. In such cases all the representative areas were taken for examination. Since the histological type of most cases of hepatoma belongs to the trabecular type, cytological types including cellular atypism, bile capillary, and bile pigment were carefully examined. Summarizing the entire status of a hepatoma, a grade was determined as a majority for a particular case. There were 4 grades: Grade I well differentiated (Photo 1), Grade II moderately differentiated (Photos 2–5), Grade III poorly differentiated (Photos 6–10), and Grade IV undifferentiated (Photo 11), according to Edmondson (*3*).

TABLE I. Number of Cases in Each Cytohistological Grade of Hepatoma and Serum AFP

Grade	I	II	III	IV	Total
AFP +	0	23	26	3	52 (67%)
AFP −	1	15	8	2	26 (33%)
Total	1 (1%)	38 (49%)	34 (43%)	5 (7%)	78(100%)

As shown in Table I, 52 (67%) of 78 cases with hepatoma were AFP-positive. Of 78 cases, 38 (49%) were Grade II, and 34 (43%) were Grade III hepatomas.

* Osaka University, Hokkaido University, Kurume University, Yamaguchi University, Wakayama Medical College, Okayama University, Sapporo Medical College, and Tokyo Medical and Dental University.

In each grade, the highest incidence of AFP-positive was in Grade III, where it was 26 (76%) of 34 cases. Next was Grade II hepatoma, with 23 (61%) of 38 cases. Although cases of Grade IV hepatoma were small in number, the incidence of AFP-positive was about the same as for Grade II, being 3 (60%) of 5 cases.

Bile Pigment and AFP in Hepatoma

It was shown at the 30th Annual Meeting of the Japanese Cancer Association in 1971 (*11*) that many more and stronger luminescent hepatoma cells were found in bile-positive areas than in bile-negative areas of the same tumor on immunofluorescent study by a frozen section technique (Photos 12 and 13). It remains to be further investigated whether bile production and AFP production take place at the same time in the same cell or whether it is just a matter of affinity between bile and AFP or between bile and fluorescent horse antibody. It also remains to be determined whether bile-positive means bile-producing or just bile-accumulating hepatoma. In normal liver there is usually no bile pigment as is the case in well-differentiated adenomatous type hepatoma of Grade I. On the other hand, definite bile pigment can be found in hepatoma cells in some cases, usually moderately differentiated type hepatomas of Grade II. For these reasons, the term " bile-positive " was prefered to " bile-producing." Bile-positive then refers both to bile in tumor cells and/or bile in the capillary as bile thrombus. The amount of bile in hepatoma may be marked, as in green hepatoma, or it may be minimal, when the bile can be found by meticulous search microscopically. When even one definite bile-positive site was identified, the hepatoma was classified as bile-positive.

The cytohistological grades of hepatoma and serum AFP were further analyzed depending upon bile-positive or bile-negative results in every case (Table II). From a total of 78 cases, 34 cases (44%) were bile-positive and 44 (56%) were bile-negative. A little less than half of the cases were bile-positive. When these 2 groups were further divided into 2 groups, AFP-positive and AFP-negative cases, the largest number among the 4 groups was the bile-positive, AFP-positive case, comprising 27 (35%) of 78 cases. The second was the bile-negative, AFP-positive case, 25 cases (32%). The third was the bile-negative, AFP-negative case, 19 cases (24%), and the 4th was the bile-positive, AFP-negative case, 7 cases (9%). Bile-positive, AFP-negative cases were rather exceptional. In 2 cases of these 7 exceptional cases, quantitative determination of the serum AFP was

TABLE II. Cytohistological Grade of Hepatoma Correlated to Bile in Tumor and Serum AFP

Grade		I		II		III		IV		Total	
Bile		+	−	+	−	+	−	+	−	+	−
AFP	+	0	0	13	10	13	13	1	2	27	25
AFP	−	0	1	7	8	0	8	0	2	7	19
Total		0	1	20	18	13	21	1	4	34	44

done by the radioimmunoassay technique. Their serum concentrations were 0.06 mg/dl (Photo 3) and 0.01 mg/dl (Photo 2). These values support the view that bile-positive hepatoma is also AFP-positive as a rule. However, the remaining half of bile-negative hepatoma cases showed no association at all with AFP-positive results.

Biological Behavior of Hepatoma in Relation to Serum AFP Concentration and Bile in the Hepatoma

There are 3 main patterns of hepatoma growth in the liver; massive, nodular, and diffuse or cirrhotic type, as gross appearance of the hepatoma. The size and weight of the entire liver including the hepatoma provide another way to measure the biological behavior of the tumor in an individual case. Markedly enlarged, heavy liver is usual when growth of the hepatoma is rapid. In cases where the size and weight of the liver are well maintained, it is usually the case that growth of the hepatoma is slow. Table III shows an average weight of liver

TABLE III. Average Weight (g) of Liver in Each Cytohistological Grade, Serum AFP, and Bile in Tumor

Grade		I		II		III		IV	
Bile		+	−	+	−	+	−	+	−
AFP	+	—	—	3,055 (11)	3,067 (10)	3,035 (12)	2,471 (11)	1,900 (1)	4,290 (1)
AFP	−	—	1,600 (1)	1,740 (5)	2,362 (6)	—	1,895 (8)	—	1,045 (2)

Figures in parentheses are number of cases.

in each cytohistological grade of hepatoma, correlated to serum AFP and bile in the tumor. A total of 46 AFP-positive and 21 AFP-negative hepatoma cases were analyzed. Since Grade I and IV hepatomas were so small in number, only Grade II and III hepatomas were compared with serum AFP and bile in the tumor. Average liver weight of AFP-positive cases was above 3,000 g except for Grade III bile-negative cases, of which the average weight was 2,471 g. Average liver weight of AFP-negative cases was below 2,000 g except for Grade II bile-negative cases, where the average weight was 2,362 g. When bile-positive hepatoma cases are selected, it is the rule rather than the exception that AFP-positive cases are rapidly growing, large hepatomas and AFP-negative are slow growing, small hepatomas. Bile-negative hepatomas show no such correlation. There are a few exceptional cases, however, AFP was negative even when the liver was as large as 3,000 g in a Grade III bile-negative hepatoma. Also, AFP was positive even when the liver was as small as 1,000 g for Grade II bile-positive hepatoma.

Serum AFP Concentration and Bile in Each Cytohistological Grade of Hepatoma

In 28 cases quantitative determination of serum AFP was done. An average serum AFP concentration was then analyzed for each cytohistological grade, with

Table IV. Average Serum AFP Concentration (mg/dl) in Each Cytohistological Grade and Bile in Tumor

Grade	I		II		III		IV	
Bile	+	−	+	−	+	−	+	−
AFP +	—	—	54.4 (6)	13.2 (2)	76.2 (6)	44.9 (7)	18.5 (1)	51.1 (1)
AFP −	—	0.001 (1)	0.035 (2)	—	—	0.05 (2)	—	—

Figures in parentheses are number of cases.

consideration of the presence of bile in the hepatoma (Table IV). When Grade II and III hepatomas were compared, moderate to high serum AFP values were observed in bile-positive hepatoma and moderate to low serum AFP values were observed in bile-negative hepatoma. According to the cytohistological differentiation of hepatoma, Grade III hepatoma cases showed much higher AFP value than Grade II hepatoma in each bile-positive and bile-negative groups. The table also shows that the highest AFP value, on average, was found in bile-positive Grade III hepatoma, being 76.2 mg/dl. The second highest was observed in bile-positive Grade II hepatoma, 54.4 mg/dl. The third was in bile-negative Grade III hepatoma, 44.9 mg/dl, and the lowest average was in bile-negative Grade II hepatoma, 13.2 mg/dl. These findings indicate bile-positive correlated better to high AFP production, as well as high AFP-positive incidence, than to cytohistological grading.

CONCLUSIONS

The relation between serum AFP-positive cases (more than 1 mg/dl) and the cytohistological grading of hepatoma could not be ascertained absolutely in each individual case without exception, but, there is a definite tendency in each grade of tumor differentiation.

The incidence of AFP-positive cases as well as the quantitative value of serum AFP, is highest in poorly differentiated Grade III hepatoma cases, followed by moderately differentiated Grade II hepatoma. Well-differentiated Grade I and undifferentiated Grade IV hepatoma cases were poor AFP producers. This finding agrees with that of Purves *et al.* (*10*).

When bile-positive (producing and/or accumulating) hepatoma cases, which correspond to about half of the cases, are selected, they correlate better to AFP-positive than cytohistological grading, particularly in poorly differentiated Grade III hepatoma. Higher serum AFP values are expected in each cytohistological grade of hepatoma when bile is positive.

Finally, AFP production is highly related to rather poor differentiation of hepatoma with remaining functional differentiation of bile production.

REFERENCES

1. Abelev, G. I. α-Fetoprotein in ontogenesis and its association with malignant tumors. *Adv. Cancer Res.*, **14**, 295–358 (1971).
2. Bagshawe, A. and Parker, A. M. Age distribution of α-fetoprotein in hepatocellular carcinoma. *Lancet*, **2**, 268 (1970).
3. Edmondson, H. A. Tumor of the liver and intrahepatic bile ducts. *In* "Atlas of Tumor Pathology," Armed Forces Institute of Pathology, Washington, D. C., pp. 63–64 (1958).
4. Foli, A. K., Sherlock, S., and Adinolfi, M. Serum α-fetoprotein in patients with liver disease. *Lancet*, **2**, 1267–1269 (1969).
5. Hull, E. W., Carbone, P. P., Moertel, C. G., and O'Connor, G. T. Serum α-fetoprotein in the U.S.A. *Lancet*, **1**, 779–780 (1970).
6. Mancini, G., Carbonera, A. O., and Heremans, J. F. Immunochemical quantitation of antigens by single radial immunodiffusion. *Immunochemistry*, **2**, 235–254 (1965).
7. Mawas, C., Buffe, D., and Burtin, P. Influence of age on α-fetoprotein incidence. *Lancet*, **1**, 1292 (1970).
8. Nishi, S. Radioimmunoassay. 11th Symposium of Japanese Cancer Association, December 8, 1971.
9. Ouchterlony, O. Antigen-antibody reactions in gels. *Acta Pathol. Microbiol. Scand.*, **26**, 507–515 (1949).
10. Purves, L. R., Bersohn, I., and Geddes, E. W. Serum α-fetoprotein and primary cancer of the liver in man. *Cancer*, **25**, 1261–1270 (1970).
11. Sakurai, M. and Miyaji, T. A histopathological study on hepatoma and hepatoblastoma relating to fetal α-globulin production in autopsy cases. *Proc. Jap. Cancer Assoc., 30th Annu. Meet.*, 205 (1971).

EXPLANATION OF PHOTOS

PHOTO 1. Grade I (#8905). White. Well differentiated, thin trabecular. Eosinophilic cytoplasm with small nucleo-cytoplasmic (N/C) ratio. Almost no cellular atypism. AFP (−). < 0.001 mg/dl. Bile (−). H-E staining. × 20. (All photos are the same magnification).

PHOTO 2. Grade II (#8927). White. Moderately differentiated trabecular. Eosinophilic cytoplasm with small N/C ratio. Mild to moderate cellular atypism. AFP = 0.01 mg/dl. Bile (+).

PHOTO 3. Grade II (#8915). White. Moderately differentiated tubular. Eosinophilic cytoplasm with small N/C ratio. Mild cellular atypism. AFP = 0.06 mg/dl. Bile (++).

PHOTO 4. Grade II (#8961). Green. Moderately differentiated trabecular. Eosinophilic cytoplasm with small N/C ratio. Mild cellular atypism. AFP > 1 mg/dl. Bile (+++).

PHOTO 5. Grade II—III. The same case as in Photo 4, but different area. White. Moderate to poorly differentiated trabecular. Increased cellular atypism and N/C ratio as compared with Photo 4. Grade II majority.

PHOTO 6. Grade III (#T-256). Green. Moderate to poorly differentiated tubular. Small N/C ratio but less eosinophilic and some basophilic cytoplasm. Marked cellular atypism. AFP = 107 mg/dl. Bile (++).

PHOTO 7. Grade III (#8936). White. Moderate to poorly differentiated trabecular. Moderate N/C ratio. Less eosinophilic cytoplasm. Moderate tumor giant cells. AFP = 44 mg/dl. Bile (+).

PHOTO 8. Grade III (#9003). White. Poorly differentiated solid and trabecular. Markedly eosinophilic but increased N/C ratio. Many tumor giant cells. AFP = 0.0075 mg/dl. Bile (−).

PHOTO 9. Grade III (#T-250). White. Poorly differentiated solid. Moderately increased N/C ratio with more basophilic cytoplasm. AFP = 0.1 mg/dl. Bile (−).

PHOTO 10. Grade III (#T-242). White. Poorly differentiated trabecular. Monotonous but large N/C ratio. More basophilic cytoplasm. AFP = 82.8 mg/dl. Bile (−).

PHOTO 11. Grade IV (#9031). White. Undifferentiated embryonal type hepatoblastoma. Large N/C ratio and basophilic cytoplasm. AFP = 42.5 mg/dl. Bile (−).

PHOTO 12. Grade III (#9092). Green. Immunofluorescent study shows more and stronger luminescent cells than in Photo 13.

PHOTO 13. The same case as in Photo 12, but white area. Grade III. Histologically the same as in Photo 12, but no bile in this area. Less luminescent cells than in Photo 12.

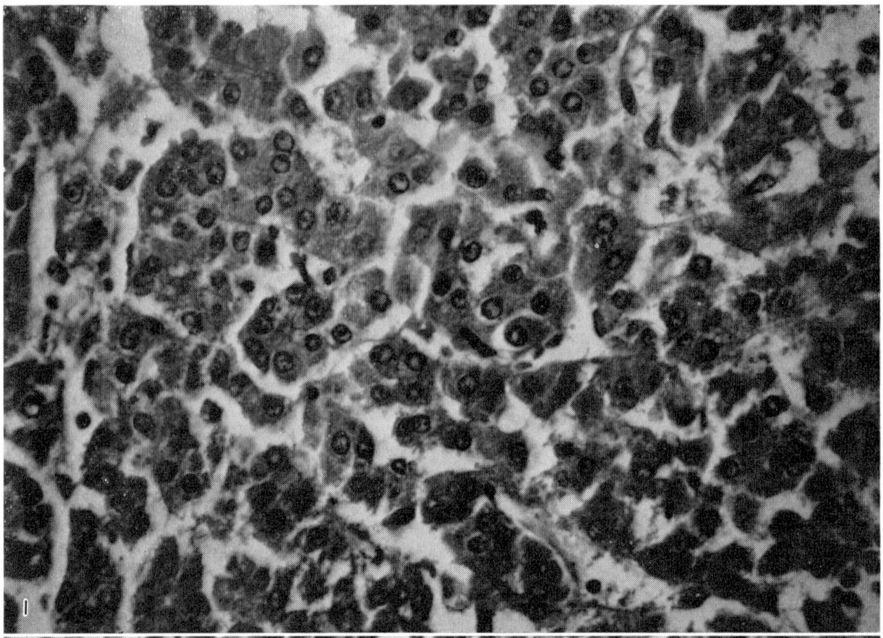
1

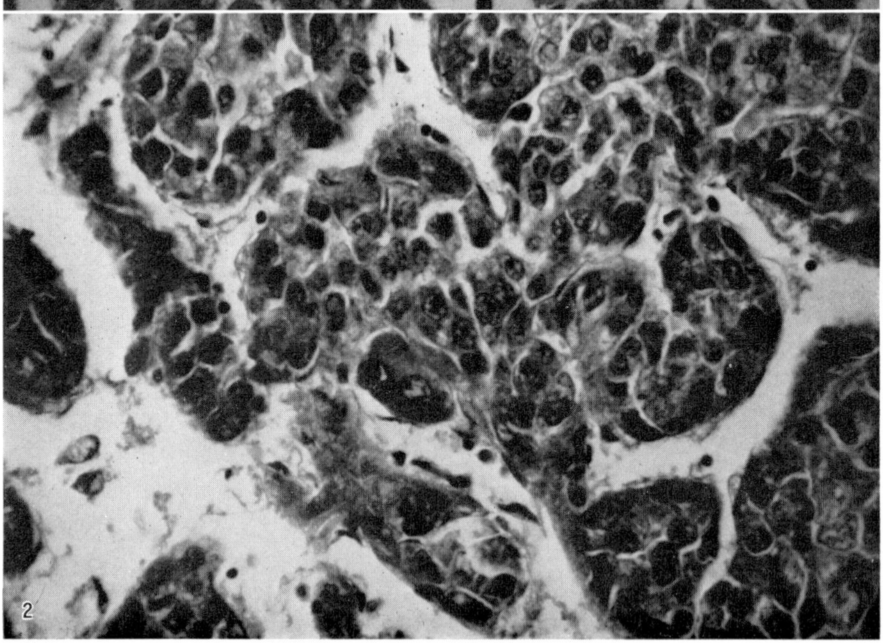
2

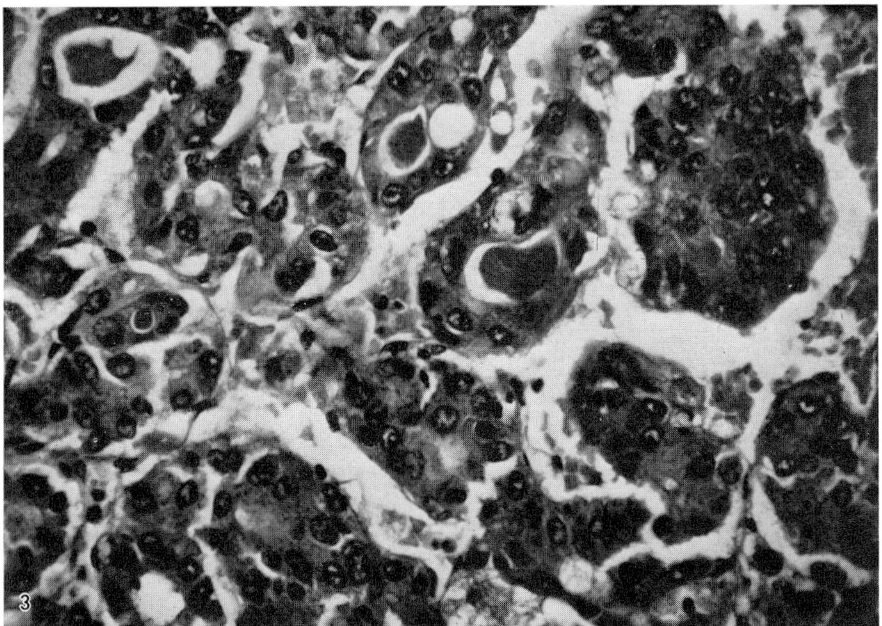

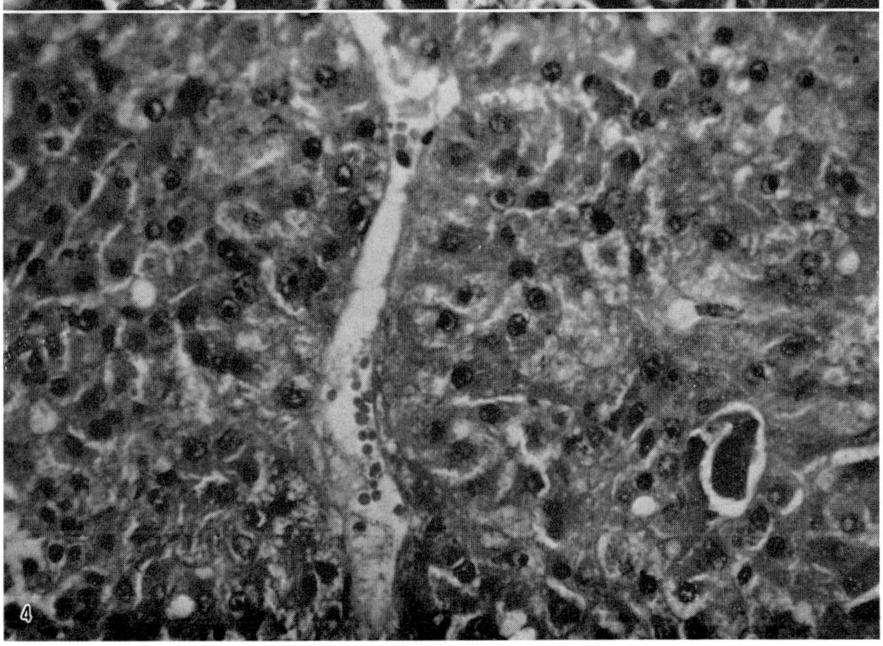

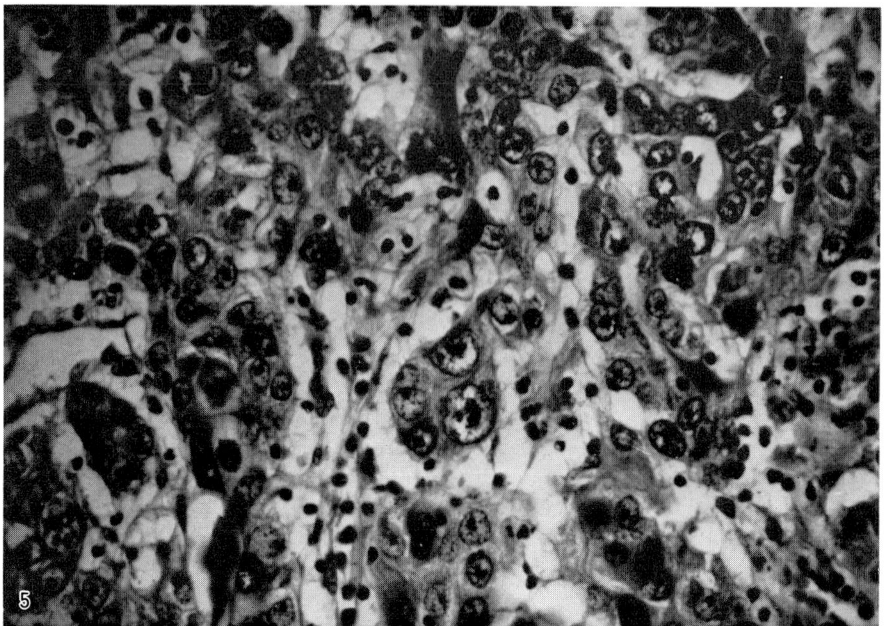

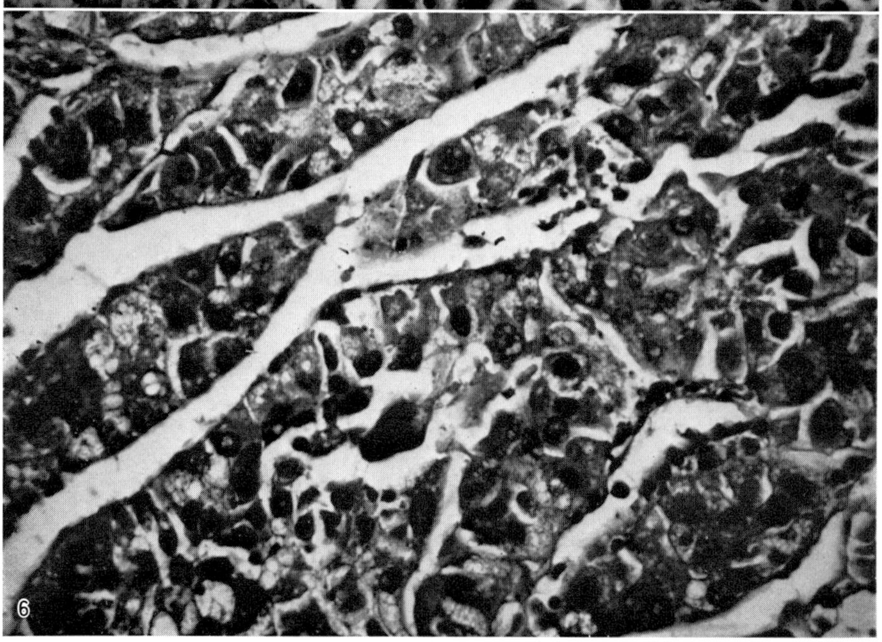

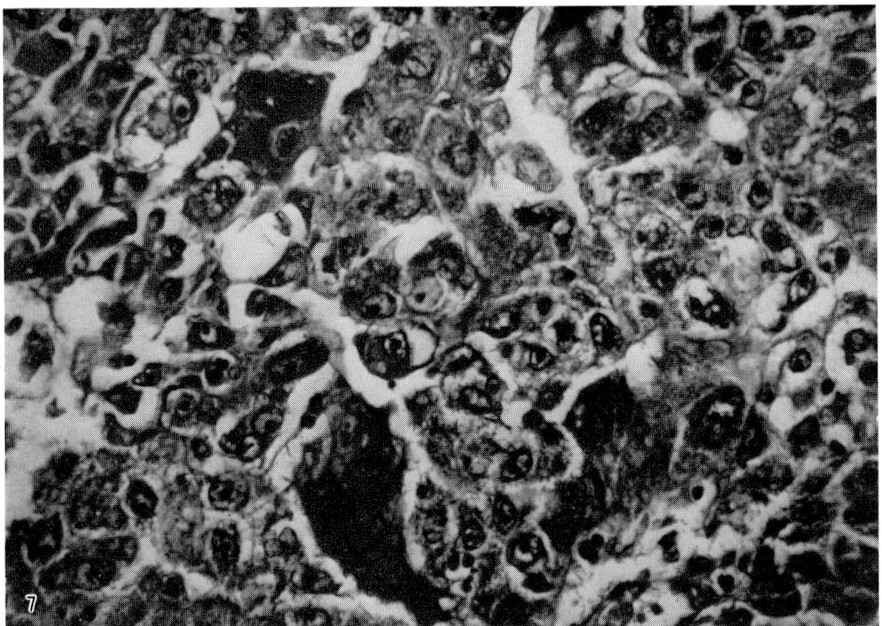
7

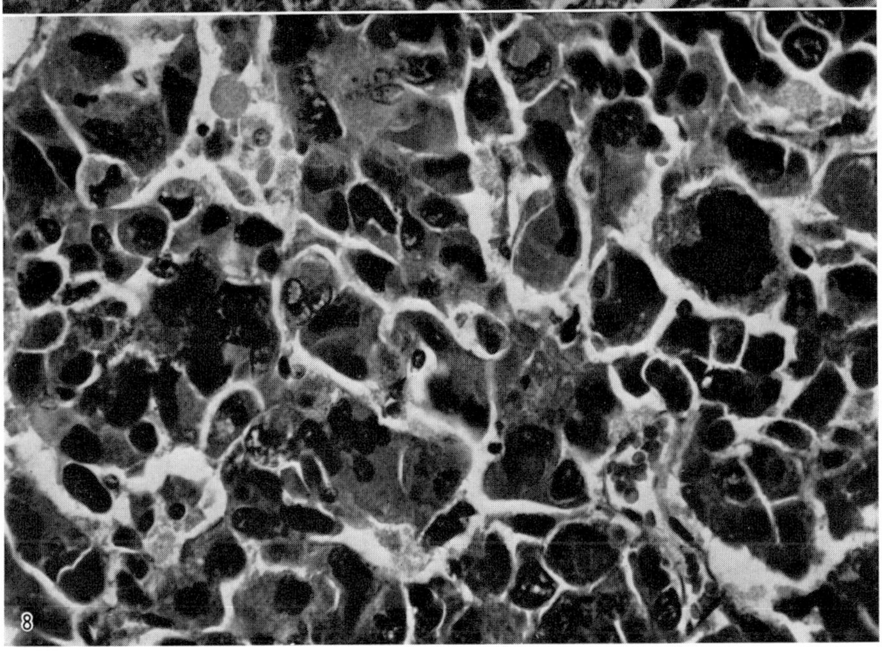
8

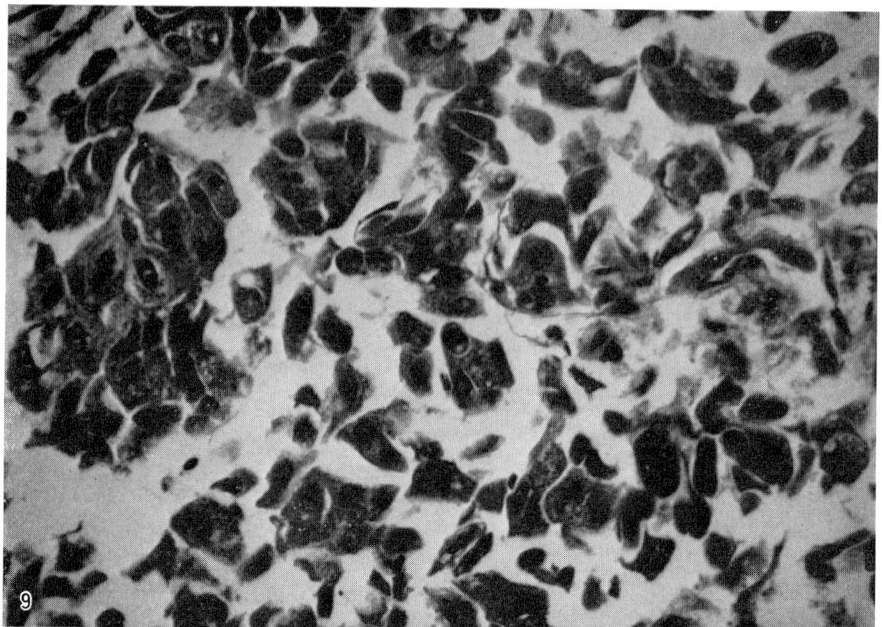
9

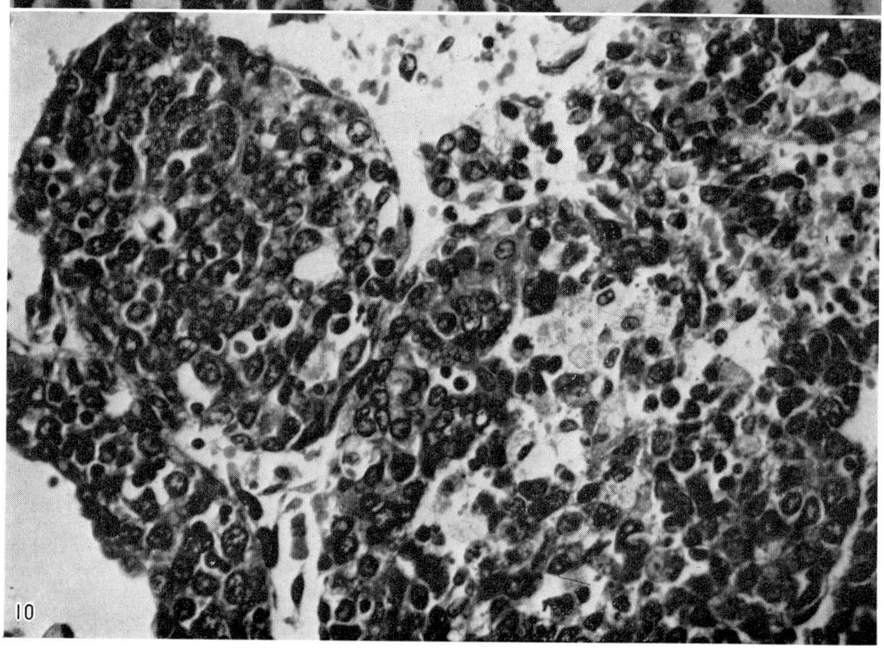
10

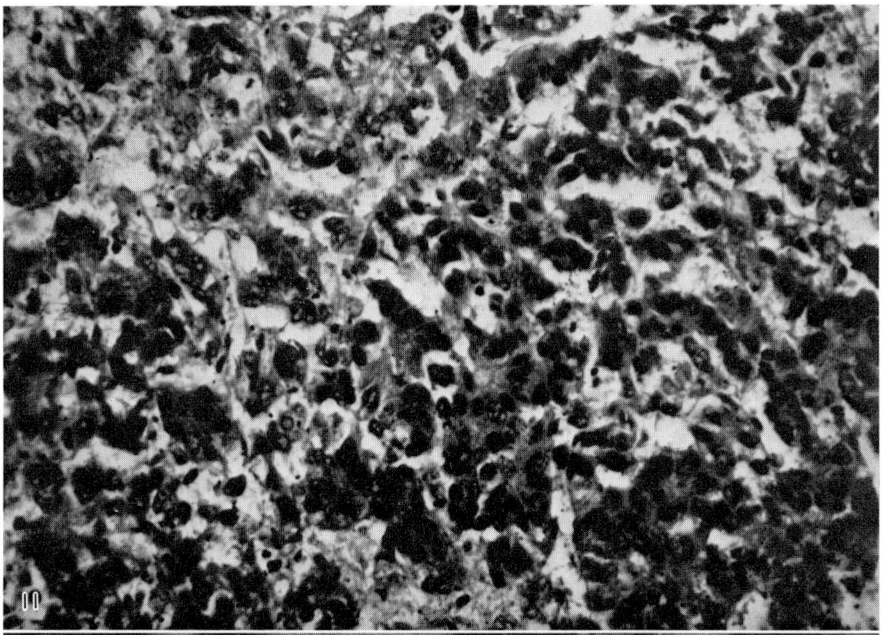
11

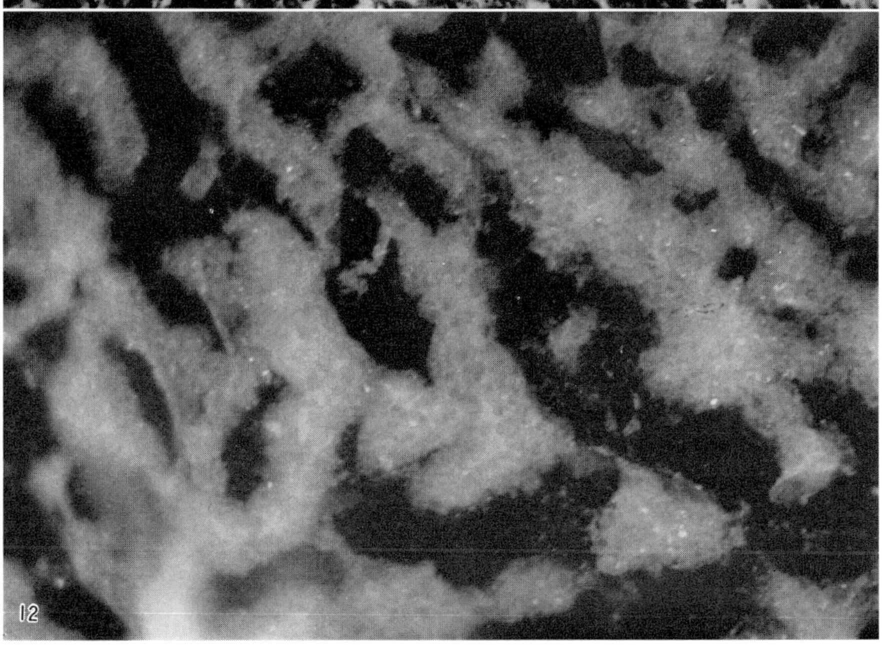
12

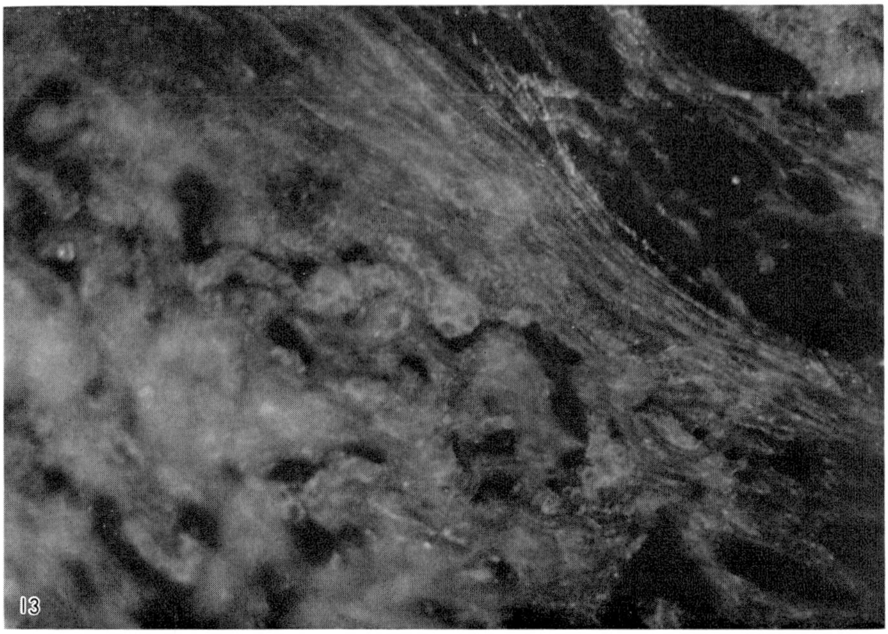
13

HISTOLOGY OF HEPATOMA IN MAN WITH REGARD TO α-FETOPROTEIN

Ken-ichi SASAKI,*[1] Akira MIYAKAWA,*[2] Michio MITO,*[3] and Yoichi KASAI*[3]

Central Clinical Laboratory, Hokkaido University Hospital,[1] *Central Clinical Laboratory, Tonan Hospital,*[2] *and Department of Surgery, School of Medicine, Hokkaido University*[3]

We examined 36 cases of hepatocellular carcinoma histologically in adults, and compared the histological features and serum α-fetoprotein (AFP) obtaining the results as follows: (1) There appeared to be a relation between cell abnormality and the quantity of AFP, *i.e.*, AFP-positive cases with primary hepatocellular carcinoma were seen in patients with every degree of differentiations of cancer, but the level tended to be higher in poorly differentiated cell population than in others. (2) Size of tumor may be one factor in AFP detectability. (3) Radioimmunoassay may be a valuable method for detecting early stages of primary hepatocellular carcinoma.

Tatarinov (*14*) and others (*1*, *10*, *11*, *15*) demonstrated the existence of α-fetoprotein (AFP) in the sera of hepatoma patients. However, the positivity rates were variable from 46 to 78%. Recently, Nishi (*8*) isolated and characterized a human fetal AFP from the sera of both fetuses and patients with hepatoma. Using pure AFP he introduced the radial immunodiffusion method and radioimmunoassay for the quantitative analysis of serum AFP. We have studied the histological features and their relation to the occurrence of AFP in patients with primary hepatoma. This article deals with the above relationship and presents some findings for clinical use.

Histological Examination

A total of 36 autopsy cases and surgical materials from hepatocellular carcinoma were selected and their histological features and serum AFP were examined. These 36 cases were composed of 30 males and 6 females. The age of these patients ranged from 27 to 68 years old. For examination of the histological features, the size of the nucleus, the amount and acidophilic quality of tumor cells, evidence of cell function, for example, bile formation, fatty degeneration, and others, *i.e.*, necrosis, vascularity and fibrous proliferation, were checked.

*[1] Kita-15-jo, Nishi-7-chome, Kita-ku, Sapporo 060, Japan (佐々木憲一).
*[2] Kita-1-jo, Nishi-6-chome, Kita-ku, Sapporo 060, Japan (宮川　明).
*[3] Kita-15-jo, Nishi-7-chome, Kita-ku, Sapporo 060, Japan (水戸廸郎, 葛西洋一).

Next, we made histological gradings after Edmondson and Steiner (*2*). Although that classification was mainly based on cytological abnormality as compared with normal liver cells, we also took the cellularity and architecture into consideration for grading. Grade I: Reserved for certain areas in Grade II carcinomas. Nuclei were small and round, cytoplasm was rich, and cohesive qualities were thin trabecular. Grade II: Nuclei were larger and more hyperchromatic, but the cytoplasm was abundant and acidophilic. The cell borders were often sharp and clear-cut. Architecture consisted of a thin or several cell-layered trabecular pattern. The lumina often contained a small amount of protein precipitate, and sometimes bile. Grade III: Nuclei were usually larger and more hyperchromatic than those of Grade II carcinomas. These nuclei occupied a relatively greater proportion of the cell. The cytoplasm was granular and acidophilic, as in Grade II, but it was usually less marked. Giant tumor cells were most numerous in this group. In general, there were 3 kinds of giant cells, (1) a large, solitary nucleus, (2) a multilobed nucleus, and (3) multinuclei, ranging from 4 to more than 10. Grade IV: The nuclei were intensely hyperchromatic and occupied a greater part of the cell. The cytoplasm was variable in amount, and often scanty. Cohesiveness was also variable: Some parts were medullary and some lost the trabecular pattern, and sometimes fibrous proliferation was widespread. The latter cases might be classified by Mori (*7*) in his third group.

The histological grading was done by considering the predominant feature of each tumor, based on the criteria described above. The histological features of hepatocellular carcinoma are variable, especially in advanced cases. Histological grading after Edmondson and Steiner was carried out in each case and the numbers of each grade are shown in Table I. As seen in the table most cases were included in Grade II or III.

TABLE I. Histological Grading of 36 Hepatoma Cases

Grade	No. of cases
Grade I+II	1
Grade II	16
Grade II+III	5
Grade III	8
Grade III+IV	3
Grade IV	3
Total	36

Quantitative Immunoassay of Serum AFP

The Ouchterlony immunodiffusion method was used to detect AFP in serum, and radial immunodiffusion (Mancini) for quantitative assay of AFP. The sera of negative cases assayed by the Ouchterlony immunodiffusion method were further quantitatively examined by radioimmunoassay. All these assays were carried out by Dr. Nishi at the Department of Biochemistry, School of Medicine, Hokkaido University.

In 23 cases in 36 hepatoma patients AFP was detected in sera by the Ouchterlony immunodiffusion method. The remaining 13 cases were negative by this method. Quantities of AFP in sera assayed by radial immunodiffusion (Mancini) were variable, ranging from 1.0 to 187.5 mg/dl.

By radioimmunoassay, more than 500 ng/ml AFP was detected in 4 of the 13 Ouchterlony-negative cases. One case (male, 65 years old) was assayed as 173 ng/ml in serum at the time of the operation, but later showed positive results by the micro-Ouchterlony immunodiffusion method at autopsy. However, 6 cases were assayed as containing negligible amounts of AFP (less than 20 ng/ml) even by radioimmunoassay.

Correlation between Histological Grade and AFP

We compared the histological grade with the quantity of AFP, as shown in Fig. 1. The AFP-positive cases (more than 500 ng/ml, *i.e.*, 0.05 mg/dl, values less than 500 ng/ml were frequently encountered in hepatitis, cirrhosis, *etc.*) were seen for Grade II, Grade III, and Grade IV. However, cases of Grade III showed AFP in every serum in our series and higher values (up to 187.5 mg/dl) than other grades. In the AFP-positive cases detected by radioimmunoassay, focal lesions were small and circumscribed and contained necrotic features.

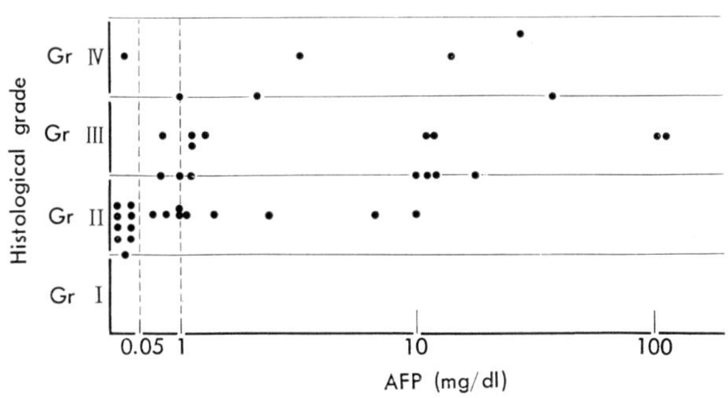

FIG. 1. Histological grade and quantity of AFP in sera

The AFP-negative cases, even by radioimmunoassay, were mostly found in the differentiated type of hepatocellular carcinoma, and only one was found in undifferentiated cases in our series.

These results suggested some relationship between the histological features and the positivity of AFP in sera of hepatoma patients, and indicated that relatively poorly differentiated cell populations of hepatocellular carcinoma might mainly produce this protein. Although there were non-AFP producing hepatoma cases, there might be some relation between the amount of tumor cells without necrosis and necrobiosis and AFP-positive results.

Although most of our cases were of advanced hepatoma, we would like to point out that some of the radioimmunologically positive cases were small enough for satisfactory surgical indication.

DISCUSSION

Gitlin and Boesman reported that the synthesizing site of AFP seemed to be in embryonal liver cells, based on studies using ^{14}C-labeled amino acids. It had been speculated that AFP detected in hepatoma patients might be synthesized in the tumor cells.

Recently, Takahashi *et al.* (*12*, *13*) and Engelhardt *et al.* (*4*) demonstrated by the immunofluorescence technique that AFP existed in the cytoplasm of hepatoma cells. These results were similar, *i.e.*, immunofluorescence appeared in variable portions of the tumor. Takahashi reported that immunofluorescence appeared bandlike or spotlike in the tumor parenchyma. Engelhardt showed that immunofluorescence was observed in the parenchymal cells surrounding the vascular spaces. These observations suggest that synthesis of AFP might be performed in the same way as albumin synthesis, because of the similarity of molecular weight and physicochemical characteristics. The difference of AFP localization in each cell or portion of the tumor is understood in terms of the synthesizing phase in each cell or the biological activity.

It was not so clear whether the amount of tumor influenced the quantity of serum AFP or not, because most cases in our study and in those of other researchers were advanced hepatoma patients. However, in our series several cases of circumscribed lesions were found. These cases were negative by Ouchterlony immunodiffusion, but were detected by radioimmunoassay.

Endo (*3*) reported that anaplastic type hepatoma cases showed higher quantities of AFP than others. Purves *et al.* (*9*) and Takahashi *et al.* (*12*) suggested that poorly differentiated types would be higher. Our results were similar to those of Purves and Takahashi. Although positive cases were seen in well-differentiated, poorly differentiated, and undifferentiated types of hepatocellular carcinoma, a higher number of cases was observed in the undifferentiated type. Cell population of the tumor might be one important factor in AFP synthesis.

Some reported that AFP-positive cases were seen in gastric cancer and other cancers (*5*). These cases were accompanied by massive liver metastasis. It is not clear whether these tumors synthesize the protein by themselves or whether reactive cells in the liver produce it.

Hirai *et al.* (*16*) reported that AFP was detected in 2 phases in DAB-hepatocarcinogenesis in rats, where the 1st phase corresponds to 3 to 10 weeks' administration of DAB, and the 2nd phase to more than 13 weeks' administration. In the 1st phase, extensive oval cell proliferation was observed in the liver parenchyma of animals. This finding was quite interesting as a precancerous phenomenon, and it may be concerned with the detection of AFP in metastatic liver carcinoma. However, these possibilities have not been fully investigated yet.

Recently, Miyakawa and Kudo (*6*) examined the histochemical differences among hepatoma, liver cirrhosis, and fulminant hepatitis. They observed that the activity of succinic dehydrogenase showed a marked decline in all of them. However, the activity of lactic dehydrogenase decreased in hepatoma, but in cirrhosis and fulminant hepatitis it was almost normal. Regarding alkaline phosphatase, activity showed a marked decrease in hepatoma, but it increased in cirrhosis and fulminant hepatitis. The activity of acid phosphatase increased but in hepatoma and cirrhosis, it decreased markedly in fulminant hepatitis. These results suggest some possibilities that the effects may be related.

Acknowledgments

The authors thank Dr. S. Nishi and Prof. H. Hirai, Department of Biochemistry, School of Medicine, Hokkaido University, for their cooperation in determination of AFP.

REFERENCES

1. Alpert, M. E., Uriel, J., and de Nechaud, B. α-Fetoglobulin in the diagnosis of human hepatoma. *New Engl. J. Med.*, **278**, 984–986 (1968).
2. Edmondson, H. A. and Steiner, P. E. Primary carcinoma of the liver: A study of 100 cases among 48,900 necropsies. *Cancer*, **7**, 462–503 (1954).
3. Endo, Y. Diagnosis of primary hepatoma by detection of serum α_1-fetoprotein (in Japanese). *Igaku-no-Ayumi (The Stride of Medicine)*, **68**, 519–520 (1969).
4. Engelhardt, N. V., Gusev, A. I., Shipova, L. Ja., and Abelev, G. I. Immunofluorescence study of α-fetoprotein in liver and liver tumors. I. Technique of AFP localization in tissue sections. *Int. J. Cancer*, **7**, 198–206 (1971).
5. Kitaoka, H., Hattori, S., and Mukojima, T. Fetoprotein and metastatic hepatoma. Relation to gastric cancer (in Japanese). *Igaku-no-Ayumi (The Stride of Medicine)*, **79**, 129–130 (1971).
6. Miyakawa, A. and Kudo, M. Some histochemical studies of hepatoma, *Lab. Clin. Conf.*, **3**, 2–7 (1972).
7. Mori, W. A study on the metastasis of hepatoma. *Transac. Soc. Pathol. Japan*, **45**, 224–236 (1956).
8. Nishi, S. Isolation and characterization of a human fetal α-globulin from the sera of fetuses and a hepatoma patient. *Cancer Res.*, **30**, 2507–2513 (1970).
9. Purves, L. R., Bersohn, I., and Geddes, E. W. Serum α-fetoprotein and primary cancer of the liver in man. *Cancer*, **25**, 1261–1270 (1970).
10. Purves, L. R., Machab, M., and Bersohn, I. Serum α-fetoprotein. I. Immunodiffusion and immunoassay results in cases of primary cancer of the liver. *S. Afr. Med. J.*, **42**, 1138–1141 (1968).
11. Smith, J. B. and Todd, D. Fetoglobulin and primary liver cancer. *Lancet*, **2**, 833 (1968).
12. Takahashi, M., Kawaguchi, A., Yasuma, T., Yanaka, M., and Kawamata, K. α-Fetoprotein by immunodiffusion and immunofluorescence and its histopathological background. *Med. Postgraduates*, **9**, 249–260 (1971).
13. Takahashi, M., Yanaka, M., and Kawaguchi, A. The diagnosis of hepatoma cells by anti-α-fetoprotein immunofluorescence. *Med. Postgraduates*, **8**, 202–204 (1970).
14. Tatarinov, Y. S. Content of embryo-specific α-globulin in fetal and neonatal sera and sera from adult humans with primary carcinoma of the liver. *Fed. Proc.*, **25**, 344–346 (1966).
15. Uriel, J. Annual Report, International Agency for Research on Cancer, Lyon, France, p. 47 (1968).
16. Watabe, H., Nishi, S., and Hirai, H. Fetal α_f-globulin and hepatoma (in Japanese). *Nippon Rinsho (Jap. J. Clin. Med.)*, **29**, Suppl. 212–217 (1971).

IMMUNOFLUORESCENCE STUDIES ON α-FETOPROTEIN IN HEPATOMA TISSUE

Mikio NISHIOKA,[*1] Takayoshi IBATA,[*1] Kaoru MIYAZATO,[*1] Kiwami OKITA,[*1] Kyozo HIRONAGA,[*2] and Teruo FUJITA[*1]

First Division, Internal Medicine, Yamaguchi University School of Medicine,[*1] *and Pharmacy Department, Yamaguchi University School of Medicine*[*2]

The immunofluorescence technique, involving fixation in 95% ethanol containing 1% glacial acetic acid, followed by embedding in paraffin, seems to be the most suitable for detecting AFP in tissue. α-Fetoprotein (AFP) in tumor cells was localized in the following 3 areas: (a) cytoplasm, (b) cytoplasmic membrane, and (c) perinuclear zone. The distribution of tumor cells containing AFP varied with the case and the specimen, and the number of these staining cells was one-fifth or less of the total. α-Fetoprotein was sometimes found in the cytoplasm of Kupffer cells but was absent in connective tissues, bile ducts, and normal hepatic cells.

Fluoroelectroimmunodiffusion was at least 30 times as sensitive as the Ouchterlony technique for the detection of serum AFP, and its great sensitivity elicited a positive reaction in sera previously found to be negative by the Ouchterlony technique.

α-Fetoprotein was detected in 33 of 37 patients (89%) with histologically confirmed primary hepatocellular carcinoma. α-Fetoprotein was also detected in 4 of 71 patients with carcinoma of the liver metastasized from the stomach. Even a patient with gastric carcinoma had AFP in his serum. Serum AFP levels were lower in these patients than in those with primary hepatocellular carcinoma.

α-Fetoprotein was present in only 1 of 31 patients with infectious hepatitis and in 5 of 195 patients with liver cirrhosis, which indicates significant possibilities for establishing the early diagnosis and treatment of primary liver carcinoma.

Since Abelev *et al.* (*2*, *3*) reported that transplantable mouse and rat hepatomas synthesize and secrete into the blood an embryo-specific α_1-globulin, and Tatarinov (*37*) confirmed the presence of α-fetoprotein (AFP) in sera from patients with primary liver carcinoma, the procedure for immunological detection of AFP in serum has been of great clinical value for the diagnosis of primary liver carcinoma. The reappearance of embryo-specific protein in primary liver car-

[*1,*2] 1,144 Kogushi, Ube 755, Japan (西岡幹夫, 井端孝義, 宮里　薫, 沖田　極, 弘長恭三, 藤田輝雄).

cinoma and the significance of this protein in relation to the malignant process have been the subject of extensive investigations (*3*, *15*, *35*). α-Fetoprotein is known to be synthesized by the fetal liver of rat and man (*11*, *38*, *39*). In patients with primary liver carcinoma, AFP seems to be the product of the tumor cell itself, but direct evidence has been lacking. However, several recent investigators (*9*, *25*, *34*) have succeeded in detecting AFP in hepatoma tissues by the immunofluorescence technique.

This article describes the difficulties in the demonstration of AFP in tissue, the contribution of immunofluorescence studies on AFP to further understanding of primary liver carcinoma, and the results of AFP tests during the past 4 years.

Problems in the Demonstration of AFP in Tissues

The main difficulty in the demonstration of AFP in tissues is due to different concentrations of AFP in the tumor cells. The concentration of AFP differs with each case, and even within the tumor itself there are different concentrations. For this reason, the indirect immunofluorescence technique has been used recently in our laboratory (*25*). This procedure is estimated to be more sensitive than the direct immunofluorescence technique and is suitable for detecting a small amount of AFP in tissues, by the application of antiserum diluted as much as possible. The application of diluted antiserum to AFP also resolved an additional source of nonspecific staining. However, in order to distinguish staining due to specific immunological reaction from nonspecific staining, many control stainings are required in the indirect immunofluorescence technique, using unconjugated immune sera as the middle layer.

An additional important point is to prepare a very potent, monospecific anti-AFP antiserum. To obtain a good supply of anti-AFP antiserum, rabbits were immunized with a supernatant (soluble in 34% saturated ammonium sulfate) of serum from a patient with primary liver carcinoma (*24*). The rabbit antiserum was absorbed first with normal human sera, then twice with mouse liver powder, and finally once with human liver homogenate to remove nonspecific materials. The absorbed antiserum formed a single precipitin line against a saline extract of fetus in the α_1-globulin region and an identical precipitin line with the patient's sera (Fig. 1). This anti-AFP antiserum was suitable for detecting AFP in tissue because of the complete absence of fluorescence in normal liver cells (Photo 1). The preparation of purified AFP antibody by the glutaraldehyde immunoadsorbent technique may be also suitable, as reported by Engelhardt *et al.* (*9*).

In the preparation of materials for the immunofluorescence study of AFP, an attempt was made to use the methods of Hamashima *et al.* (*13*) and Sainte-Marie (*33*), involving fixation in 95% ethanol containing 1% of glacial acetic acid, followed by embedding in paraffin, since AFP had an isoelectric pH of 4.7, almost the same as that of albumin (*21*). This procedure seems to be the most suitable for detecting AFP in tissues. As judged by the complete absence of fluorescence in cell nuclei and connective tissue, the convenient paraffin embeddings could be utilized in the preparation of sections for detecting AFP without solubilization of AFP in tissue or destroying their antigenicity (Photo 2). The superiority of

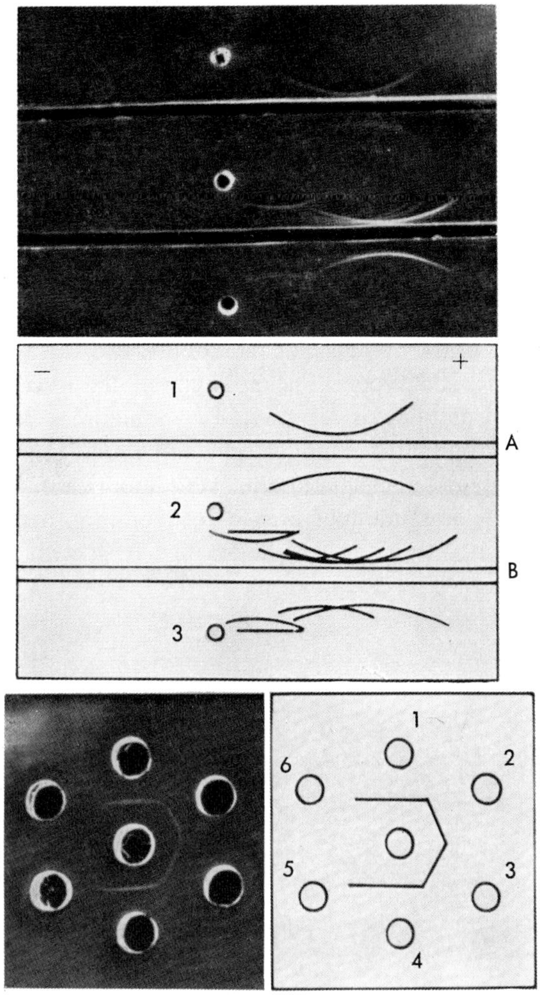

FIG. 1 (Top): Immunoelectrophoretic patterns of serum from patient with primary liver carcinoma (1), supernatant (soluble in 34% saturated ammonium sulfate) of serum (2), and of normal adult serum (3)

The lower trough contained antiserum (B) and the upper trough antiserum-absorbed by normal adult serum (A).

(Bottom): Double immunodiffusion in agar gel of the tissue extracts of fetus (1), supernatant (soluble in 34% saturated ammonium sulfate) of serum (2), patients' sera (3, 4), normal adult serum (5), and normal saline solution (6)

The center well contained absorbed antiserum.

paraffin embedding has also been confirmed by Engelhardt *et al.* (*9*). Recently Smith *et al.* (*34*) and Purtilo and Yunis (*31*) demonstrated the presence of AFP in unfixed tissue of hepatoma using the indirect immunofluorescence technique. To determine the most successful fixation method, some tissue were frozen in our laboratory (*25*) by putting them into test tubes placed in a Dry Ice-alcohol mixture at −70°. The frozen sections were cut in a cryostat at −20°. However, the frozen sections were not always suitable for detecting AFP in tissue. Difficulty was experienced in the fixation of AFP in the tissues and in washing out nonspecific conjugations.

Localization of AFP in Hepatoma Tissues

It is important to determine whether AFP is present in all tumor cells or only in particular cells and to determine its location in the cells. We have applied the indirect immunofluorescence technique in 41 autopsy specimens obtained from 10 patients with primary hepatocellular carcinoma. Fluorescence of tumor cells was found to be localized in the following 3 forms: (a) diffuse, finely granular fluorescence of the cytoplasm, (b) fluorescent line of the cytoplasmic membranes, and (c) brightly fluorescent line of the perinuclear zones (Photos 2–5). The first type was the most common. Fluorescence was in many cases found in cytoplasma as well as in the cytoplasmic membrane, and the 1st type was undistinguishable from the 2nd type. The 3rd type of fluorescence was seen in 2 patients with a small amount of serum AFP. Sometimes fluorescent granules were found in the cytoplasm of Kupffer cells and round cells, but neither connective tissues, bile ducts, nor hepatic cells were fluorescent.

Specificity of the immunofluorescence reaction was demonstrated by the negative results obtained by treatment of purified AFP with preimmune rabbit

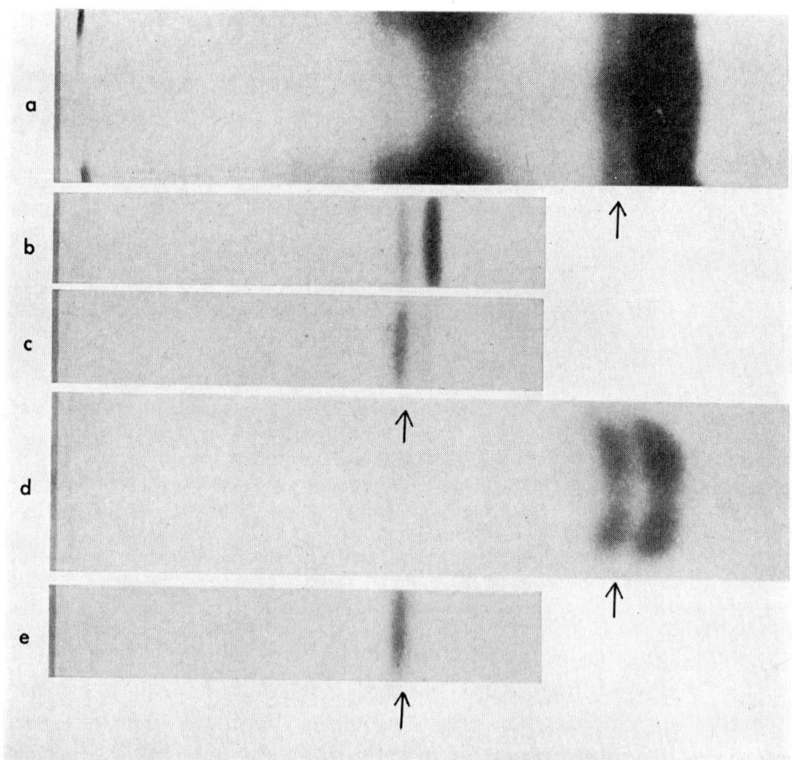

FIG. 2. Polyacrylamide gel electrophoresis of extract of fetal tissue run on a preparative disc electrophoresis gel and the preparation obtained

Arrows indicate AFP (a, d). A singe peak (e) appeared in the α_1-globulin region when the preparative fraction obtained was separated by polyacrylamide gel electrophoresis (b, c).

serum or with anti-AFP antiserum before staining with FITC*-labeled goat antiserum to rabbit γ-globulin. The purified AFP was obtained from fetal tissues by preparative disc electrophoresis (*36*) after Ornstein and Davis (*29*) (Fig. 2). Direct staining of the sections with labeled antiserum to rabbit γ-globulin was also nonreactive.

The distribution of tumor cells containing AFP varied with the case and the specimen. Sometimes there was a mass of tumor cells containing AFP (Photo 5), but the overall average of tumor cells containing AFP was one-fifth or less of the total. This strongly suggests that AFP is not a structural component or a marker of tumor cells.

Whether or not these localizations represent sites of active synthesis cannot be determined. We suggest that the tumor cells showing diffuse, finely granular fluorescence of the cytoplasm synthesize AFP, because the pattern of localization of AFP in the cytoplasm of these cells is similar to that in the cytoplasm of fetal liver, which is known to produce AFP (Photo 6). The distribution of these tumor cells is even throughout the hepatoma tissues. Interesting results have been reported by Engelhardt *et al.* (*9*), who used the direct immunofluorescence technique to detect AFP in hepatoma tissues. In their investigations, specific AFP localization was observed in a small number of tumor cells near the capillaries and blood vessels. They suggested that these cells were synthesizing AFP. Although we could not obtain similar findings, further observations are necessary for the understanding of AFP synthesis in tumor cells.

Histological Features of Tumor Cells Containing AFP

No information is available regarding the differentiating histological characteristics of tumor cells containing AFP in comparison with those not containing AFP. In one case of Grade III hepatocellular carcinoma, diffuse, finely granular fluorescence was sometimes seen in the acidophilic cytoplasm of giant cells with a large nucleus, but fluorescence was also found in other tumor cells. We found a differentiating histological characteristic of the tumor cells in only one case, which contained a small amount of serum AFP. AFP was present in the perinuclear zone of the tumor cells. Their nuclei were larger and more hyperchromic than those of tumor cells containing no AFP and occupied a greater portion of the tumor cell. The reason for this particular localization of AFP is unclear. If AFP was synthesized in these cells and secreted into the blood, AFP synthesis might depend on the state of undifferentiation of the tumor cells. This hypothesis is also supported by the observation that diffuse, finely granular fluorescence was seen in the acidophilic cytoplasm of giant tumor cells from a patient with Grade III carcinoma, as described above.

It is virtually impossible to find any difference between the histological features of tumor cells containing AFP and those not containing it. Similar difficulty was observed in fluorescence studies on fetal liver. Whether the tumor cells not containing AFP, although morphologically similar to those containing

* FITC: Fluorescein isothiocyanate.

AFP, cannot synthesize AFP, simply have not started synthesis or have completed their synthesis phase, is not yet determined.

Relationship between Fluorescence and Serum AFP Levels

There was no correlation between the levels of serum AFP and the occurrence of fluorescence in the tumor cells, except that widespread fluorescence in the cytoplasm appeared to be more frequent in one patient with high levels of AFP and that perinuclear fluorescence of the tumor cells was found in one patient with a small amount of serum AFP. Table I presents the appearance of fluorescence, serum AFP levels, and the histological gradings of primary liver carcinoma. The

TABLE I. Relationship between Localization of AFP and Levels of Serum AFP or Histological Gradings of Primary Hepatocellular Carcinoma

Patient			Histological		Serum AFP level	Fluorescence of tumor cells		
Name	Sex	Age (yrs.)	Grade	Findings	(mg/100 ml)	Cytoplasm	Cytoplasmic membrane	Perinuclear zone
J.W.	Male	61	IV	anap.	26	+	+	−
S.M.	Male	74	IV	anap.	Trace	−	−	−
Y.N.	Male	39	III	trab.	121	⧻	+	−
S.K.	Male	61	III	trab.	2.7	+	+	+
S.H.	Female	56	II	tubul.	24.0	⧻	+	−
T.N.	Male	29	II	trab.	13.0	+	+	−
Y.Y.	Female	50	II	trab.	6.0	+	±	−
K.Y.	Male	63	II	trab.	1.6	+	−	−
H.H.	Male	56	II	trab.	Trace	+	−	−
T.D.	Male	51	II	trab.	0.5	−	±	++

anap.: anaplasia. trab.: trabecular. tubul.: tubular.
− no fluorescence. ± equivocal fluorescence. ⧻ widespread fluorescence.

TABLE II. Concentration of AFP in Tissue Extracts from Patients with Primary Liver Carcinoma

	Concentration of protein[a] (mg/ml)	Concentration of AFP (mg/100 ml)	Percentage of AFP in tissue (protein mg/g)
Liver			
Tumor tissue	29.9	7.0	2.4
Necrotic tissue	9.0	6.8	7.6
Cirrhotic tissue	48.3	3.3	0.7
Lung	8.0	3.3	4.1
Kidney	20.3	4.6	2.2
Spleen	38.4	1.7	0.4
Intestine	18.3	1.5	0.8
Serum	68.7	121.0	17.6
Ascites	36.3	49.0	10.7

[a] The concentration of protein in tissue extracts was determined by the method of Warburg and Christian.

classification of Edmondson and Steiner (*7*) was used for the histological gradings of primary liver carcinoma. The concentrations of serum AFP were determined by single radial immunodiffusion with anti-AFP antiserum and 1.5% agar (Difco Specific Noble) in Veronal buffer at pH 8.6, with an ionic strength of 0.07. The AFP level of the standard serum was determined by planimetry of scans obtained by polyacrylamide gel electrophoresis of the serum of patients with primary liver carcinoma (*23*). Serum AFP was detected in 8 of 10 patients with primary liver carcinoma by single radial immunodiffusion. In 2 patients, in whom serum AFP could not be detected by single radial immunodiffusion, a trace of AFP was detected in their sera by fluoroelectroimmunodiffusion (*18*, *26*). In this procedure, based on the immunoelectrosyneresis of Bussard and Huet (*6*), following immunoelectrosyneresis in agar gel, FITC-labeled antiserum to rabbit γ-globulin was placed in the anode well, and electrophoresis was performed under the same conditions as immunoelectrosyneresis. This technique permits the detection of 0.05 mg AFP per 100 ml serum (*26*). Nine of 10 patients having AFP in their sera had specific fluorescence in the tumor cells. Even the patient with only a trace of serum AFP, undetectable by single radial immunodiffusion, had bright fluorescence in the tumor cells, which suggests that the immunofluorescence technique is more sensitive for the detection of AFP than precipitin tests. However, this inference seems contradictory to the report of Gusev *et al.* (*12*), who found no AFP in tumor cells obtained from 2 patients with low levels of serum AFP. The reason for these differences is not clear at the moment. We believe that anti-AFP antiserum should be diluted as much as possible for the detection of small amounts of AFP in hepatoma tissues using the indirect immunofluorescence technique; also, specimens should be obtained from various parts of the hepatoma material. This principle has been observed throughout our studies.

α-Fetoprotein was detected in several tissue extracts obtained from patients with primary liver carcinoma, as reported by Houstek *et al.* (*14*). As shown in Table II, higher concentrations of AFP were detected in hepatoma tissue, lung, and kidney. However, body fluids such as blood and ascites had the highest AFP level when AFP levels per 1 g of tissue protein were calculated. This suggests that tumor cells rapidly secrete AFP into the serum after synthesizing it. For this reason, it may be difficult to form a clear correlation between the levels of serum AFP and the occurrence of AFP in the tumor cells.

Relationship between Fluorescence and the Histological Gradings of Primary Liver Carcinoma

The production of AFP by experimental hepatomas was correlated with the degree of malignancy and the rapid growth of a hepatoma (*2*, *3*), but there is no clinical evidence to support these findings. The presence and level of AFP in the serum do not seem to be correlated with the degree of differentiation of the tumor or the size of the tumor in human materials. Table I presents the relationship between fluorescence and the histological gradings of primary liver carcinoma. Six patients had a histological diagnosis of Grade II carcinoma, 2 patients had Grade III, and 2 had Grade IV. Diffuse, finely granular fluores-

TABLE III. Result of AFP Test in Malignant Tumors

Diagnosis	No. of cases	No. of positive test
Hepatocellular carcinoma	37	33 (89%)
Cholangiocellular carcinoma	2	0
Metastatic liver carcinoma	71	4 (5%)
Carcinoma of esophagus	2	0
Carcinoma of stomach	15	1
Carcinoma of colon	2	0
Carcinoma of rectum	3	0
Carcinoma of lung	6	0
Carcinoma of cholecyst	1	0
Carcinoma of pancreas	3	0
Carcinoma of kidney	2	0
Carcinoma of ovary	3	1
Carcinoma of testis	3	0
Reticulosarcoma	3	0
Hodgkin's disease	3	0
Leukemia	6	0

cence of the cytoplasm of tumor cells appeared to be more common in both Grade II and Grade III carcinomas. In undifferentiated hepatoma, with a histological grading of Grade IV, widespread fluorescence of the tumor cells appeared to be less frequent. Therefore, there was no correlation between the occurrence of fluorescence and the histological gradings of primary liver carcinoma by Edmondson and Stainer (*7*).

Result of AFP Tests in Our Department during the Past 4 Years

The results of AFP tests on 162 patients with malignant diseases are presented in Table III. Diagnoses were made on the basis of biopsy and postmortem examination. α-Fetoprotein was detected in 33 of 37 patients (89%) with primary hepatocellular carcinoma. A number of investigators reported that serum AFP was present in the patients of 60 to 80% of histologically confirmed primary liver carcinoma (*1*, *4*, *8*, *17*, *20*, *22*, *27*, *28*, *32*). The high percentage in the present study resulted from the use of a more sensitive technique such as fluoroelectroimmunodiffusion for the detection of AFP. This technique is at least 30 times as sensitive as the Ouchterlony technique (*26*). Its great sensitivity elicited a positive reaction in sera previously found negative by the Ouchterlony technique. The Ouchterlony technique and single radial immunodiffusion have been most popular in the detection of serum AFP, but the lowest limit of sensitivity of these techniques is only about 1.0 to 0.5 mg AFP per 100 ml serum. Alpert *et al.* (*4*) also reported that the frequency of AFP-positive patients increased using counterimmunoelectrophoresis, which is more sensitive than the Ouchterlony technique.

Tatarinov (*37*) and Abelev *et al.* (*1*) suggested that AFP tests could be used in the differential diagnosis of primary liver carcinoma from metastatic liver carcinoma. The AFP tests have been negative in sera from patients with carcinoma of the liver metastasized from the stomach but positive in some patients with embryonic tumors of the ovary and testis (*1, 17, 19*). However, Bourreille *et al.* (*5*) detected AFP in serum from a patient with carcinoma of the liver metastasized from the stomach. In our study, AFP was detected in 4 of 71 patients with carcinoma of the liver metastasized from the stomach. Kitaoka *et al.* (*16*) also detected AFP in similar patients. In general, serum AFP levels were lower in patients with carcinoma of liver metastasized from the stomach. Whether or not AFP is synthesized in these patients by the tumor itself is an interesting subject. In observations from Dakar (*27*), AFP was detected in carcinoma of the liver metastasized from the pancreas. We detected AFP in a man with gastric carcinoma. The present report seems to be the first to describe AFP-positive gastric carcinoma (*10*). Postmortem examination revealed differential carcinoma of the stomach. Neither hepatic lesion nor embryonal carcinoma of the testes was demonstrated. These facts indicate the possibility of AFP synthesis by a tumor of nonhepatic origin other than embryonal carcinoma of the testis and ovary.

The results of AFP tests on patients with non-neoplastic liver diseases are presented in Table IV. The AFP was detected in only 1 of 51 patients with infectious hepatitis and 5 of 195 patients with liver cirrhosis. The diagnoses were made on the basis of liver biopsy but the patients are still living more than 1 year after AFP was detected in their sera. They had a small amount of AFP, and AFP was present only transiently in their sera. It is to be noted that 1 of 5 patients with liver cirrhosis had hyperplastic nodules, known to precede the development of hepatoma (*30*). An attempt to follow up these cases may elicit important information for the early diagnosis and treatment of primary liver carcinoma.

TABLE IV. Result of AFP Test in Hepatic Diseases

Diagnosis	No. of cases	No. of positive
Infectious hepatitis		
Adults	51	1
Children	2	0
Infants	3	0
Chronic hepatitis		
Adults	82	0
Children	1	0
Cirrhosis		
Adults	195	5 (2%)
Drug-induced hepatitis	10	0
Obstructive jaundice	16	0
Distomiasis	1	0
Well's disease	1	0
Amyloidosis	2	0

REFERENCES

1. Abelev, G., Assecritova, I., Kraevsky, N., Perova, S. D., and Perevodchikova, N. I. Embryonal serum α-globulin in cancer patients; Diagnostic value. *Int. J. Cancer*, **2**, 551–558 (1967).
2. Abelev, G. I., Perova, S. D., Khramkova, N. I., Postinikova, Z. A., and Irlin, I. S. Production of embryonal α-globulin by transplantable mouse hepatomas. *Transplantation*, **1**, 174–180 (1963).
3. Abelev, G. I. Production of embryonal serum α-globulin by hepatomas. *Cancer Res.*, **28**, 1344–1350 (1968).
4. Alpert, E., Hershberg, R., Schur, P. H., and Isselbacher, K. J. α-Fetoprotein in human hepatoma: Improved detection in serum, and quantitative studies using a new sensitive technique. *Gastroenterology*, **61**, 137–143 (1971).
5. Bourreille, J., Metayer, P., Sauger, F., Matray, F., and Fondimare, A. Existence d'alpha foetoprotéine au cours d'un cancer secondaire du foie d'origine gastrique. *Presse Med.*, **78**, 1277–1278 (1970).
6. Bussard, A. and Huet, M. J. Description d'une technique combinant simultanément l'électrophorèses et la précipitation immunologique dans un gel: l'électrosynérèse. *Biochim. Biophys. Acta*, **34**, 258–260 (1959).
7. Edmondson, H. A. and Steiner, P. E. Primary carcinoma of the liver. A study of 100 cases among 48,900 necropsies. *Cancer*, **7**, 462–503 (1954).
8. Endo, Y., Eto, S., Iino, S., Fujiwara, K., Miyake, K., Kanetaka, T., Yamanaka, M., Suzuki, H., Suzuki, T., Oda, T., Yoshitoshi, Y., Juji, T., Yokochi, T., and Miura, T. The diagnosis of primary liver carcinoma by fetoglobulin. *Acta Hepatol. Japon.*, **10**, 143–146 (1969).
9. Engelhardt, N. V., Gusev, A. I., Shipova, L. J., and Abelev, G. I. Immunofluorescent study of α-fetoprotein in liver and liver tumours. I. Technique of AFP localization in tissue sections. *Int. J. Cancer*, **7**, 198–206 (1971).
10. Fujita, T. Unpublished.
11. Gitlin, D. and Boesman, M. Sites of serum α-fetoprotein synthesis in the human and in the rat. *J. Clin. Invest.*, **46**, 1010–1016 (1967).
12. Gusev, A. L., Engelhardt, N. V., Masseyeff, R., Camain, R., and Basteris, B. Immunofluorescence study of α-fetoprotein in liver and liver tumours. II. Localization of AFP in the tissues of patients with primary liver cancer. *Int. J. Cancer*, **7**, 207–217 (1971).
13. Hamashima, Y., Harter, J. G., and Coons, A. H. The localization of albumin and fibrinogen in human liver cells. *J. Cell. Biol.*, **20**, 271–279 (1964).
14. Houstek, J., Masopust, J., Kithier, K., and Radl, J. Hepatocellular carcinoma in association with a specific fetal α-globulin, fetoprotein. *J. Pediatr.*, **72**, 186–193 (1968).
15. Hull, E. W., Carbone, P. P., Gitlin, D., O'Gara, R. W., and Kelly, M. G. α-Fetoprotein in monkey with hepatoma. *J. Natl. Cancer Inst.*, **42**, 1035–1044 (1969).
16. Kitaoka, H., Hattori, N., and Mukojima, T. Fetoprotein and metastatic cancer (in Japanese). *Igaku-no-Ayumi (The Stride of Medicine)*, **79**, 129–130 (1970).
17. Masopust, J., Kithier, K., Rádl, J., Koutecky, J., and Kotál, L. Occurrence of fetoprotein in patients with neoplasma and non-neoplastic diseases. *Int. J. Cancer*, **3**, 364–373 (1968).
18. Matsuhashi, C. Studies of fluoroelectroimmunodiffusion (in Japanese). *Igaku-no-Ayumi (The Stride of Medicine)*, **73**, 169–171 (1970).

19. Mawas, C., Kohen, M., Lemerle, J., Buffe, D., Schweisguth, O., and Burtin, P. Serum fetoprotein (fetuin) in children with malignant ovarian or testicular teratomas. Preliminary results. *Int. J. Cancer*, **4**, 76–79 (1969).
20. Mukojima, T., Shimodaira, K., Hattori, N., Hasegawa, H., and Kitaoka, K. The diagnosis of primary liver carcinoma by α-fetoprotein. *Acta Hepatol. Japon.*, **11**, 325–333 (1970).
21. Nishi, S. Isolation and characterization of a human fetal α-globulin from the sera of fetuses and a hepatoma patient. *Cancer Res.*, **30**, 2507–2513 (1971).
22. Nishi, S. Primary liver cancer and fetal α-globulin. 1. A clinical study. *Phys. Chem. Biol.*, **15**, 261–265 (1971).
23. Nishioka, M., Hironaga, K., and Fujita, T. Polyacrylamide gel electrophoresis of sera from patients with primary liver carcinoma. *Clin. Chim. Acta*, **31**, 439–446 (1971).
24. Nishioka, M., Ibata, T., Miyazato, K., Okita, K., and Fujita, T. Utilization of solubility of α-fetoprotein in 34% ammonium sulfate in the preparation of antiserum and its test. *Digestion*, **4**, 65–71 (1971).
25. Nishioka, M., Ibata, T., Okita, K., Harada, T., and Fujita, T. Localization of α-fetoprotein in hepatoma tissues by immunofluorescence. *Cancer Res.*, **32**, 162–166 (1972).
26. Nishioka, M., Okita, K., Okamoto, Y., Kodama, T., and Fujita, T. Comparison of various precipitin tests in the detection of α-fetoprotein in serum. *Digestion*, **6**, 205–209 (1972).
27. O'Conor, G. T., Tatarinov, Y. S., Abelev, G. I., and Uriel, J. A collaborative study for the evaluation of a serologic test for primary liver cancer. *Cancer*, **25**, 1091–1098 (1970).
28. Okita, K. Study on α-fetoprotein. Diagnostic value. *Acta Hepatol. Japon.*, **11**, 194–200 (1970).
29. Ornstein, L. and Davis, B. J. "Disc Electrophoresis," preprint. Distillation Products Industries, New York (1962).
30. Popper, H., Sternberg, S. S., Oser, B. L., and Oser, M. The carcinogenic effect of aramite in rats. A study of hepatic nodules. *Cancer*, **13**, 1035–1046 (1960).
31. Purtilo, D. T. and Yunis, E. J. α-Fetoprotein, its immunofluorescent localization in human fetal liver and hepatoma. *Lab. Invest.*, **25**, 291–294 (1971).
32. Purves, L. R., Machab, M., and Bersohn, I. Serum fetoglobulin and primary hepatic cancer. *Lancet*, **1**, 921–922 (1968).
33. Sainte-Marie, G. A paraffin-embedding technique for studies employing immunofluorescence. *J. Histochem. Cytochem.*, **10**, 250–256 (1962).
34. Smith, J. A., Francis, T. I., Edington, G. M., and Williams, A. O. Immunofluorescent localisation of human α-fetoprotein in fetal and neonatal livers and cultured cells from hepatocellular carcinoma. *Brit. J. Cancer*, **25**, 343–349 (1971).
35. Stanislawski-birencwajg, M., Uriel, J., and Graber, P. Association of embryonic antigens with experimentally induced hepatic lesions in the rat. *Cancer Res.*, **27**, 1990–1997 (1967).
36. Takeo, K., Suzuno, K., Shimizu, J., and Nakamura, S. Purification of spinach aldolases by preparative disc electrophoresis. *Phys. Chem. Biol.*, **14**, 308–310 (1970).
37. Tatarinov, Y. S. Detection of embryo-specific α-globulin in the blood serum of a patient with primary liver cancer. *Vopr. Med. Khim.*, **10**, 90–91 (1964).

38. Van Furth, R. and Adinolfi, M. *In vitro* synthesis of the fetal α-globulin in man. *Nature*, **222**, 1296–1299 (1969).
39. Wise, R. W. and Oliver, I. T. Sites of synthesis of plasma proteins in the fetal rat. *Biochem. J.*, **100**, 330–333 (1966).

EXPLANATION OF PHOTOS

PHOTO 1. A section of liver cirrhosis

The hepatic cells and the connective tissue appeared dark with no fluorescent granules. ×560.

PHOTO 2. Section of a primary hepatocellular carcinoma (Patient Y.N.)

The giant-sized cytoplasm was fluorescent; nuclei and connective tissue were nonreactive. ×560.

PHOTO 3. Same case as in Photo 2

The cytoplasm and the cytoplasmic membrane were fluorescent. ×560.

PHOTO 4. Section from Patient T.D.

A brightly fluorescent line in the perinuclear zone was found. The cytoplasm had equivocal fluorescence. ×130.

PHOTO 5. Section from Patient S.H.

Fluorescence was found in a mass of tumor cells. ×560.

PHOTO 6. Section of fetal liver

Diffuse, finely granular fluorescence of the cytoplasm was found. Some of the hemopoietic cells had equivocal fluorescence. ×560.

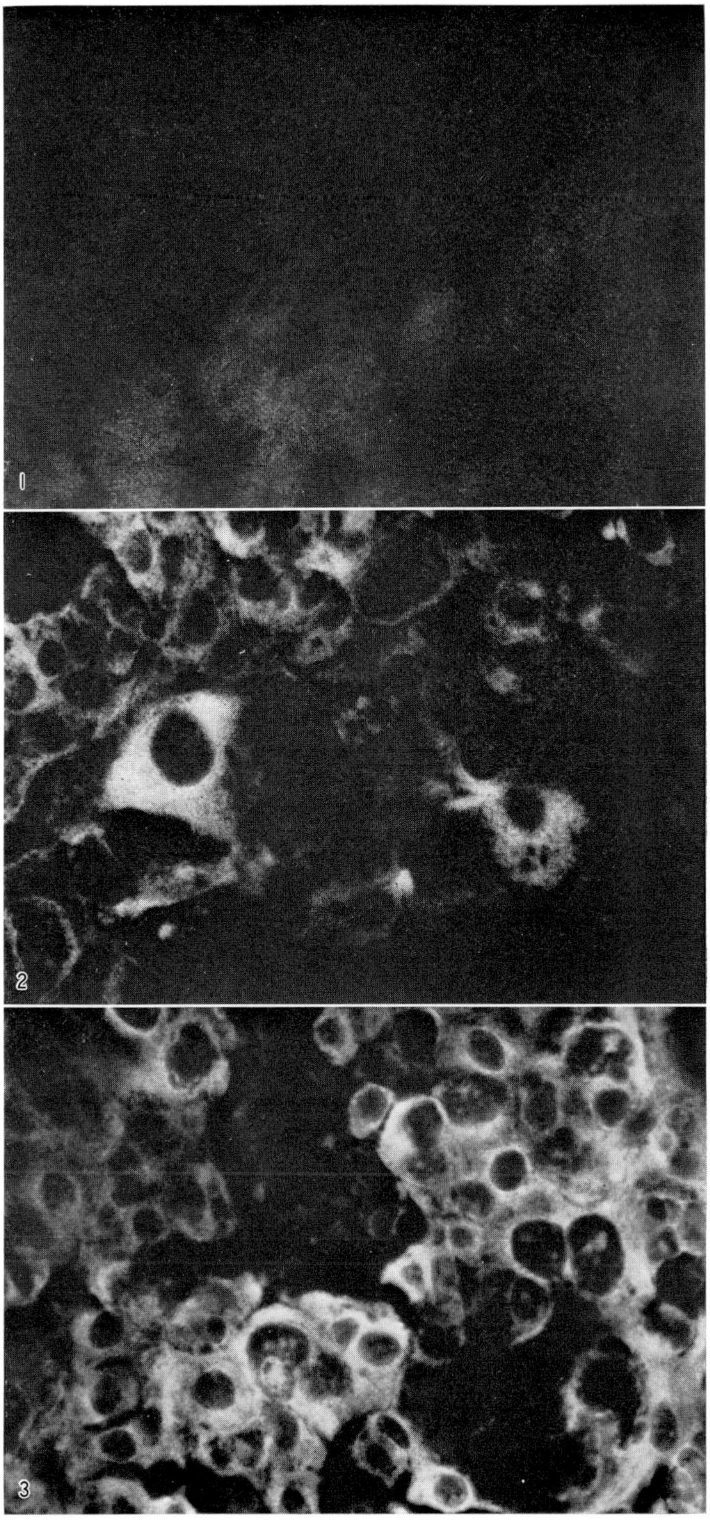
1
2
3

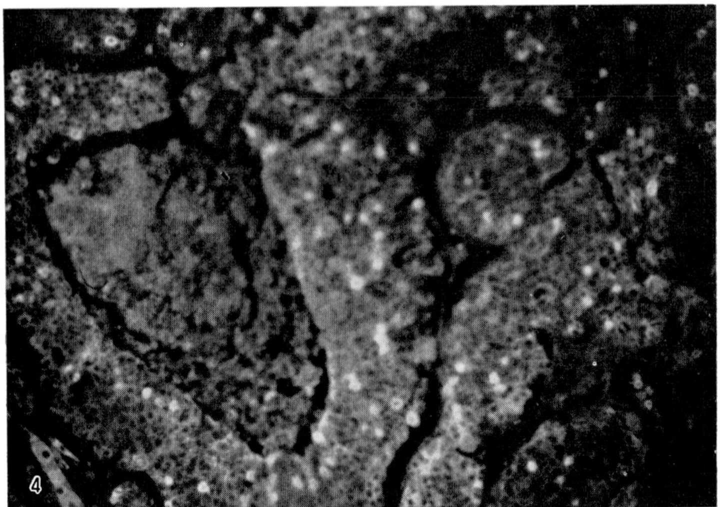
4

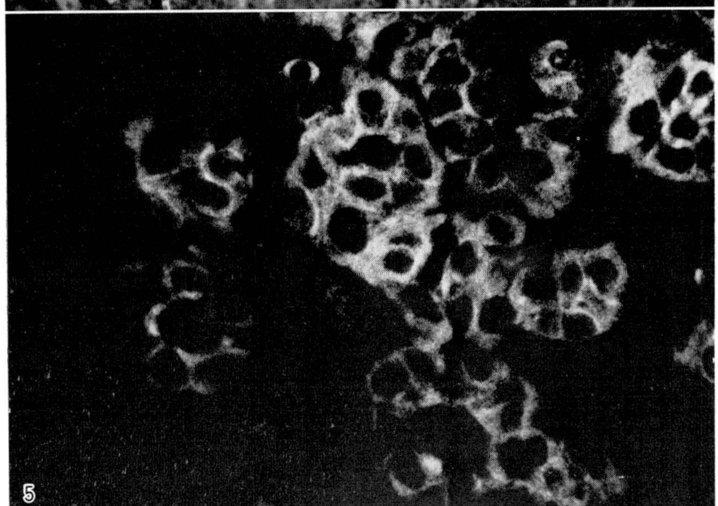
5

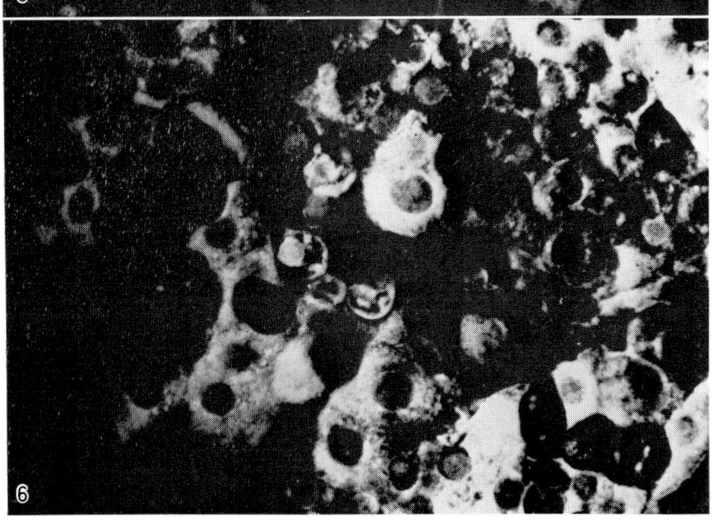
6

GANN Monograph on Cancer Research 14, 1973

α-FETOPROTEIN BY THE IMMUNOFLUORESCENT ANTIBODY TECHNIQUE IN PRIMARY LIVER CARCINOMA AND ITS HISTOPATHOLOGICAL BASIS

Masayoshi TAKAHASHI,[*1,*3] Akie KAWAGUCHI,[*1] Kunishi KAWAMATA,[*1] and Tsuguro YASUMA[*2]

Clinical and Research Laboratories, Central Hospital of the Japanese National Railways,[*1] *Department of Pathology, School of Medicine, Juntendo University,*[*2] *and Department of Pathology, School of Medicine, Kyorin University*[*3]

The specificity of diagnosis of primary liver carcinoma by detection of α-fetoprotein (AFP) in the sera or ascites was confirmed by double gel immunodiffusion. The detection rate was elevated from 74.1 to 93.6% by the introduction of radioimmunoassay. Included in 25 AFP-positive cases are a huge metastatic liver carcinoma which originated from gastric adenocarcinoma and an ovarian embryonal carcinoma. Some correlation between AFP quantity and histological malignancy has been recognized. For quantitative studies of serum AFP, single radial immunodiffusion and radioimmunoassay were carried out.

The most differentiated and anaplastic hepatomas were negative or less productive of AFP, while the intermediate types of Grade II and Grade III malignancies showed variable degrees of AFP production. Hepatomas with the highest AFP production belonged to these groups. By means of the immunofluorescent antibody technique, AFP production was specifically verified within the cytoplasm of hepatoma cells either as collections of granular fluorescence or as bright masses of greenish yellow fluorescence. The specificity of the fluorescence was confirmed by marked inhibition of the fluorescence in a blocking test. This technique can be applied to cytodiagnosis of ascitic fluids and needle aspirates.

The accuracy of immunoserological detection of α-fetoprotein (AFP) as a tool for the diagnosis of primary hepatocellular carcinoma has been highly evaluated by many researchers since this embryo-specific α-globulin was found by Tatarinov (*31*, *32*) in the serum of patients with hepatoma. As a routine screening method, Ouchterlony's double gel diffusion is now widely used in laboratories. There are some variations in diagnostic rate, ranging from 50.0 to 87.5%, probably

[*1] Yoyogi 2, Shibuya-ku, Tokyo 151, Japan (高橋正宜, 川口昭恵, 河又国士).
[*2] Hongo 2, Bunkyo-ku, Tokyo 113, Japan (安間嗣郎).
[*3] 6 Shinkawa, Mitaka, Tokyo 181, Japan (高橋正宜).

TABLE I. Immunodiffusion Assay for AFP

Histological grading of hepatoma	No. of cases	AFP-positive	
		Double diffusion	Radio-immunoassay
I	4	1	1 (3)[a]
II	7	6	1
III	7	7	
IV	3	1	1
Hepatoblastoma	1	1	
Clinical	5	4	
Total	27	20 74.1%	23 (25)[a] 85.2% (93.6%)

Control cases

Disease	No. of cases	AFP-positve
Chronic hepatitis	31	0
Liver cirrhosis	30	0
Gastric carcinoma	13 (14)	0 (1)
Cholecystitis	7	0
Metastatic liver carcinoma	5	1[b]
Cholangiogenic carcinoma	3	0
Portal hypertension	3	0
Pulmonary carcinoma	1	0
Embryonal carcinoma	2	1
Pulmonary blastoma	1	0
Neuroblastoma	1	0
Leukemia	5	0
Lymphoma	4	0
Sarcoidosis	2	0
Collagen disease	2	0
Others	89	0
Total	201	2

[a] Range of reactive increase included. [b] Metastasis from gastric carcinoma.

because of different procedures of immunization (*4*, *5*, *8*, *21*, *25*, *28*); Abelev (*1*) used embryonic serum in about the 13th to 19th week of intrauterine life, and Uriel (*33*) used serum from a patient with primary hepatocellular carcinoma. At any rate, the specificity of double immunodiffusion has been accepted; false positives were very rarely reported in large immunological surveys of sera from patients with viral hepatitis, liver cirrhosis, liver abscess, and cancers in various other organs. Alpert (*4*) noted 2 positives from a case of hepatitis and a case of liver cirrhosis, but he added the comment that subclinical hepatoma could not be ruled out for these cases. Recently, metastatic liver carcinoma originating from gastric carcinoma has been noted to be responsible for AFP positivity (*11*, *21*). In the authors' laboratories, 2 positive cases due to extrahepatic tumors were detected; 1 was a gastric adenocarcinoma that resembled trabecular type of hepatoma histologically and that developed huge metastatic tumors in the liver, and the other was embryonal carcinoma originating in the ovary (Table I). The latter should not be considered to be false positive, since antigenic reversion in the most undifferentiated embryoma may be the cause of extrahepatic AFP production, as already remarked by Abelev (*2*); he reported 13 positive cases out of 56 testicular tumors.

The antiserum used in our laboratories is a horse antiserum against human AFP which was made in the Research Laboratory of the Green Cross Corporation, Osaka, according to the method of Hirai and Nishi (*11*, *24*); as the 1st step, rabbits were immunized against embryonic serum, and secondly this antiserum, absorbed by normal adult serum, was precipitated with the patient's serum. The horse antiserum was that immunized by the above specific antigen-antibody precipitate. Experimentally, Gitlin and Boesman noted the hepatic origin of AFP synthesis using ^{14}C-labeled amino acids in human and rat fetuses. There may be some questions whether AFP is produced by hepatoma cells and/or liver cells with hepatoma, and whether its production is related to gradings of histological malignancy or not. In addition to quantitative immunodiffusion assay and radioimmunoassay, the immunofluorescent antibody technique was introduced to clarify these questions.

Correlation of AFP Production with Gross Anatomical Findings

The gross findings of primary hepatocellular carcinoma have been classified into nodular, massive, and diffuse types. Nodular and massive types are more common than the diffuse type. In an advanced stage, the nodular and massive types cannot be discriminated, because the latter may be represented by fusion of tumor nodules. At any rate, they grow in an expansive fashion, while a diffuse type shows infiltrative growth. Edmondson and Steiner (*7*) referred the growth types of the tumor to the histological maturity of cancer cells; a massive type is more frequently seen among the differentiated hepatomas than the undifferentiated. The number of our cases was too small to confirm this fact, but no relation between the growth type and histological malignancy was recognized. It may be conjectured that the size of the tumor relates to AFP production. Kithier *et al.* (*18*) emphasized a progressive increase of serum AFP content with progression of the illness. For determination of AFP quantity a single radial immunodiffusion method has come to be routinely used, since the purification of AFP became successful (*3*, *22*). In practice, the so-called agar gel immunoplates containing 2, 5 or 10% antisera were made, and calibration lines were made from the ring diameters of diffusion after 48 hr. This quantitative immunoassay is technically limited to the range above 1 mg/dl.

Although our cases reported herein were in a fairly advanced stage, hepatomas involving large areas of the liver, *i.e.*, more than half of the organ, revealed a tendency to yield more AFP than those involving small portions of the liver. On the other hand, there were several cases showing no AFP production or low AFP levels despite marked involvement of the liver by cancer. So far as practical quantitative immunoassay is concerned, there was no definite correlation of serum

TABLE II. Interrelation between AFP and Gross Findings

Name	Sex	Age (yrs.)	AFP Single radial (mg/dl)	AFP Radioimmunoassay (ng/ml)	Cirrhosis	Involvement	Growth type	Metastases
M.G.	M	73	Neg	140	+	Minor	Nodular	Portal
A.K.	F	51	7.9		−	Minor	Nodular	Splenic vein
I.K.	M	58	5.2		+	Minor	Nodular	Abdominal wall
S.I.	F	9	54.0		+	Minor	Nodular	Portal, lungs
S.N.	M	68	3.0		+	Half	Nodular	Portal, lungs
T.M.	M	68	3.8		+	Half	Diffuse	Portal, stomach
U.H.	M	47	Neg	720	+	Half	Diffuse	Portal
Y.Y.	M	56	12.0		−	Half	Nodular	Lungs, kidney
I.M.	M	56	135.0		+	Half	Massive	None
N.O.	M	48	Unavailable		+	Half	Diffuse	Portal
K.G.	F	72	Neg	20	−	Half	Nodular	None
I.S.	F	68	Neg	660	+	Major	Massive	None
S.K.	M	54	2.8(A)		+	Major	Massive	None
K.G.	M	65	3.8		+	Major	Massive	Portal
M.H.	M	54	8.3		+	Major	Diffuse	Portal
M.M.	M	57	11.5		+	Major	Massive	Portal, lungs
O.N.	M	48	95.0		+	Major	Massive	Portal
S.M.	M	38	100.0		−	Major	Massive	None

(A): Ascites. M: Male. F: Female.

AFP production with gross pathological findings such as the extent of the tumor, growth type, presence of distant metastases, and concomitance with liver cirrhosis (Table II). Concerning the incidence of concomitant cirrhosis with hepatoma, a marked geographical difference exists between Japan and European countries. Hepatoma in Japan is frequently associated with liver cirrhosis; 60.6% were concomitant in males and 56.5% in females according to the statistical review by Ichida *et al.* (*12*). In our series of studies, most hepatomas were associated with cirrhosis, and no significant difference could be obtained between the 2 groups (Table II), while Purves pointed out that positive rate was lower in noncirrhotics (8%) than in cirrhosis-associated patients (53%) (*28*).

More sensitive than single radial diffusion are the counter-immunoelectrophoresis (*5*, *19*) and radioimmunoassay techniques (*13*, *15*, *23*, *28*). For the demonstration of AFP, counter-immunoelectrophoresis is said to be about 5 times as sensitive as the conventional Ouchterlony's method, and 0.5 μg/ml of AFP is detectable (*19*). Furthermore, the application of radioimmunoassay has made it possible to detect AFP ranging from 1 to 10 ng/ml. Ishii and his associates (*13*) emphasized a marked improvement of detection rate from 80.0% by the single radial diffusion method to 92.7% by radioimmunoassay.

Correlation of AFP with Grades of Histological Malignancy

Since AFP synthesized in embryonic liver cells and hepatoma cells is also produced in extrahepatic embryonal cancer cells, its synthesis was explained as a proliferation of dedifferentiated hepatoblasts (*2*), *i.e.*, antigenic reversion, and as the withdrawal of an inhibiting factor on AFP synthesis in cancerization (depression in gene circuit) (*26*, *27*). However, these are still only hypotheses, because AFP synthesis has not been observed in the most undifferentiated tumor cells in infants such as nephroblastoma and neuroblastoma except for the embryonal type of germinal tumors arising from the testis or ovary. There have been a few reports referring to serum AFP quantity and histological malignancy; the more rapidly growing and the more undifferentiated hepatomas were thought to yield more AFP. Mito and his associates (*20*) described that Grade IV anaplastic hepatomas produced much more AFP than others. On the other hand, Purves *et al.* (*28*) recognized that AFP production was lowest in anaplastic (16 mg/dl), intermediate in well-differentiated (25 mg/dl), and highest in poorly differentiated tumors (32 mg/dl). The difference in these values seems to be too small to draw a conclusion on a statistical significance. In their papers, gradings of malignancy were classified by the criteria of Edmondson and Steiner (*7*) which was based on cellular atypism as described by Broders (*6*). Grade I carcinoma is characterized by abundant, eosinophilic and granular cytoplasm which is quite similar to that of hyperplastic liver cells in nodular, adenomatous hyperplasia. Since the nuclear cytoplasmic ratio is low, malignancy is often doubtful and is determined by the coexistence of Grade II carcinoma and the tendency to vascular invasion. Grade II carcinoma retains abundant, granular cytoplasm with an acidophilic staining reaction. However, there are moderate variations in the size of the nuclei, moderate nuclear hyperchromatism, and a slight increase in the nuclear cytoplasmic ratio. The cytoplasmic border is fairly distinct and bile droplets are often discernible in the cells as well as in the bile canaliculi. Grade III carcinoma shows marked nuclear hyperchromatism, variations of the nuclei in size and shape, high nuclear cytoplasmic ratio, and rather indistinct cytoplasmic borders, Tumor giant cell formation showing a large solitary nucleus and a single multilobed nucleus and/or multiple nuclei occurs quite frequently. The staining reaction of the cytoplasm is basophilic, with a granular appearance. Grade IV carcinoma has smaller nuclei than Grade III carcinoma, but these nuclei are intensely hyperchromatic, oval to spindle-shaped like those of pulmonary oat cell carcinoma, and vary considerably in size. The cytoplasm is scant and basophilic. The nuclear cytoplasmic ratio is markedly increased. Giant cell formation and bile droplet deposition, which are characteristics of Grade III carcinoma, are rarely encountered in this group. Some hepatomas disclosed variations of cellular differentiation from place to place, but their gradings were classified by the predominant type in the whole tumor.

Histological malignancy was compared with the serum AFP quantity, which was measured by single radial immunodiffusion, as already described. By double gel diffusion 3 of 4 highly differentiated hepatomas were negative, and 1 positive case showed a low value of 4.2 mg/dl (Table III). It should be noted that 1 of 3 negatives turned essentially positive on investigation by radioimmunoassay with a value of 640 ng/ml. The other 2 cases remained within the limits of reactive increase as shown with values of 110 ng/ml and 140 ng/ml, respectively. One of these, however, disclosed an increase of AFP value up to 640 ng/ml before death. We applied the double antibody technique supplied by the Dinabot Radioisotope Laboratories to the cases which were negative in the single radial diffusion method. The principle of this method is based on the competition of ^{125}I-labeled and unlabeled AFP (patient's AFP, being examined) for their specific antibody, followed by isotopic dilution. Fairly well-differentiated Grade II hepatoma also showed relatively low values, below 7.9 mg/dl except for 1 case that yielded a high value of 100 mg/dl. Since the latter included some portions classified as Grade III malignancy, this case could be discussed within the Grade III group. One negative case out of 7 Grade II hepatomas showed 660 ng/ml of AFP by radioimmunoassay. The Grade III hepatomas were all positive by conventional double gel diffusion and revealed a marked variation of serum AFP value, ranging from 3.8 mg/dl to 135 mg/dl. It was noteworthy that the cases producing a large amount of AFP belonged to this group; histologically, the tumor cells possessed basophilic, granular cytoplasm and prominent nucleoli. On the other hand, Grade IV hepatomas having scant, indistinct cytoplasm demonstrated lower values of serum AFP than Grade III hepatomas; 2 of 3 anaplastic carcinomas which were negative by double gel diffusion were studied by radioimmunoassay. One case turned positive, and showed 720 ng/ml AFP, but another was essentially negative (2 ng/ml). Thus, it is most probable that AFP-nonproducing hepatoma is present. We have experienced a case of hepatoblastoma in an adult with pulmonary metastases. This case was a type of mixed tumor which showed a sarcomatous component and formation of mature bony tissues in addition to tumorous proliferation of epithelial hepatocytes. Metastatic lesions to the lungs as well as a primary tumor in the liver were fairly well differentiated to be classified as Grade II hepatoma. Pathologically, the so-called hepatoblastoma includes another type of tumor which is characterized by proliferation of anaplastic embryonal hepatoblasts. Mukojima (*21*) described that 2 cases of embryonal hepatoblastoma out of 40 hepatomas yielded a large quantity of AFP. The production of AFP depends on the predominance of AFP-productive hepatoblasts and not on the sarcomatous component.

α-Fetoprotein by the Immunofluorescent Antibody Method

The immunofluorescent antibody technique is valuable to demonstrate AFP production cytologically (*29*). Localization of the specific fluorescence indicates AFP production *in situ* and its intensity parallels the amount of AFP. Practically, anti-AFP serum was adjusted with carbonate buffer to pH 9.1 and 1% protein concentration. Fluorescein isothiocyanate (FITC) in the amount of 1/50 of the protein content was mixed with the anti-AFP serum using a magnetic stirrer for 6 hr at 4°. Unreacted dye was removed by molecular sieves using Sephadex G-25 and the conjugate was purified by filtration through DEAE-cellulose columns. The first fraction, obtained by elution with 0.05 M phosphate buffer (pH 6.4), was collected and then dialyzed at 4°. The purified FITC-labeled antiserum was absorbed with normal adult liver powder. It was diluted to a protein concentration of 5 μg/ml prior to use. Tissue specimens fixed with cold acetone were embedded in paraffin with a low melting point, strictly below 58°. The staining solution was dropped on tissue sections or smears which were washed well with staining buffer at pH 7.0. After incubation of 1 hr at 37°, the tissue sections were washed well with the staining buffer and then examined fluoromicroscopically. Intense fluorescence in the cytoplasm of hepatoma cells, appearing either homogeneous or somewhat granular, consists of condensations of finely granular structures (Photos 1 and 2). Most of the positive cases in Grade II and Grade III hepatomas revealed massive fluorescence with high intensity throughout the cancer cell nests. In a case that belonged to a group producing high AFP values, fluorescence could be found in the cytoplasm as well as the nucleoli. There were a few cases showing fluorescence in zonal areas; masses of hepatoma cells yielding greenish fluorescence were scattered in cancer cell nests. In a slightly positive case, spotty fluorescence was demonstrated in single cells or in small groups of cells (Photo 2). This may indicate partial production of AFP among hepatoma cells or a rapid turnover of protein metabolism; the cancer cells seem not all to be in the same stage of protein metabolism and nonfluorescent cancer cells may come to be productive of AFP in a different stage (Photo 3).

TABLE III. Interrelation between AFP and Histology

Name	Sex	Age (yrs.)	Single radial (mg/dl)	Radioimmunoassay (ng/ml)	Immunofluorescence	Grade	Type
M.R.	F	11	—	640	—	I	Adenomatous
M.G.	M	73	—	140	—	I	Trabecular
K.K.	M	64	—	110–640	—	I+II	Trabecular
S.N.	M	68	4.2		+ focal	I+II	Adenomatous
I.S.	F	68	—	660, 2400(A)	Unavailable	II	Trabecular
A.Y.	M	48	3.7		+	II	Adenomatous
S.K.	M	54	2.8(A)		++	II	Trabecular
I.K.	M	58	5.2		+ zonal	II	Alveolar
A.K.	F	51	7.9		+ zonal	II	Alveolar
O.D.	M	48	7.3		Unavailable	II	Alveolar
S.M.	M	38	100.0		Unavailable	II+III	Alveolar
T.M.	M	68	3.8		—	III	Adenomatous
K.G.	M	65	3.8		+	III	Alveolar
M.H.	M	54	8.3 7.8(A)		++	III	Trabecular
Y.A.	M	48	14.0		Unavailable	III	Alveolar
S.I.	F	9	54.0		++	III	Trabecular
O.N.	M	48	95.0 65(A)		++	III	Alveolar
I.M.	M	56	135.0 30(A)		+	III	Trabecular
N.M.	M	46	Unavailable		+ zonal	IV	Alveolar
K.G.	F	72	—	20	—	IV	Alveolar
U.H.	M	47	—	720, 860(A)	+ (A)[a]	IV	Alveolar
M.M.	M	56	11.5 6.0(A)		++	IV	Alveolar
Y.Y.	M	56	12.0		Unavailable		Hepatoblastoma
O.T.	M	65	4.8 1.0(A)		Unavailable		Gastric cancer

(A): Ascites. M: Male. F: Female. [a] Hepatoma cells in ascites.

TABLE IV. Comparative Determination of Fluorescence by Microspectrophotometry (MMSP, Olympus)

Case No.		Cancer tissue	Liver tissue	Stromal tissue
3487 (M.H.)	Before blocking	82.7	61.5	42.3
	After blocking	61.0	58.0	37.9
3468 (S.K.)	Before blocking	106.1	62.0	35.0
	After blocking	58.1	59.8	31.0
5269 (O.N.)	Before blocking	80.8	56.8	42.5
	After blocking	58.5	54.8	41.5
41 (Normal)	Before blocking		41.7	36.0
	After blocking		46.0	38.0
42 (Normal)			50.0	40.5
43 (Normal)			54.0	42.5
2870 (Gastric cancer)		38.0		35.7

Intensity is represented by arbitrary units.

A comparative study of immunofluorescence and the histology of hepatomas led to the conclusion that intense fluorescence was shown in hepatoma with fairly abundant, basophilic, finely granular cytoplasm. Intense fluorescence tended to occur in hepatoma with slight to moderate differentiation (Grades II and III) in association with high AFP values (Table III). Takahashi and his associates (*30*) confirmed the specificity of the fluorescence from a control study for other cancers. However, it must be mentioned that 2 cases of gastric adenocarcinoma out of 34 malignant neoplasms of various sites showed a slight positive fluorescence. The liver cells adjacent to hepatoma occasionally yield greenish yellow, dull fluorescence which may be confused with that from hepatoma cells. In order to verify whether the fluorescence is specific or nonspecific, like absorption and primary fluorescence, a blocking test was carried out (Photos 4 and 5); nonlabeled antiserum was dropped onto tissue sections and incubated for 6 hr or more in a moist chamber at 37°. The tissue sections were washed well with cold staining buffer, and then stained. There was an evident decrease in immunofluorescence after the blocking test, while stromal tissue and normal liver cells remained unchanged; it could be quantitatively measured in arbitrary units by means of fluorescent microspectrophotometry (Table IV). FITC is quite a stable dye under fluoromicroscopy and its fluorescence spectrum revealed a maximum peak to be present at a wave length of 495 nm. Scanning was also available at a speed of 125 μ/min and with a measuring spot of 8.1 μ. Brownish yellow, nonspecific fluorescence by red cells and Kupffer cells could be easily excluded at this wave length. The application of the fluorescence antibody technique to cytodiagnosis for ascites and needle aspirates was mentioned as valuable because of its specificity in cell identification (*29*).

Acknowledgments

The authors are greatly indebted to Prof. Hideo Ueda, Director of the Central Hospital of the Japanese National Railways, for his encouragement. They are also grateful to Prof. H. Hirai and Drs. S. Nishi and H. Watabe at the Department of Biochemistry, School of Medicine, Hokkaido University, for making purified AFP available to them.

REFERENCES

1. Abelev, G. I., Assecritova, S. V., Kraevsky, N. A., Peroda, S. D., and Perovodchikova, N. I. Embryonal serum α-globulin in cancer patients; diagnostic value. *Int. J. Cancer*, **2**, 551–558 (1967).
2. Abelev, G. I. Production of embryonal α-globulin by hepatomas: Review of experimental and clinical data. *Cancer Res.*, **28**, 1344–1350 (1968).
3. Adinolfi, A., Adinolfi, M., and Cohen, S. Isolation and characterization of human fetal α-globulin (α_1F) from fetal and hepatoma sera. *Biochim. Biophys. Acta*, **251**, 197–207 (1971).
4. Alpert, M. E., Uriel, J., and de Nechaud, B. Alpha$_1$-Fetoglobulin in the diagnosis of human hepatoma. *New Engl. J. Med.*, **278**, 984–986 (1968).
5. Alpert, M. E., Hershberg, R., Schur, P. H., and Isselbacher, K. J. α-Fetoprotein in human hepatoma; improved detection in serum, and quantitative studies using a new sensitive technique. *Gastroenterology*, **61**, 137–143 (1971).
6. Broders, A. C. Squamous-cell epithelioma of the lip; a study of 537 cases. *J. Am. Med. Assoc.*, **74**, 656–664 (1920).
7. Edmondson, H. A. and Steiner, P. E. Primary carcinoma of the liver. *Cancer*, **7**, 462–503 (1954).
8. Endo, Y., Eto, S., and Oda, T. Clinical significance of α_1-fetoglobulin (in Japanese). *Naika* (*Internal Medicine*), **24**, 24–28 (1969).
9. Gitlin, D. and Boesman, M. Fetus-specific serum proteins in several mammals and their relation to human α-fetoprotein. *Comp. Biochem. Physiol.*, **21**, 327–336 (1967).
10. Hirai, H. Recent progress in cancer research and immunology; embryospecific α-globulin and hepatoma (in Japanese). *Sogo Rinsho* (*Clinic All-Round*), **19**, 891–899 (1970).
11. Hirai, H. Serological diagnosis of hepatoma; embryo-specific α-globulin (in Japanese). *Shinryo* (*Postgraduate Course*), **23**, 2190–2196 (1970).
12. Ichida, F., Nakagawa, T., Maniwa, H., Watanabe, K., Inoue, K., Kazuoka, T., Tanaka, Y., and Ogawa, H. Primary liver carcinoma (in Japanese). *Naika* (*Intrnal Medicine*), **17**, 243–246 (1966).
13. Ishii, M., Ikehara, H., Tozawa, T., Inoue, E., and Shinko, T. Radioimmunoassay of α-fetoprotein and its clinical significance (in Japanese). *Igaku-no-Ayumi* (*The Stride of Medicine*), **79** (2), 77–79 (1971).
14. Ishii, M., Ikehara, H., Inoue, E., Tozawa, T., Miki, S., Shinko, T., and Miyaji, Y. Liver cell carcinoma and α-fetoprotein (in Japanese). *J. Adult Dis.*, **1**, 339–343 (1971).
15. Ishiguro, T., Matsukura, S., and Muranaka, H. Purification of α-fetoprotein and radioimmunoassay (in Japanese). *Jap. J. Clin. Pathol.*, **19** (Suppl.), 157–158 (1971).
16. Kanayama, M., Koizumi, S., Makino, J., Matsuda, Y., and Harada, M. Limit of α-fetoprotein detection in primary liver carcinoma (in Japanese). *Igaku-no-Ayumi* (*The Stride of Medicine*), **80**, 17–18 (1972).
17. Kahan, B. and Levine, L. The occurrence of a fetal α_1-protein in developing mice and murine hepatomas and teratomas. *Cancer Res.*, **31**, 930–936 (1971).

18. Kithier, K., Houštěk, J., Masopust, J., and Rádl, J. Occurrence of a specific fetal protein in a primary liver carcinoma. *Nature*, **212**, 414 (1966).
19. Kohn, J. Method for the detection and identification of α-fetoprotein in serum. *J. Clin. Pathol.*, **23**, 733–735 (1970).
20. Mito, M., Kasai, Y., Miyakawa, A., Nishi, S., and Nagase, K. Hepatoma and liver cirrhosis in relation to α-fetoprotein (in Japanese). *J. Adult Dis.*, **1**, 153–156 (1971).
21. Mukojima, T., Shimodaira, K., Hattori, S., Hasegawa, H., and Kitaoka, K. Diagnosis of primary liver carcinoma; single radial diffusion method (in Japanese). *Acta Hepatol. Japon.*, **11**, 325–333 (1970).
22. Nishi, S. Isolation and characterization of a human fetal α-globulin from the sera of fetuses and a hepatoma patient. *Cancer Res.*, **30**, 2507–2513 (1970).
23. Nishi, S. and Hirai, H. Diagnosis of hepatoma by α-fetoprotein (in Japanese). *Jap. J. Clin. Pathol.*, **19** (Suppl.), 155–156 (1971).
24. Nishi, S. and Hirai, H. α_f-Globulin in fetus and the serum of hepatoma patients. *Phys. Chem. Biol.*, **14**, 301–302 (1970).
25. Okita, K. Studies on α-fetoprotein. *Acta Hepatol. Japon.*, **11**, 194–200 (1970).
26. Pitot, M. C. and Cho Y. S. Control mechanisms in the normal and neoplastic cell. *Progr. Exp. Tumor Res.*, **7**, 158–223 (1965).
27. Pitot, M. C. and Heidelberger, C. Metabolic regulatory circuits and carcinogenesis. *Cancer Res.*, **23**, 1694–1700 (1963).
28. Purves, L. R., Bersohn, I., and Geddes, E. W. Serum α-fetoprotein and primary cancer of the liver in man. *Cancer*, **25**, 1261–1270 (1970).
29. Takahashi, M., Tanaka, M., and Kawaguchi, A. Anti-α-fetoglobulin immunofluorescence method for demonstration of hepatoma cells (in Japanese). *Med. Postgraduates*, **8**, 202–207 (1970).
30. Takahashi, M., Kawaguchi, A., Yasuma, T., Tanaka, M., and Kawamata, K. α-Fetoprotein by immunodiffusion and fluorescence antibody methods and histopathology of hepatoma (in Japanese). *Med. Postgraduates*, **9**, 249–260 (1971).
31. Tatarinov, JuS. Detection of embryo-specific α-globulin in the blood serum of a patient with primary liver cancer. *Vopr. Med. Khim.*, **10**, 90–91 (1964).
32. Tatarinov, JuS. Content of embryo-specific α-globulin in fetal and neonatal sera and sera from adult humans with primary carcinoma of the liver. *Vopr. Med. Khim.*, **11**, 20–24 (1965).
33. Uriel, J., de Nechaud, B., Stanislawski-birencwaig M., Masseyeff, R., Leblanc, L., Quenum, C., Loisillier, F., and Grabar, P. Le diagnostic du cancer primaire du foie par des methodes immunologiques. *Presse Med.*, **76**, 1415–1417 (1968).

EXPLANATION OF PHOTOS

PHOTO 1. Intense fluorescence in Grade III hepatoma with a trabecular pattern. The cytoplasm is massively and homogeneously fluorescent. The serum AFP value is 54 mg/dl.

PHOTO 2. Fluorescence appearing in broad cytoplasm as collections of granular structures. The serum AFP value is 4.2 mg/dl.

PHOTO 3. Zonal fluorescence in anaplastic Grade IV hepatoma. The remainder of a large, alveolar cancer cell nest is nonfluorescent.

PHOTO 4. Bright fluorescence before a blocking test.

PHOTO 5. Inhibition of the fluorescence after a blocking test.

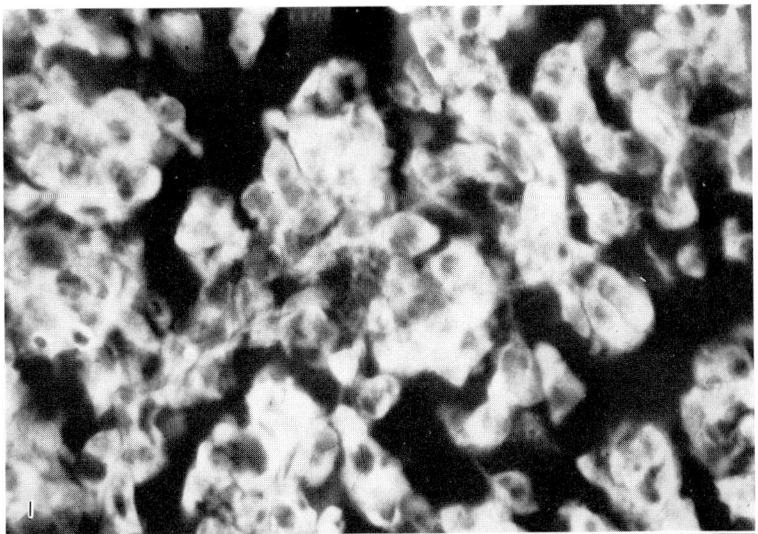

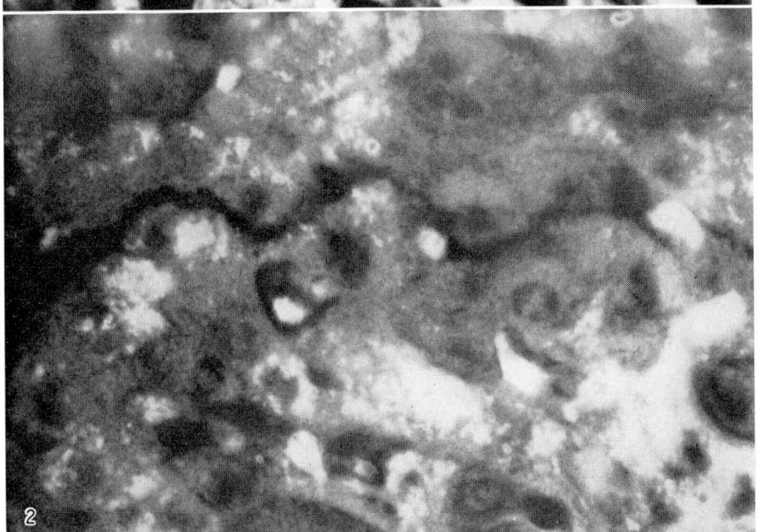

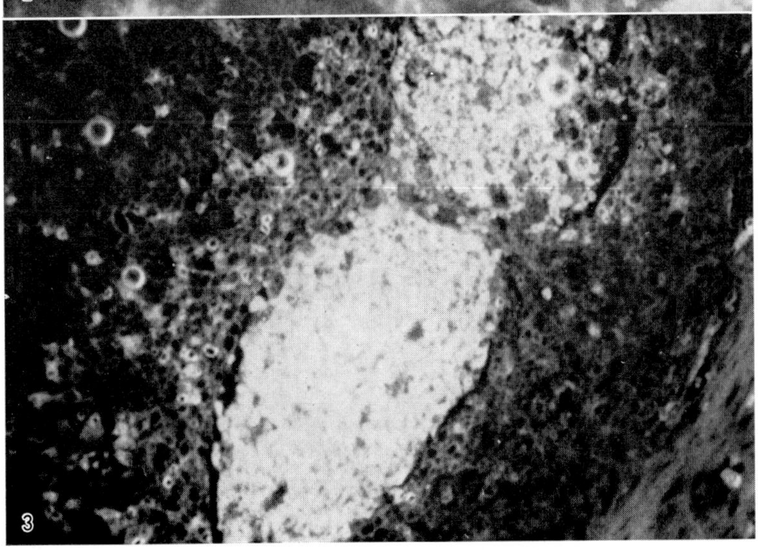

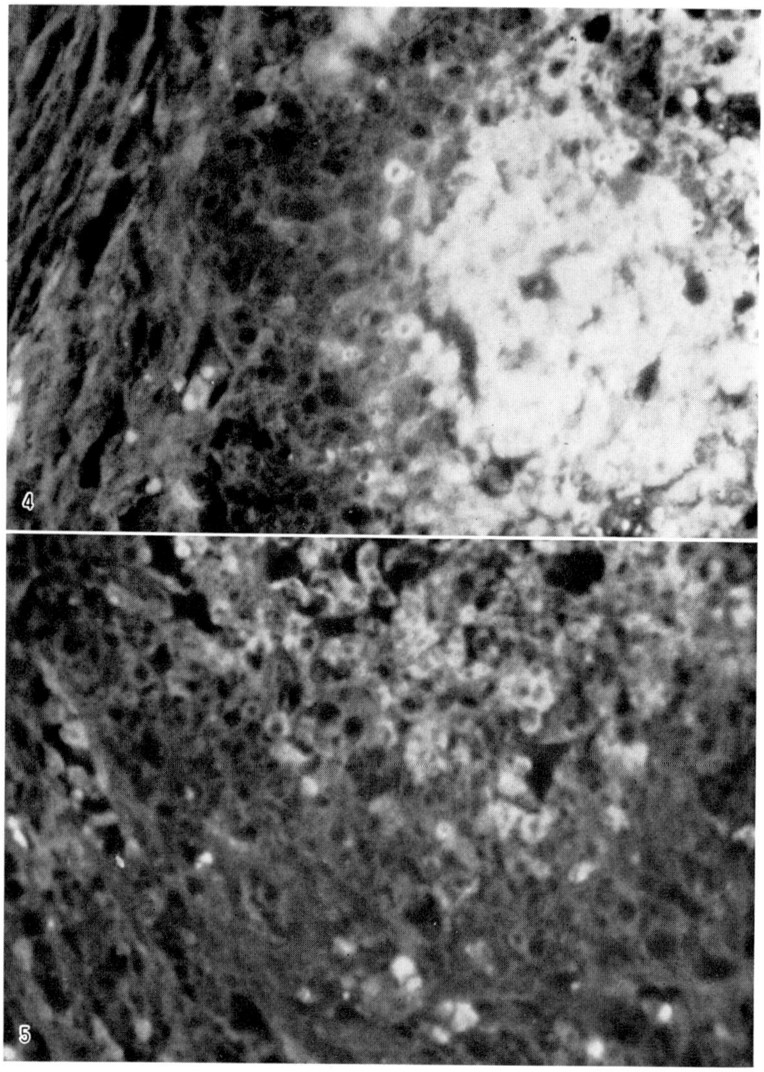
4
5

EXPERIMENTS IN HEPATOMA AND AFP

GANN Monograph on Cancer Research 14, 1973

SIGNIFICANCE OF α-FETOPROTEIN APPEARANCE IN THE EARLY STAGE OF AZO-DYE CARCINOGENESIS

Tamenori ONOÉ,*1 Kimimaro DEMPO,*1 Aiko KANEKO,*1 and Hiroyuki WATABE*2

*Department of Pathology, Sapporo Medical College,**1 *and Department of Biochemistry, School of Medicine, Hokkaido University**2

The present study has been carried out mainly to elucidate the significance of the appearance of AFP in the sera of rats in the early stage of hepatocarcinogenesis by azo-dye feeding.

In the early stage after commencement of azo-dye feeding, a striking fluctuation of various cell populations occurred in hepatic tissue through the experimental course, and transformation of the oval cells to hepatocytes was clarified from the results of morphological and radioautographic studies. By the serological examination α-fetoprotein (AFP) was transiently detected in the sera during the period when the transitional cells and small hepatocytes proliferated prominently, but it was no longer detectable when the small hepatocytes gained the same appearances as normal adult hepatocytes. Since AFP was detected in the sera concurrently with the appearance of small hepatocytes transformed from the oval cells, it is conceivable that AFP may be produced by the immature hepatocytes. In addition, it was demonstrated that in almost the same time as the transient appearance of AFP the isozyme patterns of aldolase and acid phosphatase deviated from those of normal adult liver to more immature patterns.

The appearance of AFP and these enzymatic changes in rats fed with an azo-dye-containing diet indicate that the renewed small hepatocytes possess at least partly common properties with those of fetal liver and hepatomas. If the precancerous state could be defined as a state of cellular function deviating in the direction of dedifferentiation in the ontogenetic process, it may be possible to say that some of the renewed small hepatocytes possess the properties of the precancerous state.

Since the induction of hepatomas in rats by ingestion of *o*-aminoazotoluene was reported originally by Yoshida in 1932, numerous works concerning the histological changes in hepatic tissues during the course of azo-dye feeding have been

*1 Minami-1-jo, Nishi-17-chome, Chuo-ku, Sapporo 060, Japan (小野江為則, 伝法公麿, 金子愛子).

*2 Kita-15-jo, Nishi-7-chome, Kita-ku, Sapporo 060, Japan (渡部博之).

carried out both by Yoshida and by other investigators (*4*, *14*, *23*, *26*, *29*, *30*), and the following observations on the process of cancerization were generally accepted, even though some exceptional observations were reported by other investigators in the same field (*5*, *6*): Diffuse hyperplasia of hepatocytes appeared in the initial stage, followed by nodular or adenomatous proliferation of the hepatic cells, and the production of hepatomas occurred in some of the areas of the nodules in a later stage. This progressive alteration of hepatic tissues might be explained by the summation theory, proposed by Nakahara (*16*, *17*) and others (*2*, *15*): *i.e.*, the stepwise, irreversible changes in structure and metabolic function of the individual cell towards hepatoma cells may be caused by the effects of overtime of the carcinogenic agent, and the final conversion to completely cancerized cells should be considered as the summation of the short-term effects of the agent when used continuously for a long period. If such stepwise transformations occur in the course of carcinogenesis, submanifestative, irreversibly transformed cells should appear at the intermediary stages. Although these ' precancerous ' cells would presumably be characterized by their functional or structural properties, different from those of normal hepatocytes and similar to those of cancer cells to some extent, such changes of precancerous cells have scarcely been investigated until recently.

In connection with this problem, studies on aldolase isozyme patterns in precancerous cells, reported recently by Endo *et al.* (*3*), are of great interest. These authors noticed that a definite, irreversibly altered isozyme pattern of aldolase, which was clearly different from that of normal adult liver tissues and similar to that of hepatoma tissues, appeared in the rat liver in the early stage of hepatocarcinogenesis, when hepatomas were not yet detectable by histological examinations. This irreversible change of pattern was observed in rat liver on azo-dye feeding within only 2 months. From the results of our experiments concerning the relation between the initiation of the histological change of hepatic tissues and the transient appearance of α-fetoprotein (AFP) in sera during the course of azo-dye feeding (*9*, *10*, *11*, *28*), especially in the early stage, it is possible to consider that there is a critical time for the alteration from normal to cancerous character, within 2 months of the feeding of the agent. The present study has been carried out mainly to elucidate the significance of the appearance of AFP in the early stage of carcinogenesis by azo-dye feeding.

Fluctuation of Various Cell Populations in Hepatic Tissue

Terayama (*27*), and Miller and Miller (*20*) reported that 3′-methyl-4-dimethylaminoazobenzene (3′-Me-DAB) is metabolized exclusively in the hepatocytes of rat liver to produce toxic metabolites. The primary change after the commencement of 3′-Me-DAB administration was degenerative alteration in the hepatocytes and the grade of degeneration could be expressed by the decrease of enzyme activities localized in hepatocytes, such as glucose-6-phosphatase (G-6-Pase). Figure 1 indicates the activities of G-6-Pase and acid phosphatase during the early stage of 3′-Me-DAB feeding. A marked decrease in both enzyme activities was observed 1 to 3 weeks after ingestion.

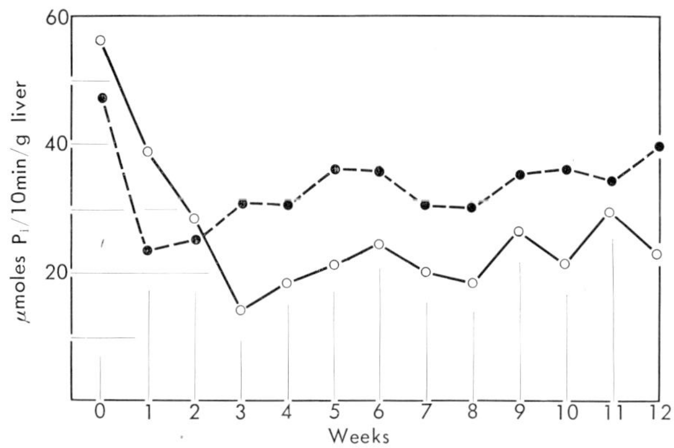

FIG. 1. Activities of glucose-6-phosphatase and acid phosphatase during 3′-Me-DAB administration
○ glucose-6-phosphatase; ● acid phosphatase.

Histologically, the degenerated hepatocytes began to disappear from the periportal areas of the hepatic lobules after 3 to 4 weeks, and simultaneously cholangiolar cells (the so-called oval cells) began to proliferate in the periportal areas occupying half of each lobule. On the other hand, marked megalocytosis of the remaining hepatocytes, whose cytoplasm was strongly eosinophilic, was observed around the central veins. Photo 1 illustrates a light micrograph of the rat liver tissue at this stage. The oval cells markedly proliferated in the periportal areas of the hepatic lobules, while megalocytic cells remained in the central areas.

The ultrastructural appearance of these megalocytic hepatocytes was characterized by marked hypertrophy of the smooth endoplasmic reticulum (SER) and diminution of the rough endoplasmic reticulum (RER), as shown in Photo 3. The activity of a drug metabolizing enzyme in hepatic tissue in this period did not show any elevation, despite the marked hypertrophy of the SER (*21*). Recently, Hutterer *et al.* (*7*) have divided hepatocellular response to chemical agents into the following 3 stages: (1) state of induction; (2) a steady state; (3) state of decompensation. The hepatocytic response to 3′-Me-DAB was evidently the hypertrophic hypoactive response of the SER, corresponding to the 3rd stage, the state of decompensation.

In these megalocytic hepatocytes, hepatocytes with giant nuclei were frequently observed. The occurrence of these giant cells may be explained as follows: When hepatocytes suffer severe and prolonged damage, caused by azo dye, and some of them show necrosis, the remainder should become hyperfunctional cells to compensate for the decline of the total function. If they do not possess the ability to complete cell division, some of them would become megalocytic, responding to regenerative stimuli. The nucleoli in these cells, as shown in Photo 3, frequently showed segregation, which suggests a disturbance in RNA synthesis (*24*). Thus, the original hepatocytes existing at the beginning of azo-dye ingestion ultimately seemed to disappear from the hepatic tissue.

The oval cells, mentioned above, were sometimes taken for fibroblasts because of their appearance on light microscopy. From findings by electron microscopy

(Photo 4), however, it became evident that they are of a cholangiocellular character. Their proliferation reached a maximum in the 4th week, and tended to decrease thereafter.

Small basophilic cells, whose cytoplasm was more abundant than that of the oval cells, began to be frequently observed among and adjacent to the oval cells in this period. They increased in number gradually, while they became hardly distinguishable from normal hepatocytes in respect to morphological appearance (Photo 2). This increase in number and size was followed by a decrease in the oval cells, as well as the degenerated original hepatocytes. The reciprocal change in the number of hepatocytes and of oval cells is supposed to be the result of differentiation and maturation of the oval cells to hepatocytes, as will be described later.

Fluctuation of various cell populations occurred throughout all of the hepatic lobes and to almost the same degree in each individual animal. While the proportions of original hepatocytes, oval cells, and renewed small hepatocytes fluctuated strikingly, the proportions of other types of cells, such as littoral cells and bile duct cells, showed negligible changes.

The present authors tried to determine the alteration of cell population in rat liver during azo-dye carcinogenesis semiquantitatively, by cutting off and weighing the portions occupied by each of the different cell types on the light microscopic photograph (*9*). Figure 2 shows the time course of the change of proportions of original hepatocytes, oval cells and renewed hepatocytes. At the same time, the appearance of AFP in the sera was examined by the double diffusion method of Ouchterlony (*22*) or by Mancini's single radial immunodiffusion method (*18*) (Fig. 3).

As shown in Fig. 2, the original hepatocytes gradually disappeared from the hepatic tissues after 3′-Me-DAB ingestion, being replaced by renewed hepatocytes. On the other hand, as shown in Fig. 3, AFP appeared transiently in the sera of rats around the 6th week, and its appearance seemed to be retarded slightly relative to the proliferation of the oval cells, and concurrent with the appearance of the renewed hepatocytes. AFP was always observed in the sera of rats whose

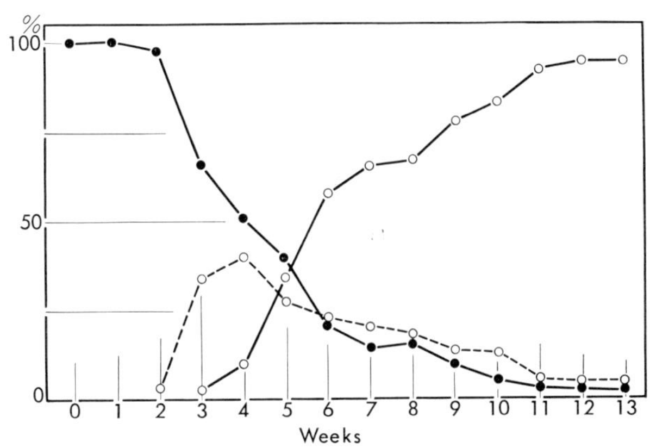

FIG. 2. Cell types in rat liver during 3′-Me-DAB administration
● original hepatocyte ; ○ renewed hepatocyte ; – –○– – oval cell.

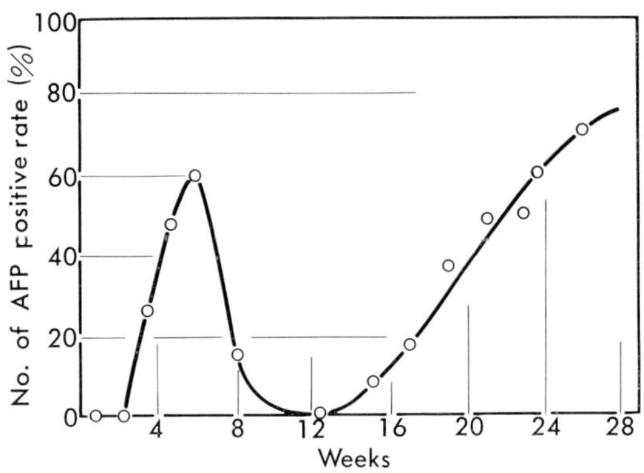

FIG. 3. Number of AFP-positive rats during 4-dimethylaminoazobenzene carcinogenesis

hepatic biopsy specimens showed a marked proliferation of small hepatocytes. Direct evidence for the presence of AFP in the renewed hepatocytes by the immunofluorescence method could not be obtained in the present experiment. However, it is easily conceivable that the immature hepatocytes may produce AFP on differentiation from oval cells to hepatocytes, as fetal hepatocytes do in certain periods of the ontogenic process. Thus the oval cells seemed to play an important role as blast cells of hepatocytes in azo-dye carcinogenesis.

Transformation of Oval Cells

Ultrastructurally, a few oval cells were in a cluster, forming a small lumen, and were surrounded by a distinct basement membrane, as shown in Photo 4a. In the cytoplasm of most of the oval cells the development of organelles was scanty, as shown in Photo 4a. Their morphological features were similar to those of the cholangiolar cells which form the connecting tubules between the bile canaliculi and the interlobular bile ducts. Some of these cells, though rarely, possessed small secretory vesicles and small mucinous secretory granules of high density in the cytoplasm, adjacent to the surface facing the lumen, as indicated by arrows in Photo 4b, and these aspects closely resembled those of the undifferentiated cells found in the crypt epithelium of the small intestine. When the oval cells markedly proliferated in hepatic lobules, mitotic figures were frequently observed histologically and oval cells having ^{3}H-thymidine grains were more frequently observed in the radioautograph after a single injection of ^{3}H-labeled thymidine.

Transformation of the oval cells to hepatocytes could be observed by light microscopy, but was more easily followed by electron microscopy. The canals of Hering, where the terminal ductules of the bile ducts join the parenchyms to receive bile from the system of canaliculi between the hepatocytes, are hardly detected in a normal liver, while they were easily observed in hepatic tissues in the period when the oval cells actively proliferated (Photo 5). Some of the oval cells had a direct contact with the original hepatocytes. In the majority of cases,

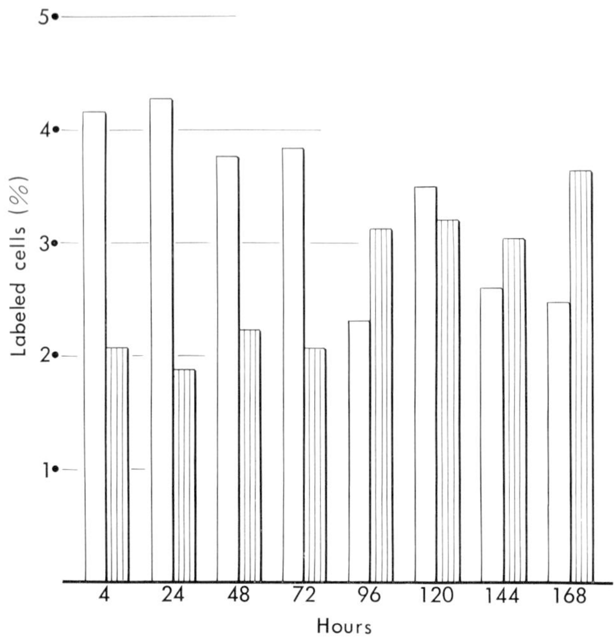

FIG. 4. Percentage of labeled oval cells and hepatocytes from the liver of rats following the injection of ^{3}H-thymidine, after feeding 3′-Me-DAB for 45 days □ oval cell; ▥ hepatocyte.

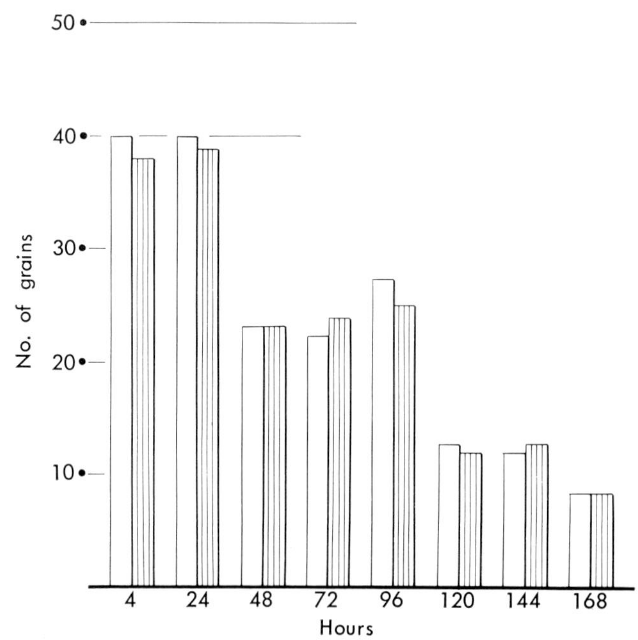

FIG. 5. Grain counts of labeled oval cells and hepatocytes from the liver of rats after the injection of ^{3}H-thymidine, after feeding 3′-Me-DAB for 45 days □ oval cell; ▥ hepatocyte.

however, the transitional cells were detected between the oval cells and the original hepatocytes (Photo 6). The transitional cells possessed ultrastructurally cytoplasmic characteristics of various degrees between the specific structural characters of the latter 2 types of cells. The difficulty in distinguishing the immature hepatocytes from the oval cells could frequently be overcome by the detection of peroxisomes with nucleoids as a specific characteristic of hepatocytes (Photo 7).

Inaoka (*8*), one of our colleagues, has studied radioautographically the fluctuation of cellular components during azo-dye feeding, especially focussing his attention on the fate of the oval cells. ^{3}H-Thymidine was injected once into rats in whose livers marked proliferation of oval cells was detected. In his study, the labeling index of various kinds of cells in the hepatic tissue was calculated at definite time intervals after ^{3}H-thymidine injection. Figures 4 and 5 indicate the percentage of labeled oval cells and hepatocytes, and the grain counts of the hepatocytes after a single injection of ^{3}H-thymidine, respectively. As shown in Fig. 4, the percentage of labeled cells of both types remained almost the same for 3 days. On the 4th day, a marked change was observed; *i.e.*, the percentage of labeled oval cells decreased, while that of labeled hepatocytes increased. Since there was a reciprocal relation between the labeling rates of both types of cells with time, it could be assumed that the transition from oval cell to hepatocyte might occur during 2 successive cell divisions, considering the grain counts of both types of cells in Fig. 5.

From the results of these morphological and radioautographic studies, it is inferred that the transition or differentiation of oval cells to hepatocytes occurs actively in the early stage of azo-dye carcinogenesis.

In normal rats, regeneration of the hepatic parenchyma occurs through the division of preexisting hepatocytes. However, some explanation as to why the proliferation and differentiation of the oval cells play a leading role in the regeneration of hepatic tissue damaged by 3′-Me-DAB is necessary. As mentioned above, the azo dye is almost exclusively metabolized in hepatocytes (*1*), resulting in their inability to respond by cell division to regenerative stimuli. On the other hand, the oval cells, which are not able to metabolize the azo dye and thus produce no toxic metabolites, must not be affected at all by the azo dye. Thus, the following hypothesis is easily acceptable: When the hepatocytes suffer severe and prolonged damage caused by the metabolites, oval cells with multipotentiality proliferate, in place of hepatocytes, and then transform to hepatocytes. This phenomenon should be considered as a kind of adaptation to the azo dye.

Appearance of AFP and the Precancerous State

Finally, we would like to present some considerations regarding the significance of AFP appearance at the early stage. As stated above, since the AFP appeared in the sera at the early stage of carcinogenesis concurrently with the appearance of small hepatocytes transformed from oval cells, it is conceivable that AFP may be produced by the immature hepatocytes, as it is produced by immature hepatocytes in the fetus. In this connection, it is noteworthy that the early appearance of AFP was not observed in experiments with 2-acetylaminofluorene (AAF), where marked proliferation of oval cells was not observed following the administration of 0.025% AAF.

On the other hand, results reported separately by one of the present authors indicate the existence of a relationship between the early appearance of AFP and cancerization of hepatocytes (*28*). Namely, of 22 rats in whose sera AFP appeared in the early stage, 20 (91%) developed hepatomas after 19 weeks. In addition, it was demonstrated that the transient appearance of AFP was observed at almost the same stage when a deviation of the isozyme pattern of aldolase from that of normal adult liver was recognized (*3*, *10*). A similar deviation was also found in the isozyme pattern of acid phosphatase in the same period, as indicated in Fig. 6. Namely, the present authors found that 3 types of acid phosphatase, tentatively designated as A, B, and C, exist in normal rat liver, of which 2 types of enzyme (A and B) are located in parenchymal cells and the other (C) essentially in reticuloendothelial cells. In addition, it has been suggested that the former

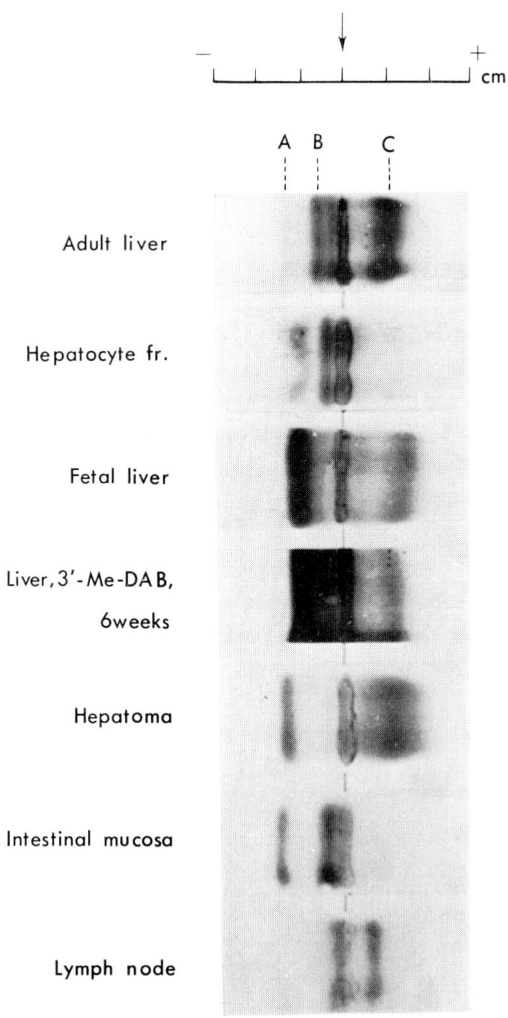

FIG. 6. Electrophoretic patterns of acid phosphatase

2 types of enzyme are related to the differentiation of hepatocytes, since type B was predominent in adult rat liver and the other (A) appeared preferentially in fetal and newborn livers and also in hepatocellular carcinomas (*12*). Examinations of the hepatic tissues after 6 weeks of 3′-Me-DAB ingestion, in which the small hepatocytes were markedly proliferating, revealed an increase in type A and a decrease in type B, while the amount of type C showed almost no change during this period (*11*). This result strongly suggests that the isozyme of type A may be derived from the undifferentiated small hepatocytes, as in the case of AFP.

The appearance of AFP and these enzymic changes in rats fed with a 3′-Me-DAB-containing diet indicate that the renewed small hepatocytes possessed at least common properties with those of fetal livers and hepatomas. If the precancerous state could be defined as a state of cellular function deviating in the direction of dedifferentiation in the ontogenetic process, it may be fairly safe to say that the small hepatocytes possess the properties of the precancerous state.

In the present experiments, the appearance of AFP was transient, while the alterations in isozyme patterns seemed to be irreversible. This discrepancy may be resolved by using more sensitive methods for detecting AFP and for isolation of the renewed hepatocytes. If techniques are improved, we could determine whether there was continuous production of AFP by the renewed hepatocytes and their progeny throughout the entire course, though the amount must be very small in the intervening period. It is not probable, however, that most of the renewed hepatocytes maintain the properties of precancerous cells for a long period. The majority of them may revert to the state of normal hepatocytes as regards function and structure, while minor populations may retain their state of dedifferentiation as precancerous cells. In the advanced stage, very small populations of these, which continue to possess the properties of precancerous cells, may form small hyperplastic foci which become larger later. Finally, some of their progeny in large hyperplastic nodules may develop into cancer cells as described by other investigators (*13*, *19*, *25*), although this process is not yet clarified.

Further investigations will be performed in order to elucidate the characteristics of the precancerous hepatocytes after the first peak of AFP appearance.

Acknowledgments

The authors express their gratitude to Professor Takashi Hayashi, Department of Microbiology, Sapporo Medical College, for valuable suggestions for improving this manuscript. This work was partly supported by a Grant-in-Aid for Cancer Research from the Ministry of Education, which is gratefully acknowledged.

After this article was submitted for publication, the authors obtained the additional results concerning the localization of AFP by the immunofluorescence method, and also the histochemical staining of isoenzymatically changed aldolase and non-specific esterase: *i.e.*, AFP was exclusively detectable in the transitional cells and small hepatocytes transformed from the oval cells, and the isoenzyme patterns of these cells altered from those of the original hepatocytes. The results have been reported at the 31st Annual Meeting of the Japanese Cancer Association, October, 1972.

REFERENCES

1. Baba, T. Study on the intrahepatic topographical distribution of protein-bound azo dye in rat by means of ^{14}C-labeled *p*-dimethylaminoazobenzene radioautography. *GANN*, **52**, 253–256 (1961).
2. Druckrey, H., Schmähl, D., and Dischler, W. L. Dosis-Wirkungs-Beziehungen bei der Krebserzeugung durch 4-Dimethylamino-stilben bei Ratten. *Z. Krebsforsch.*, **65**, 272–288 (1963).
3. Endo, H., Eguchi, M., and Yanagi, S. Irreversible fixation of increased level of muscle-type aldolase activity appearing in rat liver in the early stage of hepatocarcinogenesis. *Cancer Res.*, **30**, 743–752 (1970).
4. Farber, E. Similarities in the sequence of early histological changes induced in the liver of the rat by ethionine, 2-acetylaminofluorene, and 3′-methyl-4-dimethylaminoazobenzene. *Cancer Res.*, **16**, 142–148 (1956).
5. H. I. H. Prince Masahito (Hitachi). Chromosome changes in rat liver cells after administration of diethylnitrosamine. *Proc. Jap. Cancer Assoc., 30th Annu. Meet.*, 3 (1971).
6. Hughes, P. E. Liver cell responses to the carcinogen, 3′-methyl-4-dimethylaminoazobenzene. *Chem. Biol. Interactions*, **1**, 301–305 (1969/70).
7. Hutterer, F., Klion, F. M., Wengref, A., Schaffner, F., and Popper, H. Hepatocellular adaptation and injury. Structural and biochemical changes following Dieldrin and methyl Butter Yellow. *Lab. Invest.*, **20**, 455–464 (1969).
8. Inaoka, Y. Significance of the so-called oval cell proliferation during azo-dye hepatocarcinogenesis. *GANN*, **58**, 355–366 (1967).
9. Iwasaki, T., Dempo, K., Kaneko, A., and Onoé, T. Fluctuation of various cell population and their characteristics during azo-dye carcinogenesis. *GANN*, **63**, 21–30 (1972).
10. Kaneko, A., Dempo, K., Iwasaki, T., and Onoé, T. Changes in the activities of glucose-6-phosphatase, aldolase, and alkaline phosphatase during azo-dye carcinogenesis. *GANN*, **63**, 31–39 (1972).
11. Kaneko, A., Dempo, K., and Onoé, T. Changes in acid phosphatase during azo-dye carcinogenesis. *GANN*, **63**, 40–48 (1972).
12. Kaneko, A., Ikeda, T., and Onoé, T. Acid phosphatases from different cell types in rat liver. *Biochim. Biophys. Acta*, **222**, 218–221 (1970).
13. Karasaki, S. The fine structure of proliferating cells in preneoplastic rat livers during azo-dye carcinogenesis. *J. Cell Biol.*, **40**, 322–335 (1969).
14. Kinosita, R. Studies on the carcinogenic chemical substances. *Nippon Byori Gakkai Kaishi* (*Transact. Soc. Pathol. Japan*), **27**, 665–727 (1937).
15. Nothdurft, H. Grundprobleme der Krebsforschung. *Z. Krebsforsch.*, **59**, 167–179 (1953).
16. Nakahara, W. Critique of carcinogenic mechanism. *Progr. Exp. Tumor Res.*, **2**, 158–202 (1961).
17. Nakahara, W. Mode of origin and characterization of cancer. *In* "Chemical Tumor Problems," Japan Society for the Promotion of Science, Tokyo, pp. 287–330 (1970).
18. Mancini, G., Carbonara, A. O., and Heremans, J. F. Immunochemical quan-

titation of antigens by single radial immunodiffusion. *Immunochemistry*, **2**, 235–254 (1965).

19. Merkow, L. P., Epstein, S. M., Farber, E., Pardo, M., and Bartur, B. Cellular analysis of liver carcinogenesis. III. Comparison of liver nodules and hepatocellular carcinomas induced in rat liver by 2-fluorenylacetamide. *J. Natl. Cancer Inst.*, **43**, 33–63 (1969).
20. Miller, E. C. and Miller, J. A. Biochemical investigations on hepatic carcinogenesis. *J. Natl. Cancer Inst.*, **15**, 1571–1590 (1955).
21. Onoé, T., Fuse, Y., and Kaneko, A. A comparative electron microscopic study on the changes of endoplasmic reticulum in rat hepatocytes induced by 3′-Me-DAB and phenobarbital. *6th Int. Congr. Electron Microscopy*, 621–622 (1966).
22. Ouchterlony, O. Antigen-antibody reaction in gels. IV. Types of reaction in coordinated systems of diffusion. *Acta Pathol. Microbiol. Scand.*, **32**, 231–240 (1953).
23. Price, J. M., Harman, J. W., Miller, E. C., and Miller, J. A. Progressive microscopic alterations in the livers of rats fed the hepatic carcinogens, 3′-methyl-4-dimethylaminoazobenzene and 4′-fluoro-4-dimethylaminoazobenzene. *Cancer Res.*, **12**, 192–200 (1952).
24. Reddy, J. and Svoboda, D. The relationship of nucleolar segregation to ribonucleic acid synthesis following the administration of selected hepatocarcinogens. *Lab. Invest.*, **19**, 132–145 (1968).
25. Reuber, M. D. Development of preneoplastic and neoplastic lesions of the liver in male rats given 0.025% N-2-fluorenylacetamide. *J. Natl. Cancer Inst.*, **34**, 697–723 (1965).
26. Sasaki, T. and Yoshida, T. Experimentelle Erzeugung des Lebercarcinoms durch Fütterung mit *o*-Amidoazotoluol. *Virchows Arch.*, **295**, 12–42 (1935).
27. Terayama, H. Aminoazocarcinogenesis—methods and biochemical problems. *In* "Methods in Cancer Research," Academic Press, Inc., New York-London, pp. 399–449 (1967).
28. Watabe, H. Early appearance of embryonic α-globulin in rat serum during carcinogenesis with 4-dimethylaminoazobenzene. *Cancer Res.*, **31**, 1192–1194 (1971).
29. Yoshida, T. "Gan no Hassei (Production of Cancer)," Nippon Isho, Tokyo-Kyoto (1948) (in Japanese).
30. Yoshida, T. Über die experimentelle Erzeugung von Hepatome durch die Fütterung mit *o*-Amidoazotoluol. *Proc. Imp. Acad.*, **8**, 464–467 (1932).

EXPLANATION OF PHOTOS

PHOTO 1. A light micrograph from the liver of a rat at the 3rd week after 3′-Me-DAB ingestion. Periportal areas (P) of hepatic lobules are occupied by a great number of oval cells. Hepatocytes around the central vein (C) are megalocytic. Some have gigantic nuclei. ×93.

PHOTO 2. A light micrograph from the liver of a rat at the 6th week. In the right upper corner, a small number of original megalocytic hepatocytes are seen in the central area, while renewed small hepatocytes occupy a large part of the lobules in this section. Oval cells are also observed among the small hepatocytes. ×93.

PHOTO 3. An electron micrograph of a megalocytic hepatocyte. The cytoplasm is packed with hypertrophied smooth endoplasmic reticulum (SER), while lamellar arrangements of rough endoplasmic reticulum are inconspicuous. A few lipid droplets are seen. Note the typical nucleolar segregation. ×10,000.

PHOTO 4. Electron micrographs of oval cells. (4a) The oval cells form a lumen (L). Their cytoplasm contains few organelles. On the surface abutting on the stroma, a distinct basement membrane (BM) is observed. ×10,000. (4b) Secretory granules of high density are seen in the cytoplasm near the cell surface. Nucleus (N). ×7,300.

PHOTO 5. A portion of the canal Hering. Among an oval cell (O) and a transitional cell (Tr), original hepatocytes (H) form small lumens. In the cytoplasm of hepatocytes packed with fine tubular or vesicular SER, conspicuously hypertrophied Golgi apparatuses are seen. ×7,300.

PHOTO 6. A higher magnification of the transitional cells in Photo 5. Compared with the oval cells, cytoplasmic organelles are more abundant. No peroxisomes are seen in the cytoplasm. ×10,000.

PHOTO 7. A renewed small hepatocyte. The cell has an appearance similar to that of the oval cell or transitional cell in Photo 5, though the organelles in the cytoplasm are more abundant. Note the presence of peroxisomes with a distinct nucleoid (indicated by arrows). ×10,000.

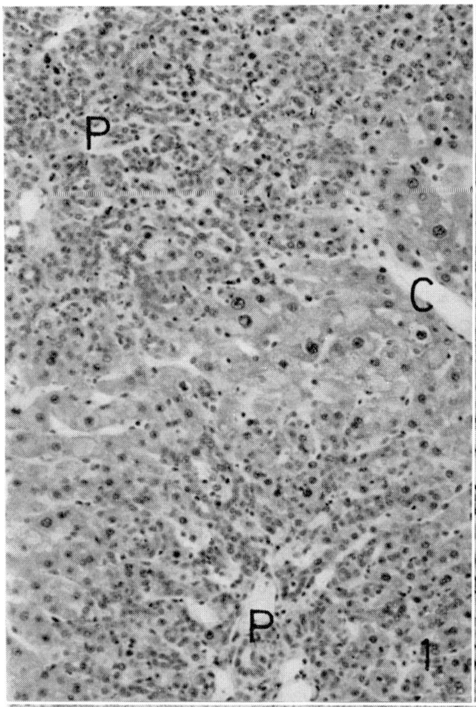
P
C
P
1

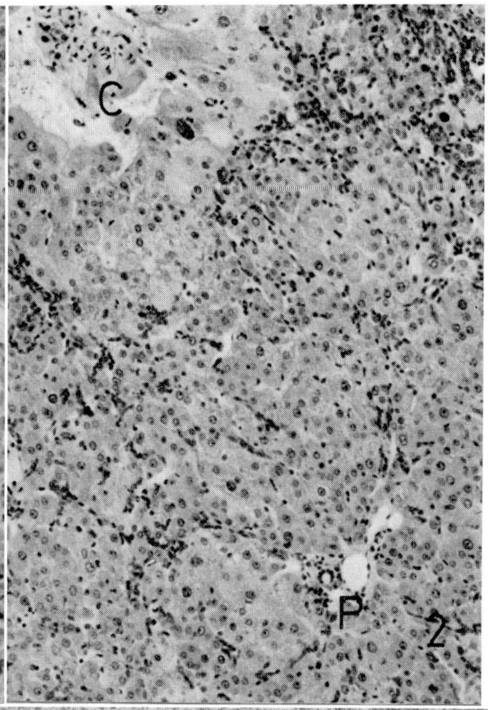
C
P
2

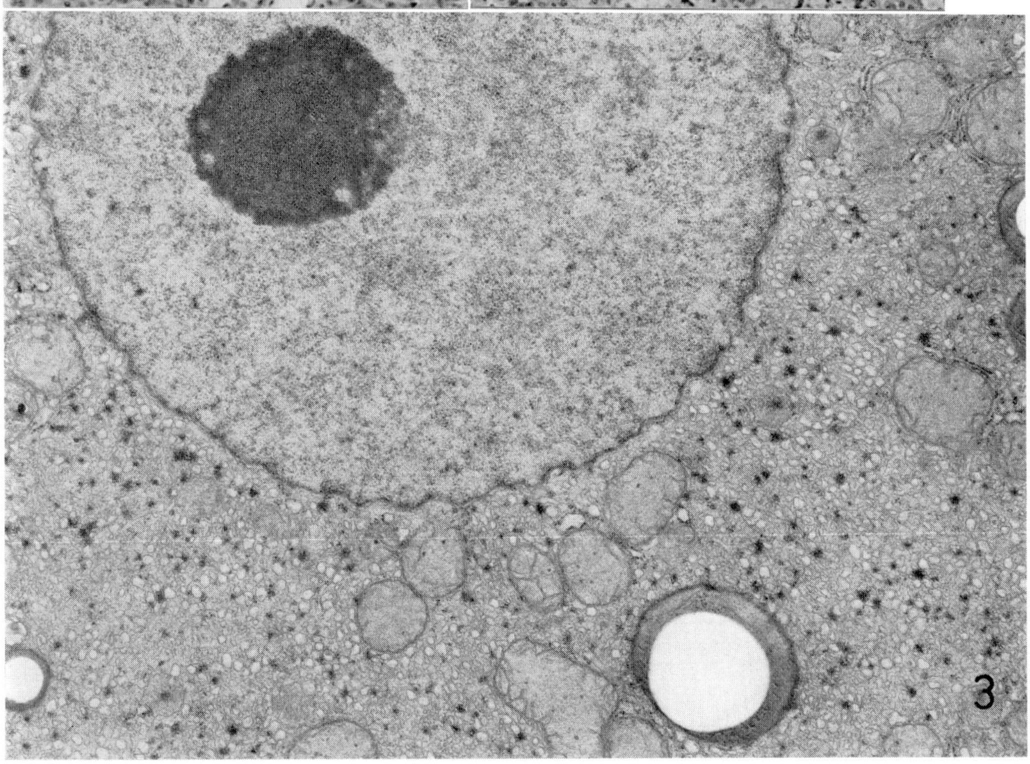
3

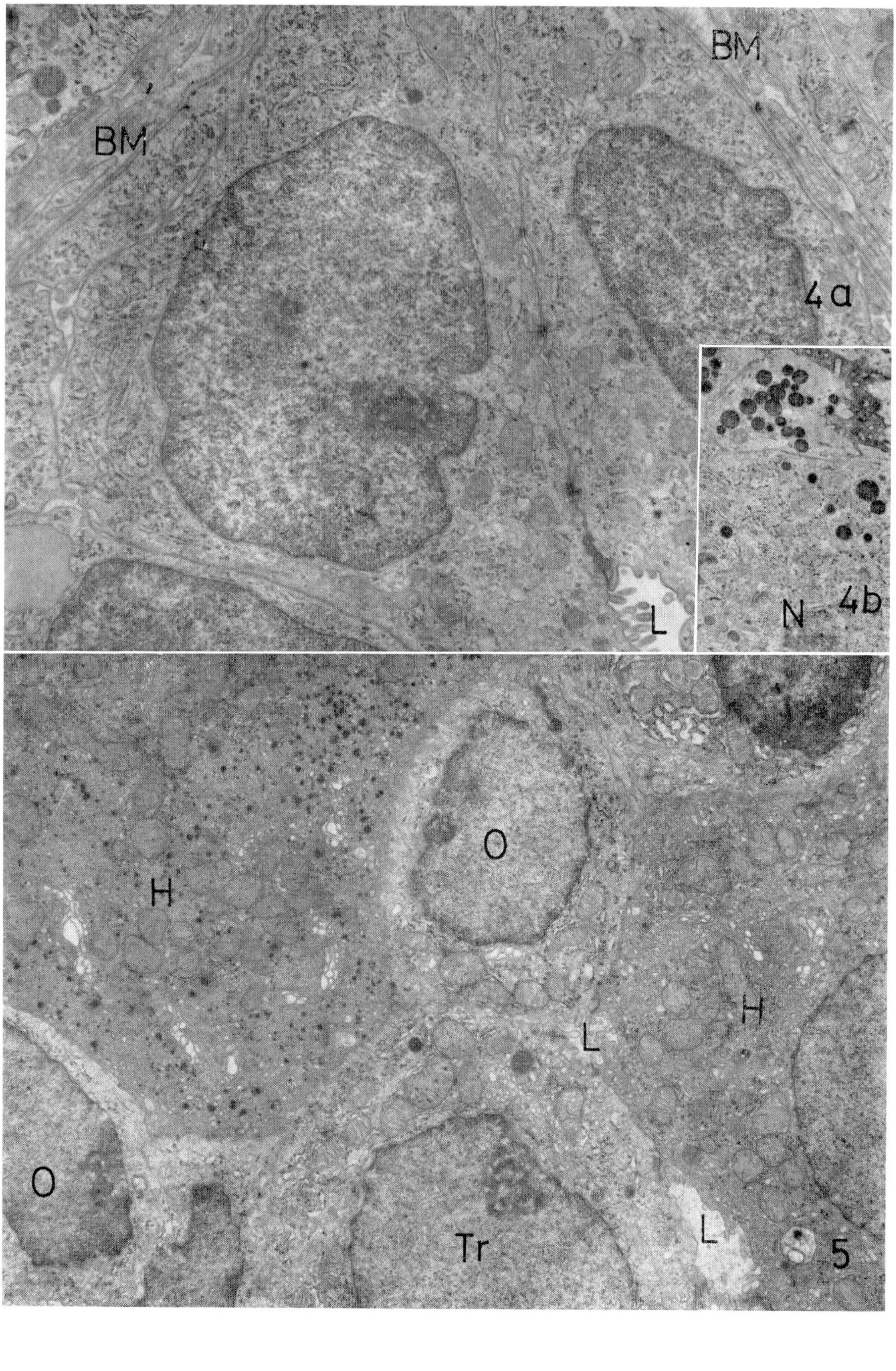
BM
BM
4a
4b
N
L
O
H
H
L
O
Tr
L
5

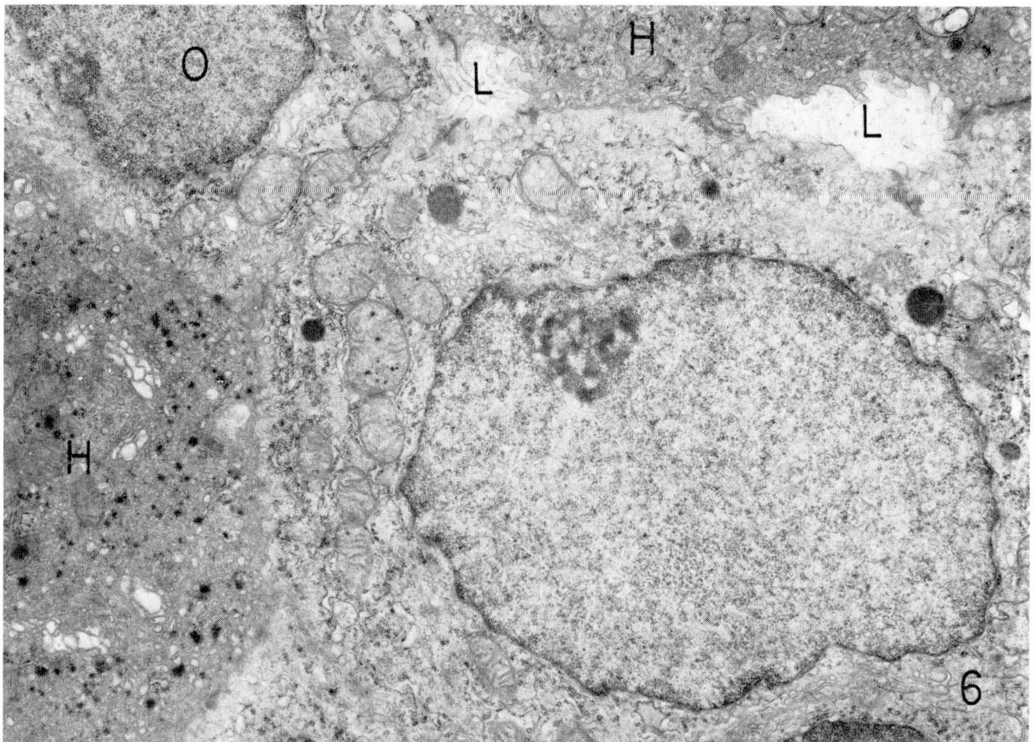
O
H
L
L
H
6

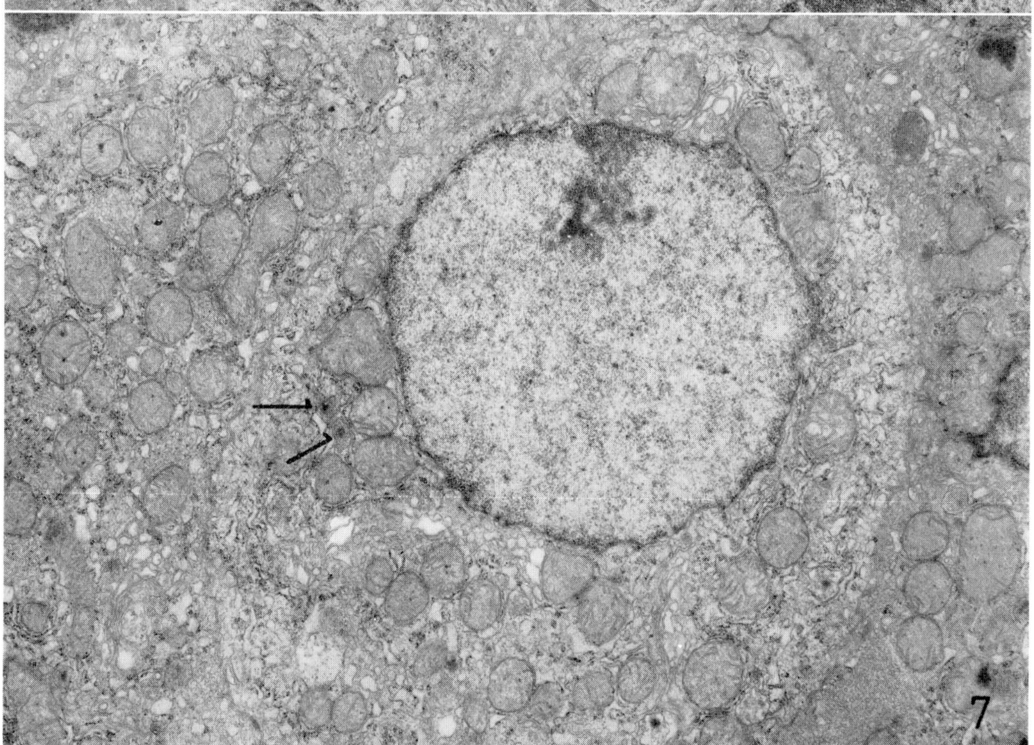
7

GANN Monograph on Cancer Research 14, 1973

α-FETOPROTEIN AND HEPATOCARCINOGENESIS IN RATS

Tomoyuki KITAGAWA, Taeko YOKOCHI, and Haruo SUGANO
*Department of Pathology, Cancer Institute**

Serum α-fetoprotein (AFP) appeared in 2 phases during hepatocarcinogenesis in rats fed 3′-methyl-4-dimethylaminoazobenzene (3′-Me-DAB) or N-2-fluorenylacetamide (FAA). The frequency of appearance of serum AFP as well as its concentration, however, varied considerably according to differences in age, sex, and strain of the animals or differences in the type or dose of the carcinogen. In general, 3′-Me-DAB was a much stronger carcinogen than FAA as regards producing serum AFP in both phases.

The early AFP was believed to be produced by oval cells. The cells composing the nodular hyperplasia or the area of hyperplasia, which replaced the major part of the liver in the next stage and had been considered the most probable forerunner of the carcinoma, did not produce AFP. The serum AFP in the late phase was produced by the carcinoma. The majority of 3′-Me-DAB-induced carcinomas belonged to the mixed-type carcinoma, which was strongly AFP-producing. Most of the FAA-induced carcinomas were the trabecular carcinoma, which was relatively weak in AFP production.

The appearance of early serum AFP was a distinct indicator of fair progress of hepatocarcinogenesis. However, it was not an absolute requisite for the later development of carcinomas.

Before the development of an overt carcinoma, numerous hyperplastic lesions with different features appear in succession in the liver during carcinogenesis (*9*, *13*, *17*, *18*, *22*, *24*, *26*, *28*, *29*, *31*, *32*, *37*). These hyperplastic lesions have long been considered possible forerunners of the carcinoma. Yet, despite numerous studies, concrete and convincing evidence is still lacking as far as their exact nature is concerned. When specific production of α-fetoprotein (AFP) by the liver carcinoma with high frequency was emphasized (*1*, *2–4*, *7*, *8*, *10*, *15*, *25*, *33*), we assumed that here was an excellent clue for characterizing the "precancerous" lesions. Watabe and Hirai (*34*, *36*) were the first to report the frequent transient appearance of serum AFP during the early weeks of hepatocarcinogenesis by azo dyes. Onoé and Fuse (*26*) pointed out the close relationship between this phenomenon and proliferation of the oval cells from which small hepatocytes were derived at this stage.

In order to determine the mechanism of the transient early appearance of serum AFP and its meaning in hepatocarcinogenesis, we checked serum AFP of

* Kami-Ikebukuro 1-37-1, Toshima-ku, Tokyo 170, Japan (北川知行, 横地妙子, 菅野晴夫).

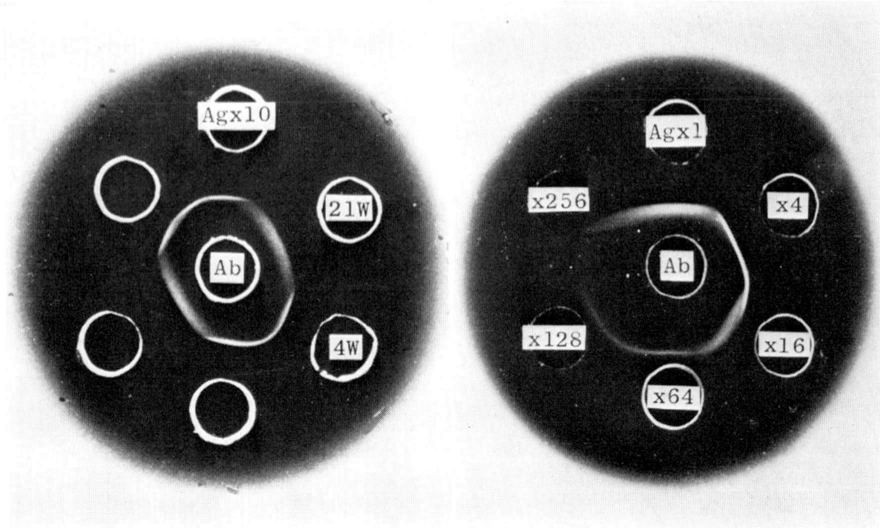

FIG. 1. (Left): Reaction in gel between anti-AFP (Ab) and 10-fold dilution of amniotic fluid (Ag×10), the serum of a carcinoma-bearing rat (21W), and the serum of a rat at the 4th week (4W)
(Right): Reaction between anti-AFP (Ab) and serially diluted antigen (amniotic fluid)

TABLE I. Experimental Groups

Group	Strain of rat	Sex	Initial body weight (g)	No. of rats used	Carcinogen
I	Donryu	Male	140–160	170	0.06% 3′-Me-DAB
II	Donryu	Male	80–100	10	0.06% 3′-Me-DAB
III	Donryu	Male	350–450	9	0.06% 3′-Me-DAB
IV	Donryu	Female	130–150	10	0.06% 3′-Me-DAB
V	Wistar	Male	140–160	10	0.06% 3′-Me-DAB
VI	Wistar	Female	140–160	10	0.06% 3′-Me-DAB
VII	Sprague-Dawley	Male	130–150	10	0.06% 3′-Me-DAB
VIII	ACI	Male	130–150	20	0.06% 3′-Me-DAB
IX	ACI	Male	130–150	10	0.09% 3′-Me-DAB
X	ACI	Male	130–150	10	0.12% 3′-Me-DAB
XI	ACI	Male	130–150	10	0.18% 3′-Me-DAB[a]
XII	ACI	Male	130–150	10	0.30% 3′-Me-DAB
XIII	Donryu	Male	140–160	130	0.03% FAA[b]
XIV	Donryu	Male	140–160	10	0.05% FAA
XV	Donryu	Male	140–160	10	0.07% FAA

[a] Up to the 4th week, then basal diet. [b] Up to the 18th week, then basal diet.

rats throughout the experimental course with correlative morphological and histochemical studies of the liver. The serum AFP was detected semiquantitatively by the micro-Ouchterlony method, using specific anti-AFP rabbit serum which was prepared in our laboratory (*19*), principally according to the method of Birencwajg (*6*) (Fig. 1). Histochemically, the activities of glucose-6-phosphatase (G-6-Pase) (by Wachstein-Meisel's method (*5*)), canalicular ATPase (ATPase) (by Wachstein-Meisel's method (*5*)), β-glucuronidase (by Hayashi-Fishman's method (*12*)), and phosphorylase (by Takeuchi's method (*5*)) were examined. The experimental schedule and the animals used are shown in Table I.

Sequential Change of Serum AFP during Carcinogenesis

The results of long-term observation of serum AFP in Group I, Donryu male rats fed with a 0.06% 3′-Me-DAB diet, and Group XIII, Donryu male rats fed with a 0.03% FAA diet, are shown in Fig. 2. In Group I, serum AFP became positive in 90% of the rats from the 3rd to 5th experimental week,

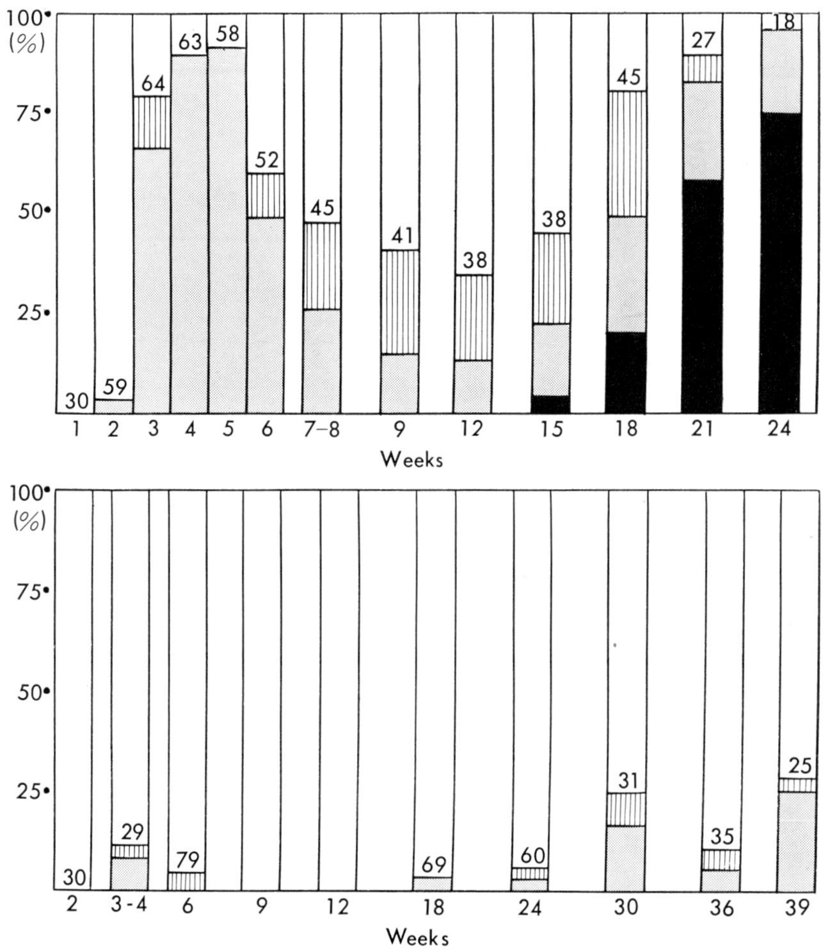

FIG. 2. Frequency of appearance of serum AFP during carcinogenesis by feeding 3′-Me-DAB (top) and FAA (bottom) in male Donryu rats, Groups I and XIII

The figures at the top of bars indicate the number of rats tested.
negative; weakly positive; moderately positive; strongly positive.

then turned negative or weakly positive in the following weeks. From the 15th week, the number of rats with positive or strongly positive serum AFP increased and, up to the 24th week, 95% of the rats showed a strongly positive reaction. In Group XIII, a similar biphasic appearance of serum AFP was observed but, in this group, the frequency and concentration of serum AFP were very low in both phases and the start of the later phase was retarded. Since the rats with positive serum AFP were sacrificed or inclined to die, the frequency of AFP-positive rats at the 36th and 39th week became lower than it might really be.

The frequency of early appearance of serum AFP differed considerably according to differences in age, sex, and strain of the animals or differences in the type and dose of the carcinogens used. It was higher in younger animals (Fig. 3,A)

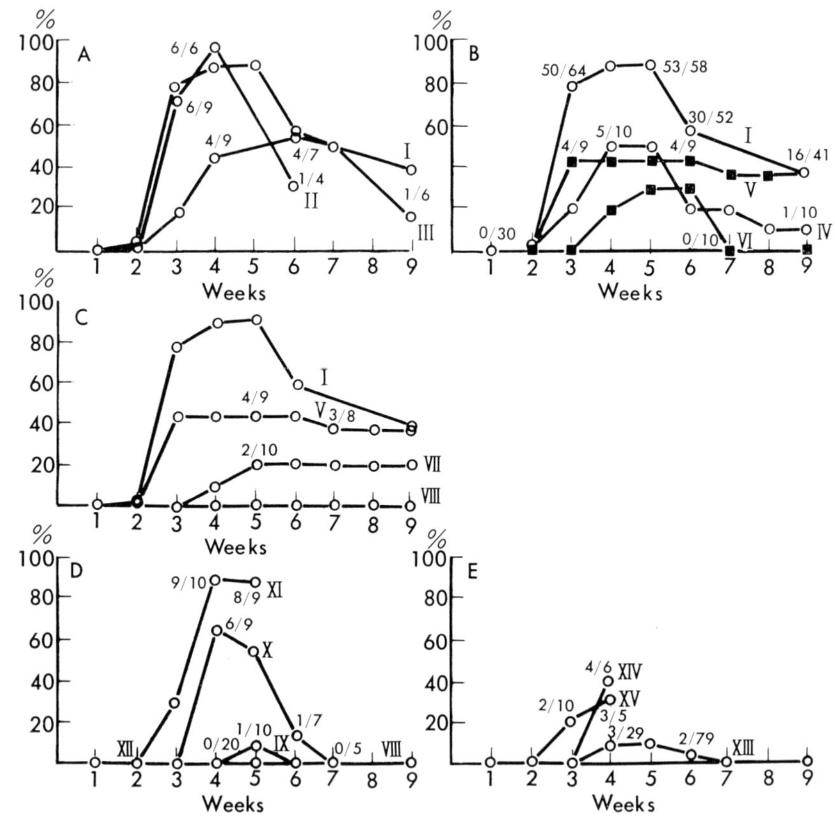

FIG. 3. Different frequencies of early appearance of serum AFP according to differences in age, sex, and strain of animals, and type or dose of carcinogen used

A: Difference by age of rats. I, Donryu ♂ (140–160 g); II, Donryu ♂ (80–100 g); III, Donryu ♂ (350–450 g), 0.06% 3′-Me-DAB.

B: Difference by sex. I, Donryu ♂; IV, Donryu ♀; V, Wistar ♂; VI, Wistar ♀; 0.06% 3′-Me-DAB.

C: Difference by strain. I, Donryu ♂; V, Wistar ♂; VII; Sprague-Dawley ♂; VIII, ACI ♂, 0.06% 3′-Me-DAB.

D: Difference by dose of 3′-Me-DAB. VIII, 0.06%; IX, 0.09%; X, 0.12%; XI; 0.18%; XII, 0.30% 3′-Me-DAB, ACI ♂ (130–150 g).

E: Difference by dose of FAA. XIII, 0.03%; XIV, 0.05%; XV, 0.07% FAA, Donryu ♂ (140–160 g).

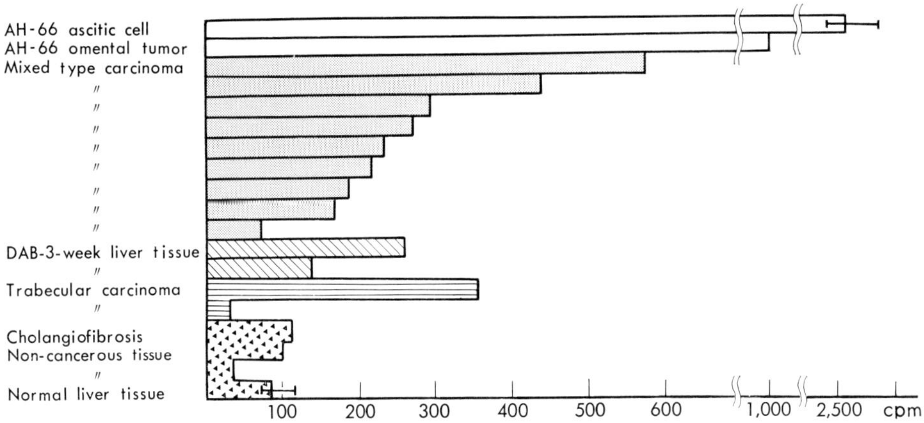

FIG. 4. *In vitro* synthesis of AFP

and in males (Fig. 3,B). Difference by strain was remarkable. Among the strains used, Donryu rats showed an outstandingly high frequency while Sprague-Dawley and ACI rats were quite low or completely negative in 0.06% 3′-Me-DAB carcinogenesis (Fig. 3,C). When ACI rats were fed 0.12 or 0.18% 3′-Me-DAB diet, serum AFP became positive in the majority during the 3rd week (Fig. 3,D). Serum AFP was never positive up to the 2nd week in rats of Group XII, all of which died during the 3rd week with severe hepatic damage. When Donryu rats were fed 0.05 or 0.07% FAA diet, almost all the rats died during the 4th week in a state of acute liver atrophy, but the frequency in appearance of serum AFP was below 40% (Fig. 3,E), and, if positive, the concentration was low.

Morphology and Histochemistry of the Liver at the Phase of Early Appearance of Serum AFP

To certify the AFP production by the liver or tumor tissue, we also performed an experiment concerning *in vitro* synthesis of AFP by tissue slices, using ^{14}C-leucine (*19*). The results are shown in Fig. 4. From this experiment, it was apparent that the liver was the source of serum AFP in the early phase of carcinogenesis. The histological change in the early phase of 0.06% 3′-Me-DAB carcinogenesis was largely similar to that described by previous workers (*9*, *26*, *28*). The characteristic change in the liver is a prominent proliferation of oval cells (*9*) and small hepatocytes, which are believed by some authors (*13*, *28*) to be derived from the oval cells, and megalocytic degeneration of the original mature hepatocytes (Photos 1 and 2). The histological and histochemical features of the liver during 0.03% FAA carcinogenesis have been described previously (*16*, *17*). In this carcinogenesis, proliferation of the oval cells and small hepatocytes was slight and the original mature liver cells became atrophic instead of megalocytic change (Photos 3 and 8).

A good correlation was observed between the serum AFP level and the intensity of oval cell proliferation in individual rats of various groups. Generally, oval cell proliferation was marked in Groups I, II, V, and XI, and slight in Groups VIII, IX, and XIII.

Histochemically, the oval cells were quite immature with a lack of enzyme activities and glycogen, while the small hepatocytes showed slight activity of G-6-Pase and β-glucuronidase that increased to a certain extent with time (Photos 4 and 5). Canalicular ATPase and phosphorylase activities were inconspicuous in both types of cell (Photo 6).

Electron microscopic observations of the oval cells and small hepatocytes gave results similar to those described by other workers (*11*, *13*, *26*). The oval cells had a pale cytoplasm and scanty organelles, resembling the cholangiole cells (Photos 7 and 8). The small hepatocytes had round nuclei and more organelles, but were still fairly immature compared with the original mature hepatocytes.

Through these correlative serological and histological observations, the oval cell was believed to be the cell producing AFP at this stage. However, the possibility of AFP production by degenerative or altered mature original hepatocytes cannot be completely ruled out at present, though it seems unlikely because serum AFP was not detected in any of the rats in Group XII which died during the 2nd week or in most of the rats in Groups XIII to XV which died during the 4th to 5th week with severe hepatic damage but without marked proliferation of oval cells. Serum AFP was not detected in animals which received hepatotoxins (*6*).

Histological and Histochemical Features of the Liver at the Phase of Disappearance of Early Serum AFP

In DAB carcinogenesis after the 6th week, and from the 3rd week in the earliest case, foci of nodular hyperplasia (*31*) appeared in the periportal area. They grew most prominently from the 6th to 9th week, so that the majority of the liver became occupied by this lesion (Photos 4, 5, and 6). By this time, almost all the original hepatocytes had disappeared (Photo 4). At this phase, active proliferation of the oval cells and small hepatocytes was no longer marked. On the contrary, the cells which had previously proliferated were compressed by nodular lesions and ran in narrow bundles around the nodules, so that the liver had a cirrhotic appearance (Photos 5 and 6). The oval cells were spindles as was seen in FAA carcinogenesis. The focal cells among small hepatocytes showed a fairly high enzymic or glycogen level but in the majority maturation was inconspicuous (Photos 5 and 6).

In FAA carcinogenesis at this stage, the area of hyperplasia (*29*) became marked and the major part of the liver was occupied by this lesion by the 12th week (Photo 9).

Histochemically, individual nodular hyperplasia or areas of hyperplasia varied from fairly mature to quite immature (Photos 5, 6, and 9). On the whole, the component cells of nodular hyperplasias or areas of hyperplasia seemed to be newly established ones, not direct descendants of oval cells or small hepatocytes.

As for the mechanism of disappearance of the early serum AFP, both factors, *i.e.*, the prominent development of nodular hyperplasia, not producing AFP, and the cessation of oval cell proliferation associated with maturation, or inactivation of previously proliferated cells, seemed important. The possibility of development of an antibody for AFP causing the disappearance of serum AFP was excluded, based on the following evidence: (a) Anti-AFP was never detected in the serum of rats after disappearance of the early serum AFP. (b) An immunosuppressive treatment with whole-body (except the liver) irradiation of 350 R and 3 injections of 2.5 mg of cortisone acetate on 5 rats at the phase of disappearance of early AFP failed to cause reappearance of serum AFP in the following 10 days. (c) Rats which were fed with a 3′-Me-DAB diet only for the initial 3 weeks and which were positive in serum AFP at the 3rd and 4th week but negative at the 5th and 6th week, became positive for serum AFP again at the 8th week when returned to the carcinogenic diet from the 6th week.

Morphology and Histochemistry of AFP-Producing Carcinomas and the Required Size for Positive Serum AFP

From the results of *in vitro* synthesis of AFP (Fig. 4) and circumstantial evidence, it was obvious that the serum AFP in the later stage of carcinogenesis was produced by the liver carcinoma. When there was no apparent carcinoma in a rat in the later stage, serum AFP was negative. When the serum AFP turned positive, there was always a liver carcinoma with a certain growth size.

In 3′-Me-DAB carcinogenesis, rats with positive serum AFP had 1, or usually several to multiple, liver carcinomas. When alone, the carcinoma measured at least 10 mm, but was usually 15 mm in diameter. The majority of 3′-Me-DAB-induced carcinomas, especially the ones which developed relatively early and grew rapidly with frequent metastasis, belonged to the mixed-type carcinoma (" mixed tumor " of Price *et al.* (*28*), " cholangiohepatoma " of Muley and Firminger (*24*)). The trabecular carcinoma (after Stewart and Snell (*32*), with a modification to include adenohepatoma in this type) appeared several weeks later and grew more slowly, so that it constituted only a small part of the cancerous tissue up to the time of death of the animals. In *in vitro* synthesis, mixed-type carcinomas of predominantly medulary pattern (Photo 10) showed relatively high counts of 300 to 575. Mixed-type carcinomas with prominent fibrosis or a cystoadenomatous pattern (Photo 11) showed a relatively low count, including one with a count below the control level. One trabecular carcinoma counted 360 while another was only 40.

In FAA carcinogenesis, most of the carcinoma was trabecular carcinoma, which became grossly apparent after the 24th week. The serum AFP was usually negative up to the 30th week, until a trabecular carcinoma became larger than 20 mm in diameter. All 12 rats carrying a carcinoma larger than 30 mm in diameter showed positive serum AFP, although there was a tendency for serum AFP concentration to decrease when a rat developed a large trabecular carcinoma later than the 39th week. The majority of trabecular carcinomas which attained a large size up to the 39th week and which were AFP-producing, were a rather malignant type of trabecular carcinoma with basophilic cytoplasm, frequent mitosis, and considerable nuclear atypism (Photo 13). However, ones with less malignant appearance, having eosinophilic cytoplasm and mild nuclear pattern, were also included (Photo 14). In FAA carcinogenesis, the serum AFP rarely became positive within 24 weeks. At that time there was a mixed-type carcinoma measuring 10 mm or more in diameter or a carcinoma with a papillary pattern (Photo 15).

The electron-microscopic features of experimental liver carcinomas have been described by previous authors (*21*, *23*, *26*). Our results were similar. Mixed-type carcinomas were composed of variable cells mimicking immature hepatocytes, oval cells, or cholangiole cells, and intestinal epithelial cells (Photo 16). Trabecular carcinomas were composed of uniform, mature cells with fairly numerous cytoplasmic organelles (Photo 17). Histochemically, all the mixed-type carcinomas were quite immature in enzymic activity, although there was an exceptional case in which G-6-Pase activity was demonstrated in tumor cells taking a papillotubular pattern (Photo 12). All the AFP-producing trabecular hepatomas found in the present experiments were also of an enzymically immature type.

DISCUSSION AND CONCLUSIONS

Serum AFP in rats during hepatocarcinogenesis by 3′-Me-DAB or FAA was checked by the micro-Ouchterlony method throughout the course. The serum AFP appeared in two phases, early from the 3rd to 5th week and late in the stage of development of large carcinoma.

The frequency of early appearance of serum AFP, as well as its concentration, varied considerably according to differences in age, sex, and strain of the animals or differences in type or dose of carcinogen. In general, 3′-Me-DAB was a much stronger carcinogen than FAA as regards producing early serum AFP.

The early AFP was believed to be produced by the oval cells diffusely proliferated in the periportal area at this stage. The meaning of the appearance of early serum AFP in hepatocarcinogenesis is rather difficult to understand fully. The problem concerning this phenomenon is similar to that of the oval cells. Since Farber (*9*) suggested the importance of oval cell proliferation in the early phase of hepatocarcinogenesis, many studies concerning the oval cell have appeared (*11*, *13*, *30*, *etc.*). However, the fate of oval cells in the following stages of carcinogenesis is still a matter of dispute. On the other hand, proliferation of this type of cell was also noticed in experiments other than carcinogenesis, such as bile duct ligation (*11*) or application of α-naphthyl isothiocyanate (*20*). Furthermore, carcinomas developed without preceding proliferation of oval cells (S. Takayama and N. Kuwabara, personal communication concerning diethyl- and dimethylnitrosamine hepatocarcinogenesis). It is highly probable that the appearance of serum AFP in the early stage is neither a specific phenomenon for carcinogenesis nor an absolute requisite for later development of the carcinoma. In the present experiments, carcinomas did develop in rats lacking serum AFP in the early phase. It was clear, however, that the appearance of early AFP was correlated with fair progress of carcinogenesis and frequent development of strongly AFP-producing carcinomas. The resemblance in histochemical and electron-microscopic features between oval cells and the cells composing the medullary portion of mixed-type carcinomas is also not to be overlooked.

The serum AFP in the late phase was produced by the carcinoma. The majority of 3′-Me-DAB-induced carcinomas were of the mixed-type. This type of carcinoma was strongly AFP-producing with a minimally required size of 10 mm diameter for positive serum AFP. Most of the FAA-induced carcinomas were trabecular. This type of carcinoma was relatively weak as regards AFP production and serum AFP was negative until a trabecular carcinoma became larger than 20 mm in diameter.

In a previous work, Abelev (*3*) found AFP in 3 out of 4 transplantable mouse hepatomas, but not in 20 transplantable cancers other than hepatoma. According to Khramkova and Guelstein (*15*), 7 out of 29 *o*-aminoazotoluene (AAT)-induced primary mouse hepatomas and 10 out of 15 transplantable mouse hepatomas were AFP-producing. Summarizing these data, Abelev (*1*, *3*) assumed a positive correlation between the degree of malignancy of a hepatoma and the production of AFP by the hepatoma. On the other hand, Birencwajg *et al.* (*7*) reported that 100 out of 122 azo-dye-induced rat liver carcinomas were AFP-producing while all 15 aflatoxin B_1-induced rat hepatomas were not AFP-producing. From this result, they suggested a positive correlation between the type of carcinogen used and AFP production by the developed carcinoma.

As far as our results are concerned, they are consistent with both Abelev's and Birencwajg's assumptions. In ascites hepatoma (*34*), however, the frequency of AFP production was much lower, being positive in 20 out of 60, and its relation to malignancy appeared reversed; Yoshida sarcoma, a highly malignant ascites hepatoma, was not AFP-producing, while LY5, LY52, LY80, and LY176, which are variants of Yoshida sarcoma and are less malignant, were AFP-producing (*14*, *34*). On the other hand, AFP was not detected in 4 out of 5 Morris minimum deviation hepatomas (*35*). We also observed a tendency for decreasing serum AFP concentration when a rat developed a large trabecular carcinoma later than the 39th experimental week. These facts seem to suggest that, first, the AFP production of a carcinoma should not be regarded as a fixed feature of the carcinoma, and second, that AFP production is a feature of liver carcinomas within a certain range of malignancy. In fact, all the trabecular carcinomas which attained large size within 39 weeks and were determined in this study as AFP-producing, were of a histochemically immature type, although in FAA carcinogenesis, trabecular carcinomas with certain enzymic maturity were not infrequently encountered (*17*, *18*).

The nodular hyperplasia or area of hyperplasia, which has been regarded as the most probable forerunner of carcinoma (*17*, *22*, *29–31*, *37*) did not produce AFP. As mentioned above, we judged that the component cells of the nodular hyperplasia or area of hyperplasia are a different type of cell, established *de novo* at this stage. Accordingly, the importance of oval cells for later development of carcinoma was not stressed. The fact that AFP was produced by the oval cells but not by the cells of the most probable " precancerous lesion " seems to offer an interesting problem in hepatocarcinogenesis.

Acknowledgments

This work was supported by a Grant-in-Aid for Scientific Research from the Ministry of Education and the Ministry of Health and Welfare.

We are greatly indebted to Mr. Tsugukatsu Nashiro and Mrs. Keiko Nakamura for technical assistance.

REFERENCES

1. Abelev, G. I. Study of the antigenic structure of tumors. *Acta Unio Int. Contra Cancrum*, **19**, 80–82 (1963).
2. Abelev, G. I., Assecritova, I. V., Kraevsky, N. A., Perova P. D., and Perevodchikov, N. I. Embryonal serum α-globulin in cancer patients: Diagnostic value. *Int. J. Cancer*, **2**, 55–58 (1967).
3. Abelev, G. I. Production of embryonal serum α-globulin by hepatomas: Review of experimental and clinical data. *Cancer Res.*, **28**, 1344–1350 (1968).
4. Alpert, M. E., Uriel, J., and Nechaud, D. B. Alpha-1-fetoglobulin in diagnosis of human hepatoma. *New Engl. J. Med.*, **278**, 984–986 (1968).
5. Barka, T. and Anderson, P. J. *In* "Histochemistry," Hoeber-Harper Co., New York (1963).
6. Birencwajg, M. S. Specific antigens of rat embryonic serum. *Cancer Res.*, **27**, 1982–1989 (1967).
7. Birencwajg, M. S., Uriel, J., and Graber, P. Association of embryonic antigens with experimentally induced hepatic lesions in the rat. *Cancer Res.*, **27**, 1990–1997 (1967).
8. Endo, Y. Diagnosis of primary liver cancer by α-fetoglobulin (in Japanese). *Acta Hepatol. Japon.*, **10**, 143–146 (1969).
9. Farber, E. Similarities in the sequence of early histological changes induced in the liver of the rats by ethionine, 2-acetylaminofluorene, and 3′-methyl-4-dimethylaminoazobenzene. *Cancer Res.*, **16**, 142–148 (1956).
10. Graber, P., Birencwajg, M. S., Oisgold, S., and Uriel, J. Immunochemical and enzymatic studies on chemically induced rat liver tumors. *UICC Monograph*, **2**, 20–31 (1967).
11. Grisham, J. W. and Porta, E. A. Origin and fate of proliferated hepatic ductal cells in the rat: Electron-microscopic and radioautographic studies. *Exp. Mol. Pathol.*, **3**, 242–261 (1964).
12. Hayashi, M., Nakajima, Y., and Fishman, W. H. The cytologic demonstration of β-glucuronidase employing Naphthol AS-BI glucuronide and Hexazonium Pararosanilin. *J. Histochem. Cytochem.*, **12**, 293–297 (1964).
13. Inaoka, Y. Significance of the so-called oval cell proliferation during azo-dye hepatocarcinogenesis. *GANN*, **58**, 355–366 (1967).
14. Isaka, I., Umehara, S., Hirai, H., and Tsukada, Y. Development of variant tumor cells of Yoshida ascites sarcoma producing α-fetoprotein. *GANN*, **63**, 63–71 (1972).
15. Khramkova, N. and Guelstein, V. Antigenic structure of mouse hepatomas. V. Organospecific liver antigens and embryonal α-globulin in mouse hepatomas induced by *o*-aminoazotoluene. *Neoplasma*, **12**, 239–250 (1965).
16. Kitagawa, T., Enomoto, M., and Oota, K. Histochemical analysis of hepatocarcinogenesis in rats fed 2-acetyl-aminofluorene (in Japanese). *Nippon Byori Gakkai Kaishi* (*Transact. Soc. Pathol. Japan*), **57**, 115–116 (1968).
17. Kitagawa, T. Histochemical analysis of hyperplastic lesions and hepatomas of the liver of rats fed 2-fluorenylacetamide. *GANN*, **62**, 207–216 (1971).
18. Kitagawa, T. Responsiveness of hyperplastic lesions and hepatomas to partial hepatectomy. *GANN*, **62**, 217–224 (1971).
19. Kitagawa, T., Yokochi, T., and Sugano, H. α-Fetoprotein and hepatocarcino-

genesis in rats fed 3′-methyl-4-(dimethylamino)azobenzene or N-2-fluorenylacetamide. *Int. J. Cancer*, **10**, 368–381 (1972).

20. Lopez, M. and Mozzanti, L. Experimental investigation on α-naphthyl isothiocyanate as a hyperplastic agent of the biliary ducts in the rats. *J. Pathol. Bacteriol.*, **69**, 243–250 (1955).
21. Ma, M. H. and Webber, A. J. Fine structure of liver tumors induced in the rat by 3′-methyl-4-dimethylaminoazobenzene. *Cancer Res.*, **26**, 935–946 (1966).
22. Maruya, H. Morphological studies on the development of liver cancer by Butter Yellow. *GANN*, **33**, 203–205 (1939).
23. Merkow, L. P., Epstein, S. M., Farber, E., Pardo, M., and Bartus, B. Cellular analysis of liver carcinogenesis. IV. Comparison of the ultrastructure of hyperplastic liver nodules and hepatocellular carcinomas induced in rat liver by 2-fluorenylacetamide. *J. Natl. Cancer Inst.*, **43**, 33–63 (1969).
24. Muley, A. S. and Firminger, H. I. Liver tumors induced in rats by *p*-dimethylaminoazobenzene-1-azonaphthalene compared with tumors induced by *p*-dimethylaminoazobenzene. *J. Natl. Cancer Inst.*, **13**, 35–55 (1952–1953).
25. de Nechaud, P. B., Economopoulos, P., and Uriel, J. Frequence d'apparition des fetoprotéins dans le sérum de malades alleints d'hépatopathies diverses. *Presse Med.*, **77**, 1945–1947 (1969).
26. Onoé, T. and Fuse, Y. Hepatocarcinogenesis by azo dyes (in Japanese). *Cell*, **2**, 25–34 (1970).
27. Ouchterlony, O. Antigen-antibody reaction in gels. *Arkiv. Kem. Mineral. Geol.*, **26B**, 14 (1949).
28. Price, J. M., Harman, J. W., Miller, E. C., and Miller, J. A. Progressive microscopic alterations in the liver of rats fed the hepatic carcinogen, 3′-methyl-4-dimethylaminoazobenzene and 4-fluoro-4-dimethylaminoazobenzene. *Cancer Res.*, **12**, 192–200 (1952).
29. Reuber, M. D. Development of preneoplastic and neoplastic lesions of the liver in male rats given 0.025% N-2-fluorenylacetamide. *J. Natl. Cancer Inst.*, **34**, 697–723 (1965).
30. Rubin, E. The origin and fate of proliferated hepatic bile ductal cells. *Exp. Mol. Pathol.*, **3**, 279–286 (1964).
31. Sasaki, T. and Yoshida, T. Experimentelle Erzeugung des Lebercarcinoms durch Fütterung mit *o*-Aminoazotoluol. *Virchows Archiv Pathol. Anat. Physiol.*, **295**, 175–200 (1935).
32. Stewart, H. L. and Snell, K. C. Histopathology of experimental tumors of the liver of the rat. A critical review of the histogenesis. *In* "The Physiopathology of Cancer," Hoeber-Harper Co., New York, pp. 85–126 (1959).
33. Tatarinov, Ju. Detection of embryospecific α-globulin in the blood sera of patient with primary liver tumor. *Vopr. Med. Khim.*, **10**, 90–91 (1964).
34. Watabe, H. and Hirai, H. Rat ascites liver cancers and α-fetoprotein (in Japanese). *Proc. Jap. Cancer Assoc., 28th Annu. Meet.*, 129 (1969).
35. Watabe, H., Hirai, H., and Satoh, H. α-Fetoprotein in rats transplanted with ascites hepatoma. *GANN*, **63** (**2**) 189–199 (1972).
36. Watabe, H. Early appearance of embryonic α-globulin in rat serum during carcinogenesis with 4-dimethylaminoazobenzene. *Cancer Res.*, **31**, 1192–1194 (1971).
37. Yoshida, T. Über die Histogenese des experimentellen malignen Hepatoms (Leberzellenkrebses) durch *o*-Aminoazotoluol. Zugleich ein Beitrag zur Frage der formativen Reizung Virchows. *GANN*, **36**, 9–44 (1942).

EXPLANATION OF PHOTOS

PHOTO 1. Marked proliferation of oval cells and small hepatocytes in the periportal area and megalocytic degeneration of the original mature hepatocytes in a rat at the 6th week in 3′-Me-DAB carcinogenesis. H-E: Hematoxylin-Eosin staining. ×68.

PHOTO 2. Higher magnification of a lesion similar to that shown in Photo 1. ×160.

PHOTO 3. Slight proliferation of oval cells, rather spindle-shaped here, in a rat fed with FAA for 6 weeks. The original mature hepatocytes are atrophic with cytoplasmic condensation in the periportal area and vacuolation in the remaining portion of the lobuli. H-E. ×68.

PHOTO 4. β-Glucuronidase-Hematoxylin staining of the liver of a rat fed with 3′-Me-DAB for 6 weeks, showing the *de novo* development of a nodular hyperplasia (NH) amidst proliferating small hepatocytes (SH) and fading original mature hepatocytes (MH). The enzyme activity is strong in MH, weak in SH, and almost lacking in NH. ×68.

PHOTOS 5 and 6. G-6-Pase (Photo 5) and ATPase (Photo 6) stainings of the liver of a rat fed with 3′-Me-DAB for 10 weeks, showing enlargement of nodular hyperplasia compressing the site of the oval cells and small cell proliferation. Note the various enzyme activities of the individual nodular hyperplasia. Occasional small hepatocytes show considerable G-6-Pase activity but not ATPase activity. ×30.

PHOTO 7. Electron micrograph of oval cells at the 4th week in 3′-Me-DAB carcinogenesis. Note a cholangiolar lumen closely related to the proliferating oval cell. ×4,000.

PHOTO 8. Electron micrograph of oval cells at the 6th week in FAA carcinogenesis. They are just like cholangiolar cells and a tendency suggesting transition to hepatocytes is scarcely seen. ×4,000.

PHOTO 9. Marked proliferation of the area of hyperplasia at the 12th week in FAA carcinogenesis. β-Glucuronidase staining. The enzyme activity is low in the area of hyperplasia and intense in the original mature hepatocytes. ×8.

PHOTO 10. 3′-Me-DAB-induced AFP-producing mixed-type carcinoma with a fairly medullary pattern. H-E. ×135.

PHOTO 11. 3′-Me-DAB-induced mixed-type carcinoma with a prominent fibrotic or cystoadenomatous pattern. H-E. ×68.

PHOTO 12. G-6-Pase staining of the carcinoma shown in Photo 11. Marked enzyme activity exists in the cancer cells with a papillotubular arrangement. ×68.

PHOTO 13. FAA-induced, AFP-producing trabecular carcinoma with a fairly malignant appearance. ×95.

PHOTO 14. FAA-induced, AFP-producing carcinoma with a fairly benign morphological appearance. H-E. ×95.

PHOTO 15. FAA-induced, AFP-producing carcinoma with a papillary pattern. H-E. ×135.

PHOTO 16. Electron micrograph of the cells of a 3′-Me-DAB-induced, AFP-producing mixed-type carcinoma. Note the resemblance to oval cells. The cells surrounding the lumen show intestinal epithelium-type metaplasia. ×4,000.

PHOTO 17. Electron micrograph of an FAA-induced, AFP-producing trabecular carcinoma. ×4,000.

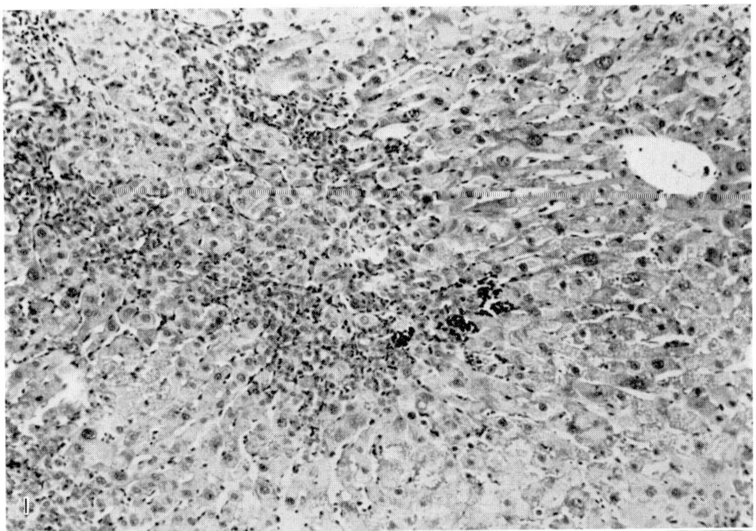
1

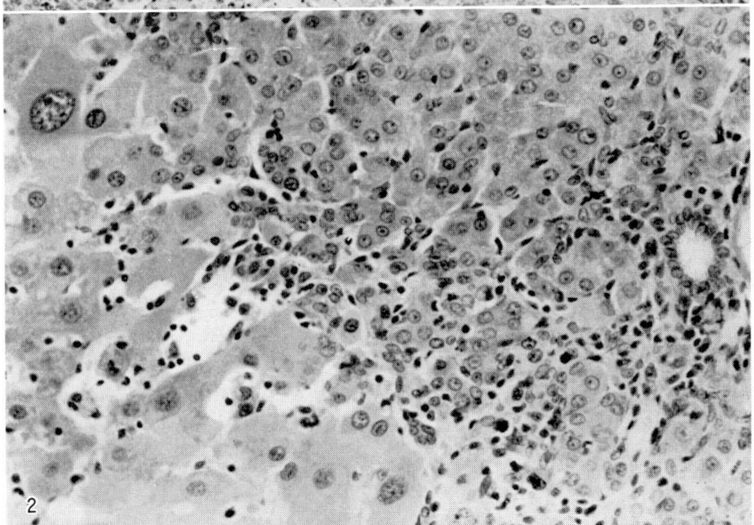
2

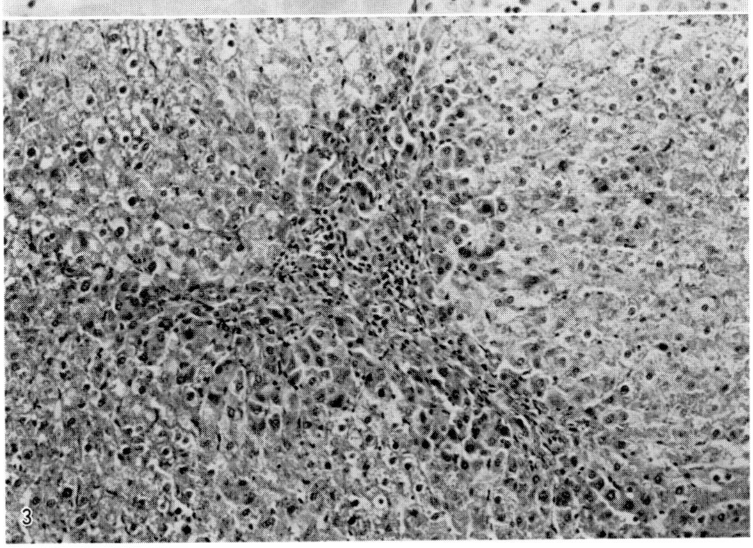
3

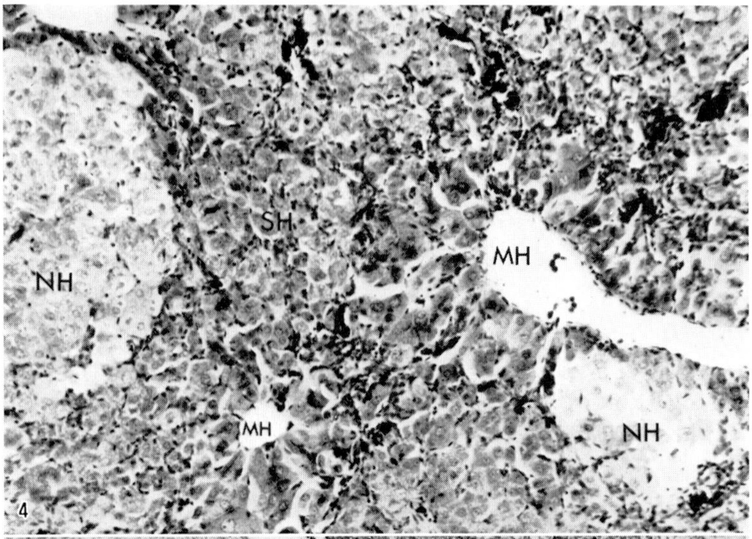
SH
MH
NH
MH
NH
4

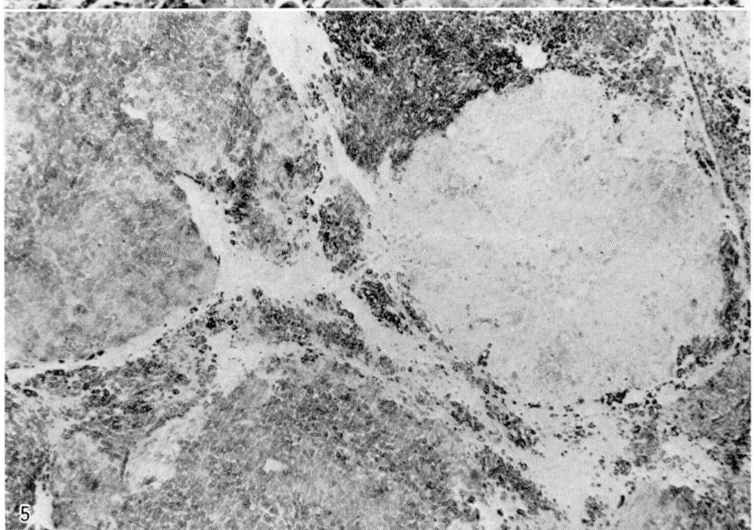
5

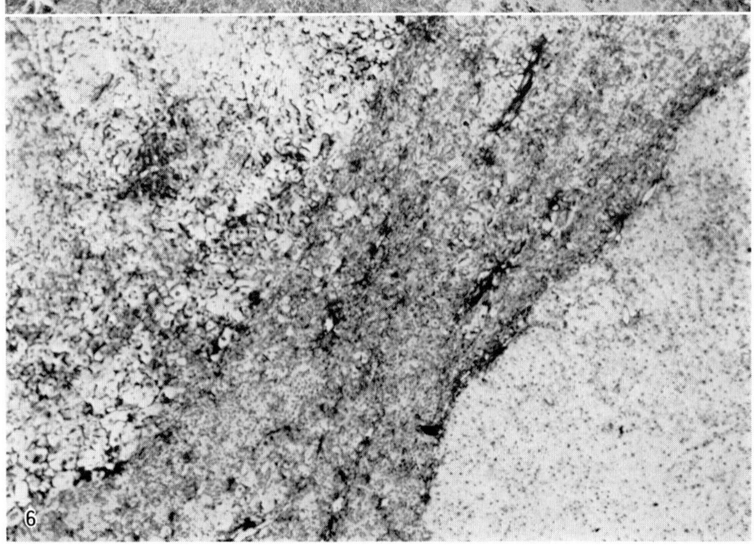
6

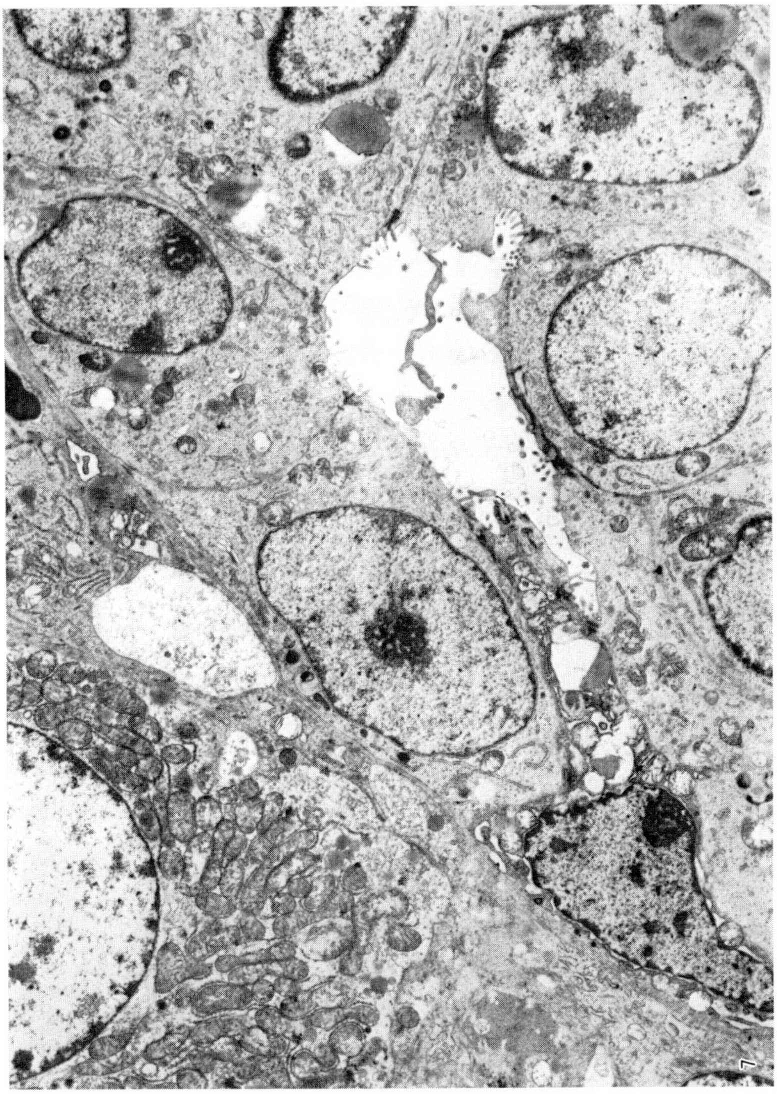

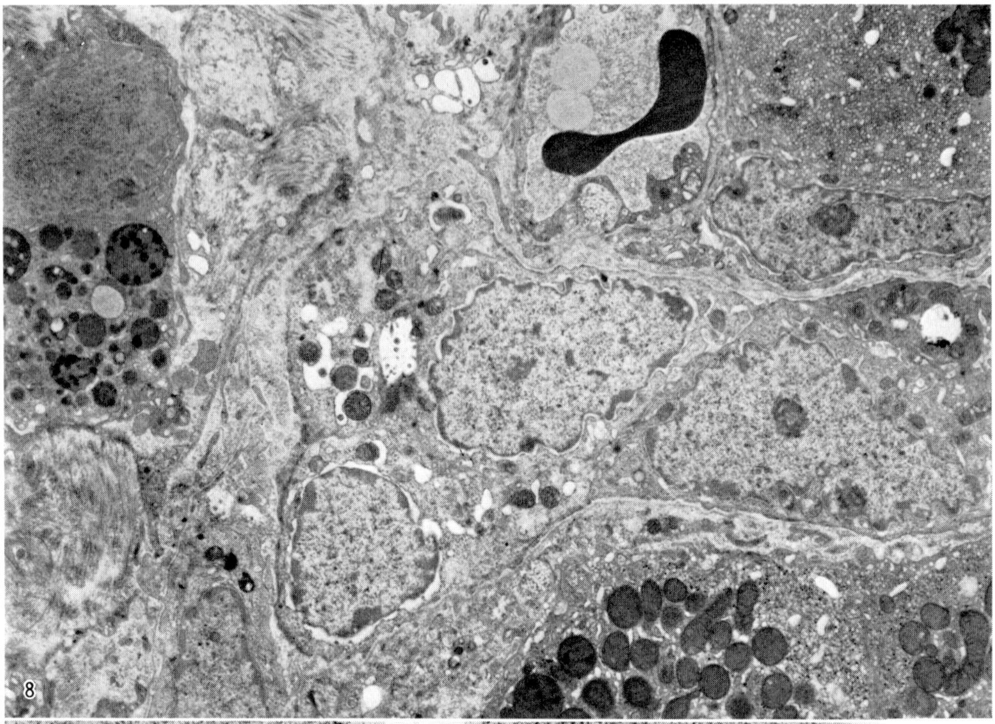
8

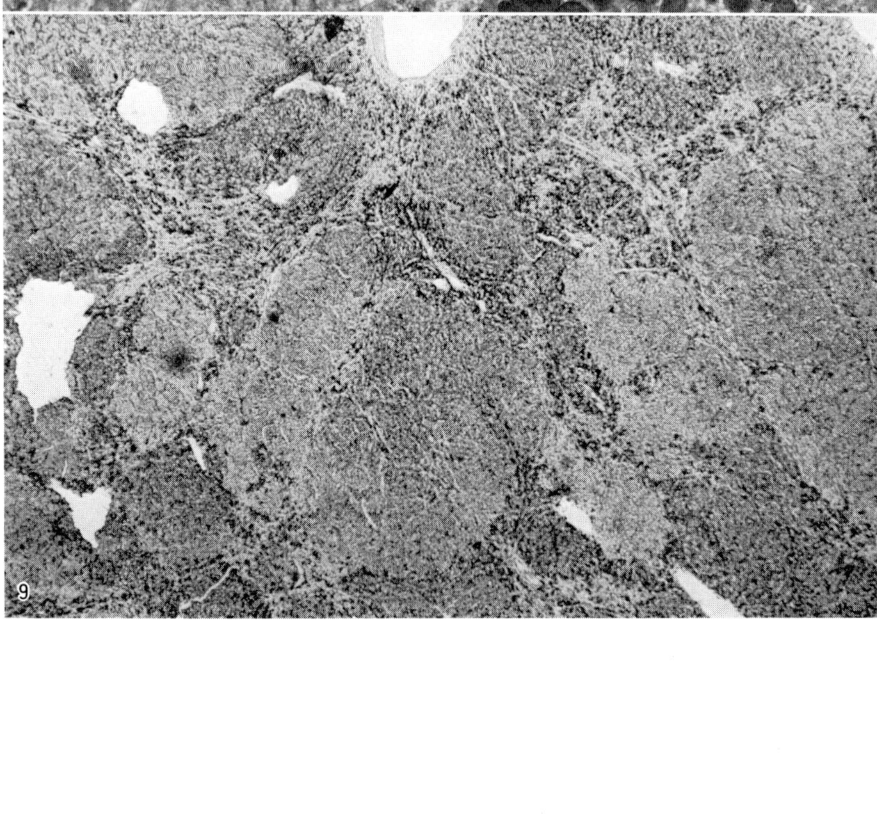
9

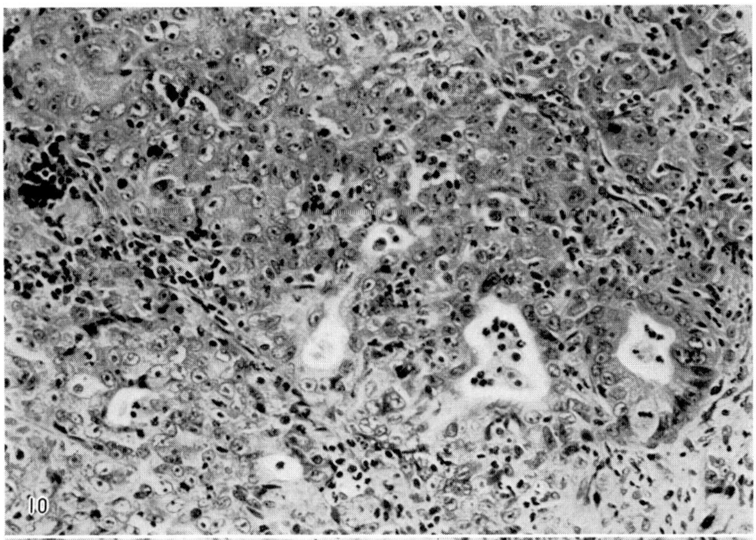
10

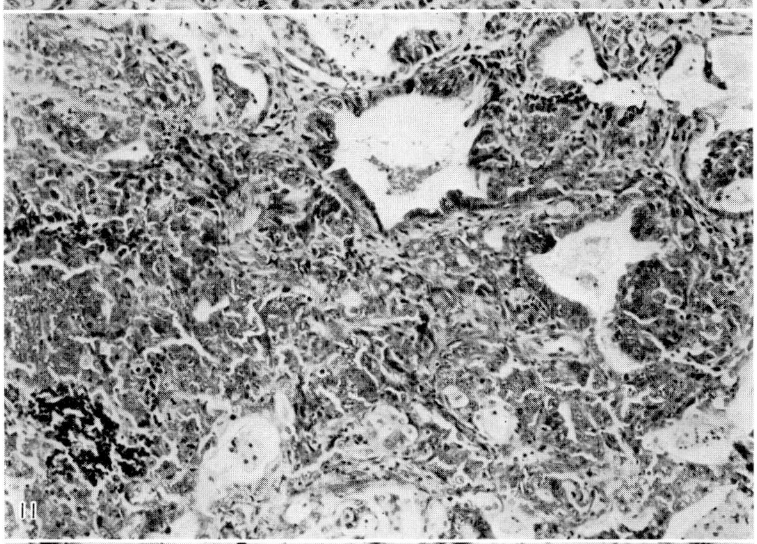
11

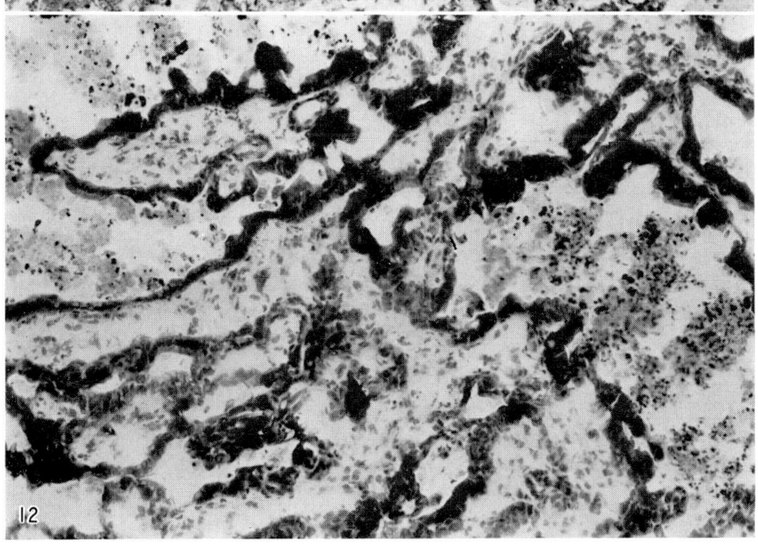
12

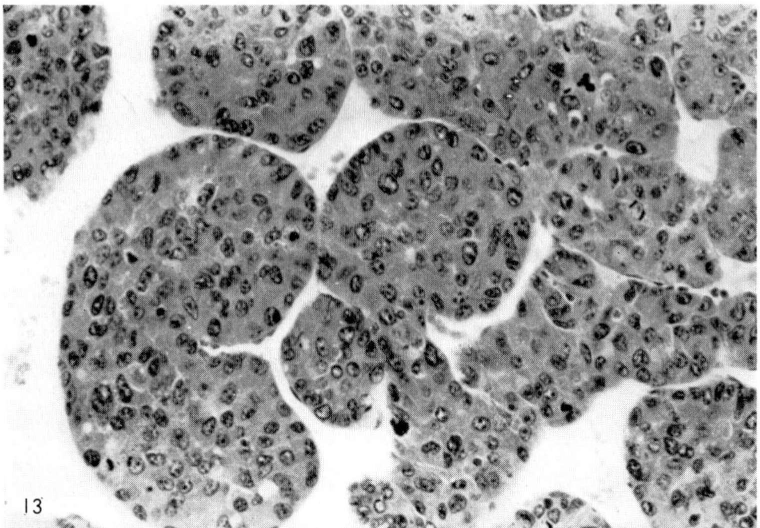
13

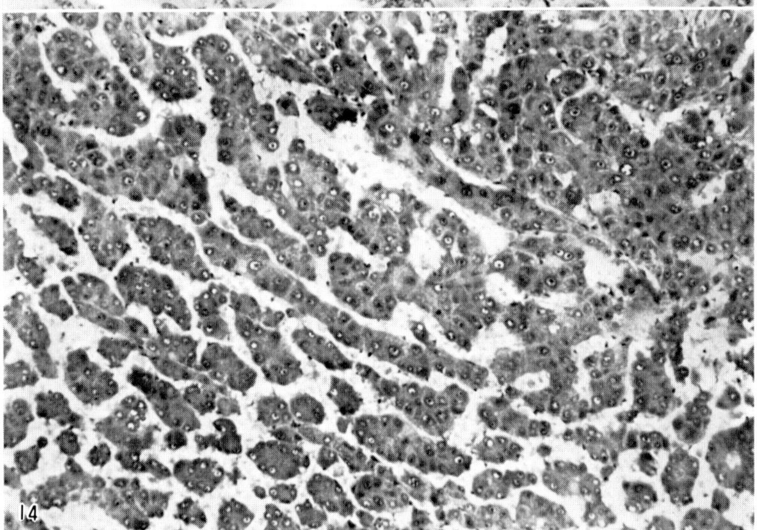
14

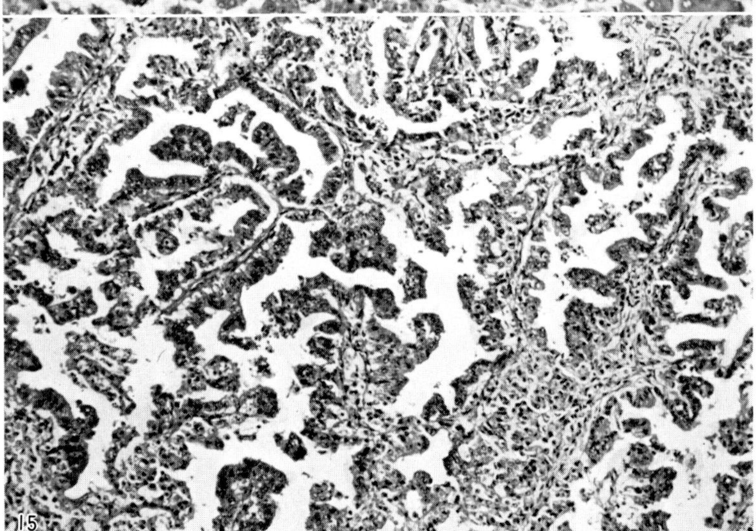
15

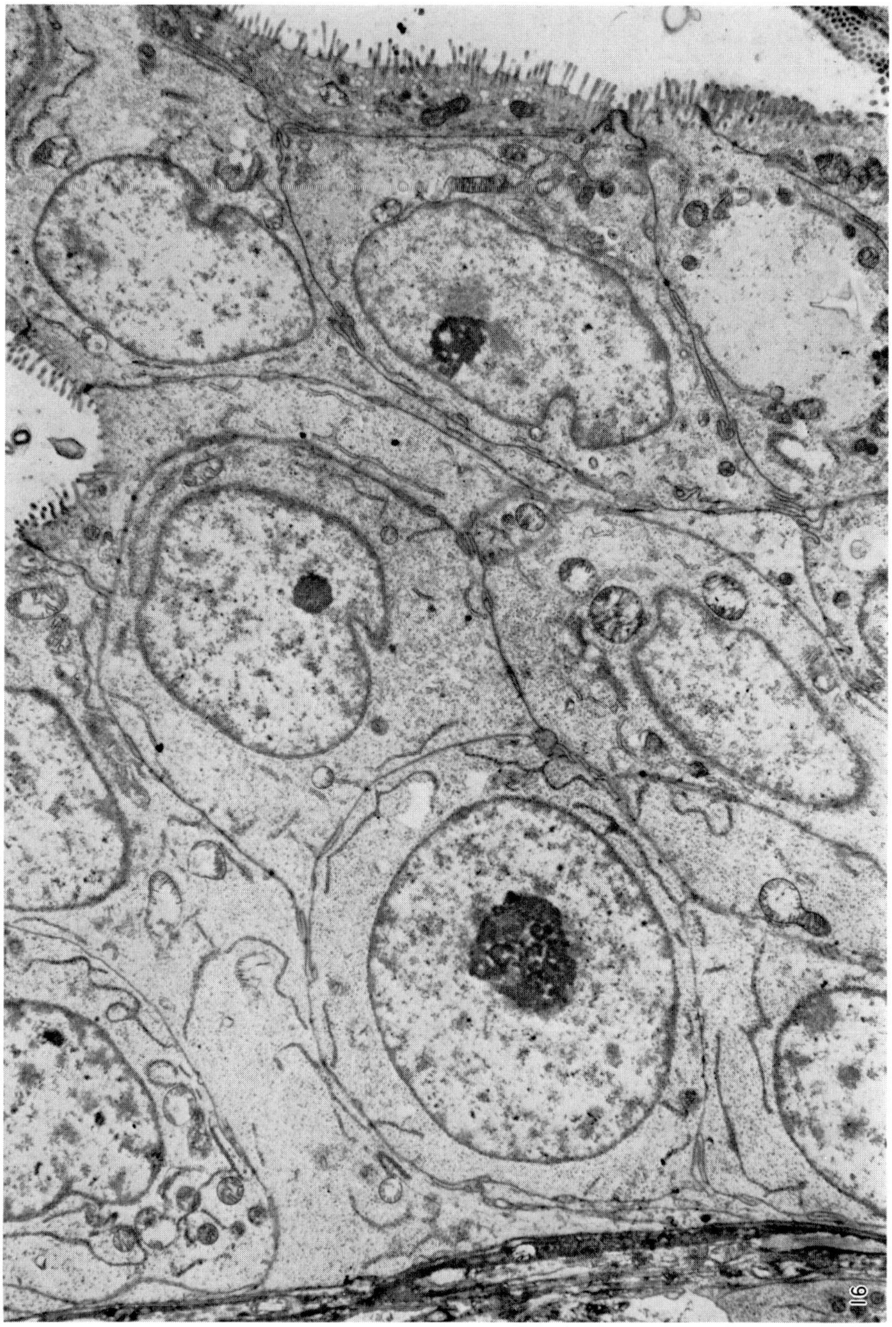
16

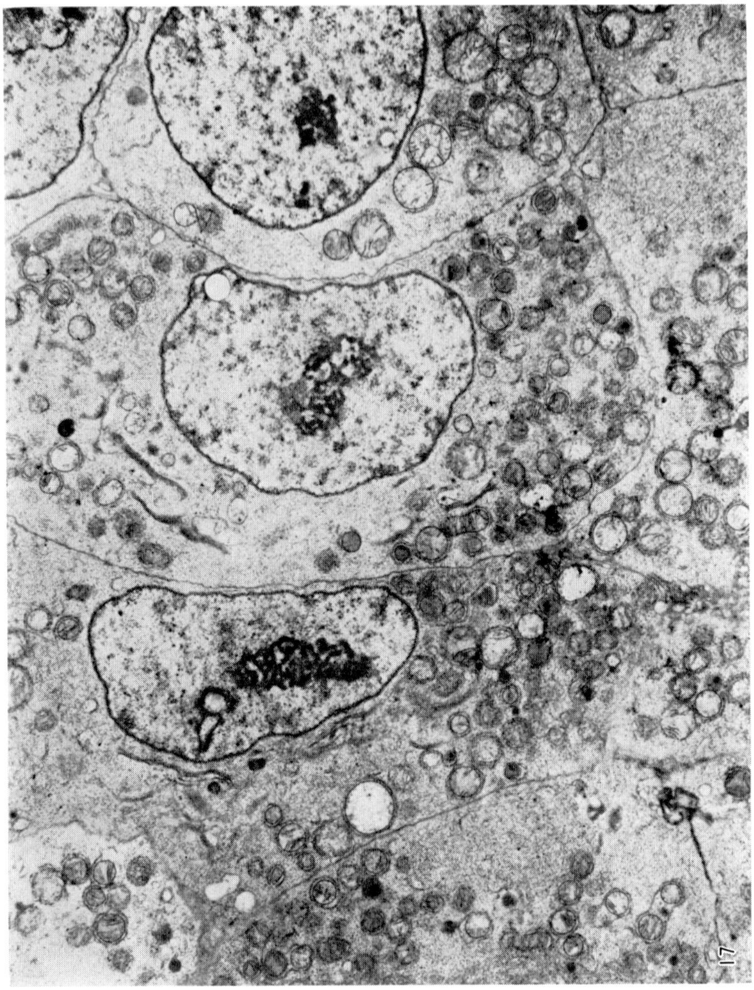

RELATIONSHIP BETWEEN α-FETOPROTEIN AND HISTOLOGICAL PATTERNS OF HEPATOMA, AND LOCALIZATION OF α-FETOPROTEIN IN HEPATOMA CELLS USING THE PEROXIDASE ANTIBODY TECHNIQUE

Toshio SHIKATA and Koko SAKAKIBARA

*Department of Pathology, Faculty of Medicine, University of Tokyo**

Studies on the relationship between serum α-fetoprotein (AFP) and histological and cytological patterns of malignant hepatoma disclosed two obvious findings. One is that well-differentiated and highly anaplastic hepatomas do not produce AFP, or if they do, the serum level of AFP is very low. Second, except for well-differentiated and poorly differentiated groups, AFP titer of the serum has a positive correlation with dedifferentiation of malignant hepatomas.

In the hepatoma cells, AFP synthesis was found to occur by the peroxidase antibody technique. AFP was stained around ribosomes on the rough endoplasmic reticulum. A secretory process was also suggested by this method.

Abelev *et al.* (*1*), Tatarinov (*7*), and other investigators have shown that α-fetoprotein (AFP) is related to hepatomas of experimental animals as well as those of human beings. Immunochemical and clinical studies concerning AFP by Hirai and Nishi (*5*, *6*) and Endo *et al.* (*4*) in Japan disclosed the chemical properties of AFP and its clinical meaning. Recently, it was revealed that AFP has been found in the serum of a few patients with malignancies other than malignant hepatoma, for instance gastric cancer. It was also detected in the serum of patients with hepatitis, and in the early stage of experimental hepatocarcinogenesis by 4-dimethylaminoazobenzene (DAB). Accordingly, attention has been largely directed to AFP synthesis on a cellular level. However, considerable difficulty exists in staining AFP by the fluorescent antibody technique, because AFP is a protein similar to albumin, and satisfactory results have not been achieved by this method.

In order to solve this problem and to clarify the production and secretion of AFP in the cells, an experiment was designed to stain AFP by the peroxidase antibody technique and to observe the results by electron microscopy.

In addition to this, the relationship between AFP in the serum and histological patterns of malignant hepatoma in human beings is also described in this report.

* Hongo 7-3-1, Bunkyo-ku, Tokyo 113, Japan (志方俊夫, 榊原耕子).

Localization of AFP in Hepatoma Cells Using the Peroxidase Antibody Technique

Hepatoma in a rat induced by 3′-methyl-4-dimethylaminoazobenzene (3′-Me-DAB) was used for this experiment. The liver of a rat fed with 3′-Me-DAB for 25 weeks and showing the 2nd appearance of AFP in the serum was selected for examination. Such a case showed small white nodes growing in some parts, and these were used as materials.

The specimen of liver was fixed with 2% glutaraldehyde for 1 hr, washed, and reacted with peroxidase-labeled anti-rat AFP serum for 12 hr at 4°. Then the peroxidase reaction and refixation with osmic acid were applied.

Anti-rat AFP serum was supplied by Dr. Nishi, Department of Biochemistry, Faculty of Medicine, Hokkaido University, and Dr. Endo, First Department of Internal Medicine, Faculty of Medicine, University of Tokyo. Peroxidase labeling was obtained according to the glutaraldehyde technique of Abrameas (*2*); crude γ-globulin precipitated by 33% saturation of ammonium sulfate was combined with horseradish peroxidase (HPO) using 1% glutaraldehyde as a coupling agent. After eliminating most of the uncoupled HPO with half-saturated ammonium sulfate, the part in which the peak of OD_{280} coincided with the peak of OD_{403} was taken by gel filtration using Sephadex G-200, and was then subjected to DEAE-cellulose column chromatography. Specific antibody activity was determined by the immunodiffusion technique.

Observation of ultrathin sections without electron staining revealed that cells showing positive peroxidase reaction are clearly distinguished from cells without positive reaction. This peroxidase reaction is considered as specific for AFP itself from the results of control experiments. Peroxidase reactions were mainly found around the rough endoplasmic reticulum. On the rough endoplasmic reticulum, the reaction was observed as an uneven, thick line along the membrane (Photos 1–3). Unstained round granules which coincided with ribosomes were found on the rough endoplasmic reticulum (Photo 2). The AFP was often found in the rough endoplasmic reticulum encompassing mitochondria (Photos 1 and 4). Moreover, stained AFP was found not only on the surface of the rough endoplasmic reticulum, but also around free ribosomes in places. In these parts, AFP was sometimes observed as granular, but further observation revealed that white and round ribosomes were found in hollows on the parts where AFP was stained, and these ribosomes were mostly observed in the form of polysomes. This finding suggests that AFP is synthesized not only on the rough endoplasmic reticulum but also by free ribosomes. The ratio of the production of AFP between ribosomes of the rough endoplasmic reticulum and free ribosomes, although slightly different in different parts of cell, is considered about 10 to 1.

In addition to areas surrounding ribosomes, the dilated cisternae of rough endoplasmic reticulum showed a slightly positive peroxidase reaction (Photo 3).

It is interesting that AFP is focally stained in some parts of the outer layer of the nuclear membrane. The AFP is also observed in some parts of the smooth endoplasmic reticulum and hepatoma cell membrane (Photo 4). No AFP is detected in the Golgi apparatus (Photo 1).

Most of the hepatoma cells showing the presence of AFP have large clear cytoplasm, a dispersed distribution of cell organellae, and a distorted nucleus. It is now being investigated which cells produce AFP in the case of the primary reaction of DAB hepatocarcinogenesis.

From the fact that AFP exists in the sera of patients with hepatoma, it has been considered that hepatoma cells produce it, but this has not been definitely proved. Although some workers, including the present authors, stain AFP by the fluorescent antibody technique, satisfactory results have not been obtained. On the other hand, AFP is found in the early stage of administration of DAB and in the case of hepatitis, and though small in number, in some cases of cancer other than hepatoma. Therefore the need to clarify which cells produce AFP is clear.

The AFP could be clearly stained by the peroxidase antibody technique, as shown in this paper. The main portion in which AFP is stained is the circumference of ribosomes on the rough endoplasmic reticulum.

From the finding of external secretory cells of pancreas and plasma cells, it has been generally considered that secretory protein is mainly produced on the rough endoplasmic reticulum and structural protein in the free ribosomes; over 90% of albumin is produced in rough endoplasmic reticulum in the liver.

Biochemical data concerning AFP synthesis have not yet been presented. Staining of AFP by the peroxidase antibody technique revealed that AFP is produced around ribosomes attached to the rough endoplasmic reticulum and a few around free ribosomes. The AFP focally exists in the outer layer of the nuclear membrane. The fact that AFP is stained in some parts of the smooth endoplasmic reticulum and cell membrane probably illustrates a secretory process.

Relationship between AFP and Histological Patterns of Hepatomas

The AFP has been detected in 70–80% of patients with malignant hepatoma. Nishi and Hirai (*6*) described that the AFP titer of the serum roughly correlated with the grade of atypism of the hepatoma cells. However, the authors had the impression that highly anaplastic hepatomas could not produce AFP and, therefore, further detailed study concerning the histological and cytological differences between hepatomas producing AFP and hepatomas not producing it was carried out.

Concerning the histological forms of malignant hepatomas, we usually classified them into thin trabecular, trabecular, solid, and trabeculotubular types. In this study, however, to compare serum AFP titer precisely, trabecular and thin trabecular types were further divided into 4 groups according to the thickness of the cell plate. In normal human liver, liver cells may exist as a tortuous plate in one cell line. However, during regeneration, it attains a thickness of two cells. In hepatoma, the thickness of the cell plate almost correlated with the growth rate. According to the growth rate, the cell plate became thicker and thicker. Finally, it was composed of a solid tumor mass with scattered blood capillaries in it. This final form is described as a solid type (Fig. 1).

The relationship between AFP titer in the serum and histological patterns is shown in Fig. 2. Well-differentiated thin trabecular hepatoma does not produce

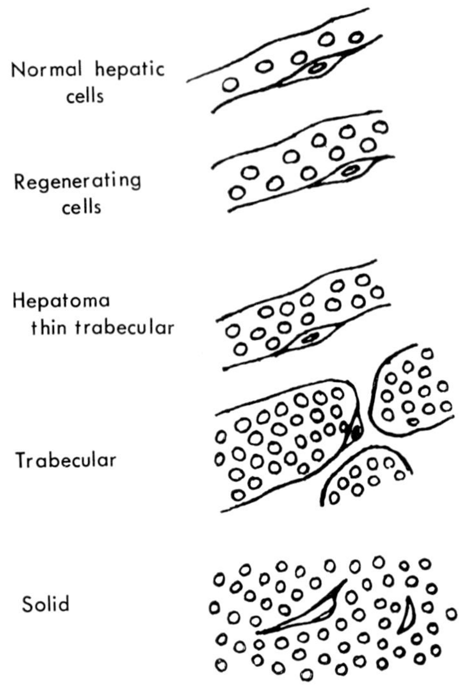

FIG. 1. Scheme of the cell cord in normal liver, regenerative nodule, and hepatoma

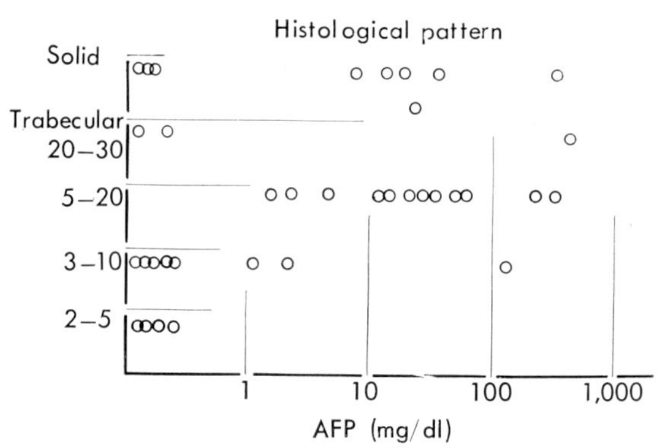

FIG. 2. Relationship between AFP titer of the serum and histological pattern

AFP, or if it does, the serum level of AFP is under 0.5 mg/dl. Hepatomas with a broad trabecular pattern produce much AFP, but some of the solid type, which are highly anaplastic, do not produce AFP.

Except for well-differentiated and poorly differentiated groups, AFP titer of the serum has a positive correlation with the thickness of cell cord.

Concerning the number of mitotic figures, we divided hepatoma into 3 groups; those showing no mitotic figure, moderate number of mitosis, and large number of mitosis. The AFP titer of serum also roughly corresponds to the number of mitosis, as shown in Fig. 3.

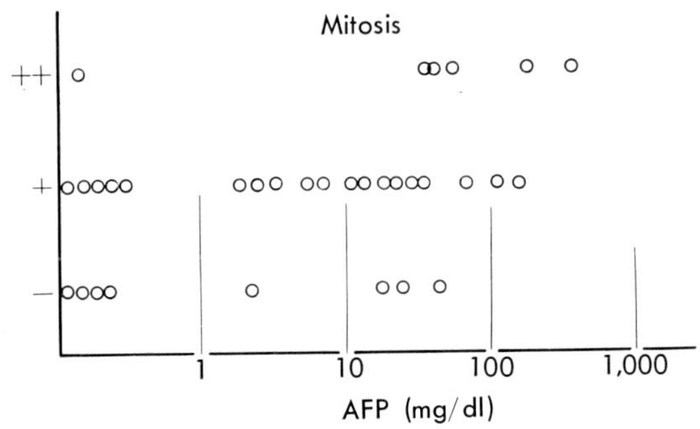

FIG. 3. Relationship between AFP titer of the serum and mitosis

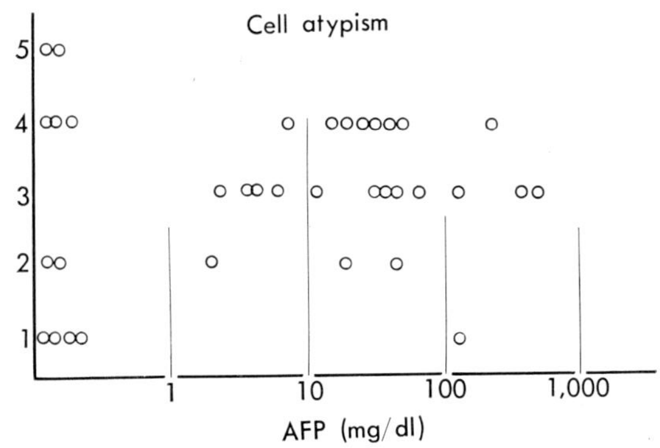

FIG. 4. Relationship between AFP titer of the serum and cell atypism

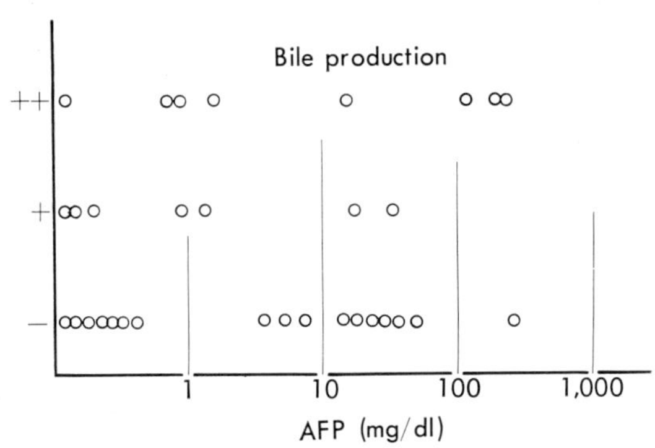

FIG. 5. Relationship between AFP titer of the serum and bile production

Cell atypism was divided into 5 groups in this study. Similar correlation was observed, as in the case of the histological classification. It was observed that hepatomas with minimal atypism and hepatomas with high grade atypism do not produce AFP (Fig. 4).

Histologically, bile production is only proved by the presence of bile pigments in the tumor cells and bile canaliculi. In well-differentiated hepatoma, bile pigment often cannot be proved to be present in the tumor cells. It is uncertain whether tumor cells produce bile or not. In any event, the relationship of bile pigments in hepatoma with AFP titer in the serum is shown in Fig. 5. No obvious correlation is observed.

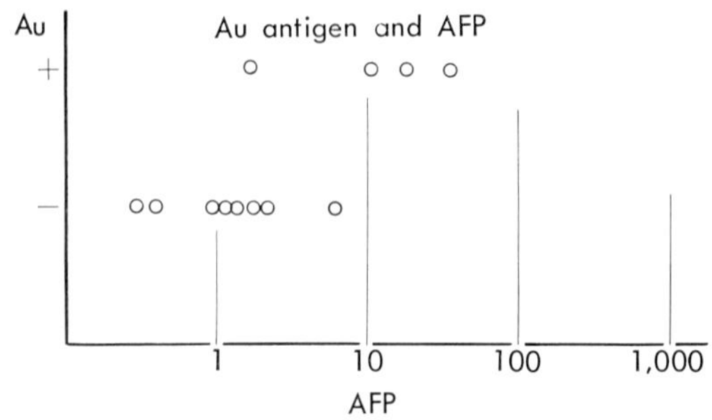

FIG. 6. Relationship between AFP titer of the serum and Australia antigen

Australia antigen in the serum was detected in 5 cases among 13 cases of malignant hepatoma. Fluoromicroscopy showed granular deposition in the cytoplasm of the liver cells with noncancerous lesions. No Australia antigen was detected in the hepatoma cell itself. The relationship between Australia antigen and AFP titer is shown in Fig. 6. Australia antigen-positive cases of hepatoma show higher titer than negative cases.

Summarizing these findings, AFP titer in the serum of patients with malignant hepatoma is correlated with histological pattern, cell atypism, and the number of mitosis of the tumors. Highly differentiated and highly anaplastic hepatoma do not produce AFP. Otherwise, the AFP titer of the serum is directly proportional to the cell and histological atypism.

Histological Classification of Malignant Hepatoma

Edmondson (*3*) made a grading of malignant hepatomas on the basis of cytological as well as histological properties. However, in a few cases, discrepancy exists between the cytological and histological atypism. Practical classification of malignant hepatomas, made by many pathologists according to Edmondson's grading, are very different from each other. We therefore propose the following new classification, according to the combination of histological patterns and cell atypism.

Histological pattern:

1. Thin trabecular.
2. Trabecular.
3. Solid.
4. Trabeculo-tubular.

Cell atypism:

Grade I.
Grade II.
Grade III.

For description of a case of malignant hepatoma, both classifications should be presented; for instance, trabecular type, with Grade II cell atypism. We believe that this classification is better than Edmondson's classification.

REFERENCES

1. Abelev, G. I., Perova, S., and Kharamkowa, N. Production of embryonal α-globulin by transplantable hepatomas. *Transplantation*, **1**, 174–180 (1963).
2. Abrameas, S. Coupling of enzymes to proteins with glutaraldehyde. *Immunochemistry*, **6**, 43–52 (1969).
3. Edmondson, H. A. Tumors of the liver and intrahepatic bile ducts. *In* "Atlas of Tumor Pathology," A.F.I.P., Washington, pp. 63–64 (1958).
4. Endo, Y., Eto, S., Iino, S., Fujiwara, K., Miyake, K., Kanetaka, T., Yamanaka, M., Suzuki, H., Oda, T., Yoshitoshi, Y., Juji, T., Yokochi, T., and Miura, K. Diagnosis of primary hepatic carcinoma by detection of α_1-fetoglobulin (in Japanese). *Kanzo (Liver)*, **10**, 143–146 (1969).
5. Hirai, H. Serelogical diagnosis of the hepatic cancer—fetal α-globulin (in Japanese). *Shinryo (Postgraduate Course)*, **23**, 2190–2195 (1970).
6. Nishi, S. and Hirai, H. α_f-Globulin of the patients with malignant hepatoma and fetus (in Japanese). *Seibutsu-Butsuri-Kagaku (Physicochem. Biol.)*, **14**, 301 (1970).
7. Tatarinov, Ju. S. Content of embryo-specific α-globulin in fetal and neonatal sera and from adult humans with primary carcinoma of the liver. *Fed. Proc.*, **25**, 344–346 (1966).

EXPLANATION OF PHOTOS

PHOTO 1. Electron micrograph of AFP production in a hepatoma cell showing peroxidase reaction

Positive reaction is observed on the rough endoplasmic reticulum encompassing mitochondria. Negative reaction in Golgi apparatus (G). N: Nucleus. ×23,000.

PHOTO 2. α-Fetoprotein around ribosomes of the rough endoplasmic reticulum

Hollow round particle (arrow) coincided with ribosomes. ×57,000.

PHOTO 3. α-Fetoprotein on the rough endoplasmic reticulum

A few peroxidase-positive granules are observed in the slightly dilated cisternae of the rough endoplasmic reticulum (arrow). ×57,000.

PHOTO 4. Distribution of AFP in a hepatoma cell

α-Fetoprotein was also detected in parts of the outer layer of the nuclear membrane (arrow), smooth endoplasmic reticulum, and some parts of the cell membrane (arrow). ×23,000.

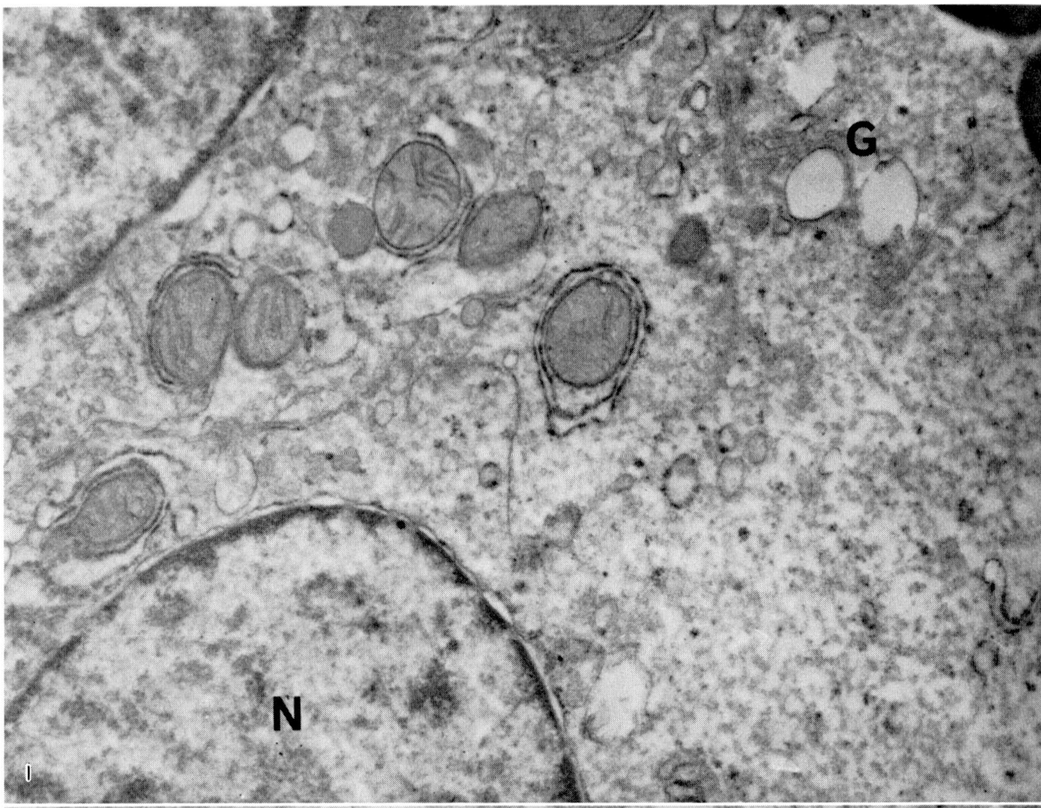
G
N
1

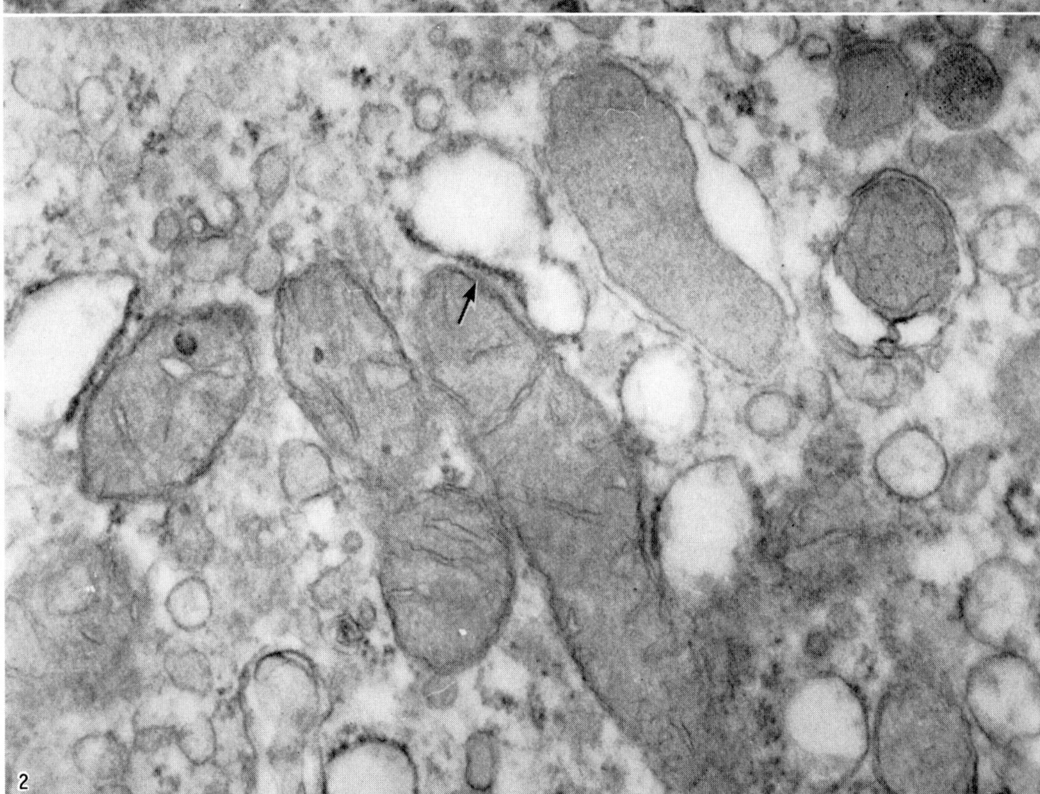
2

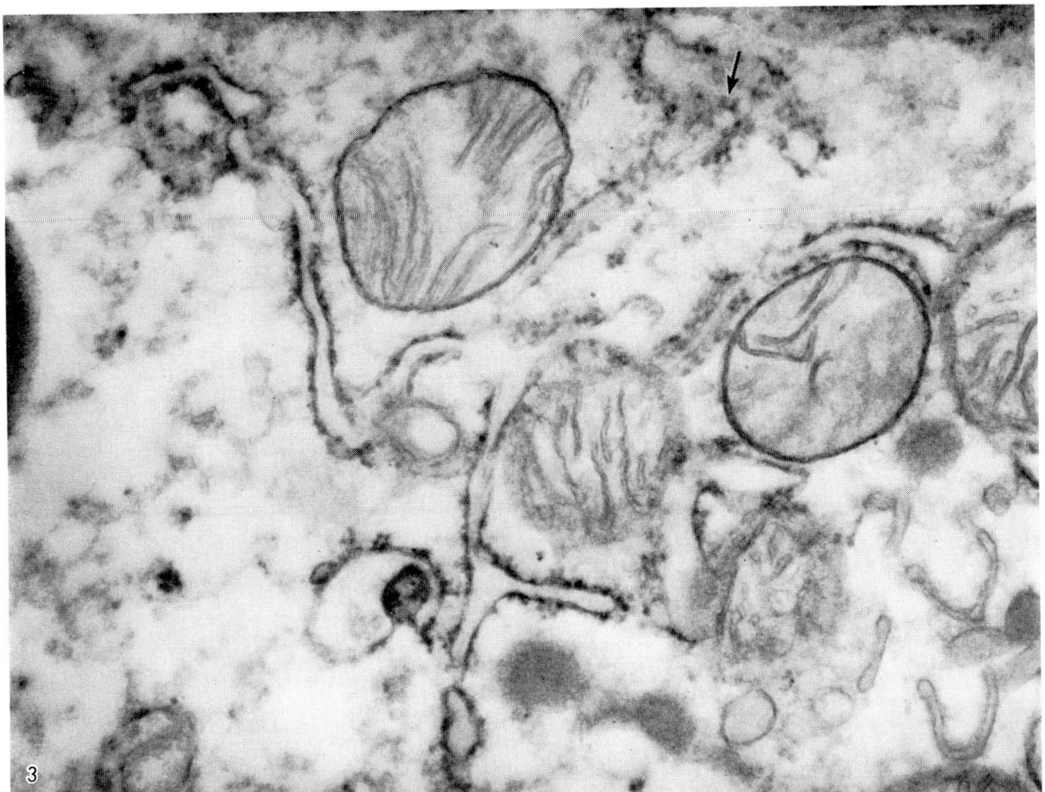
3

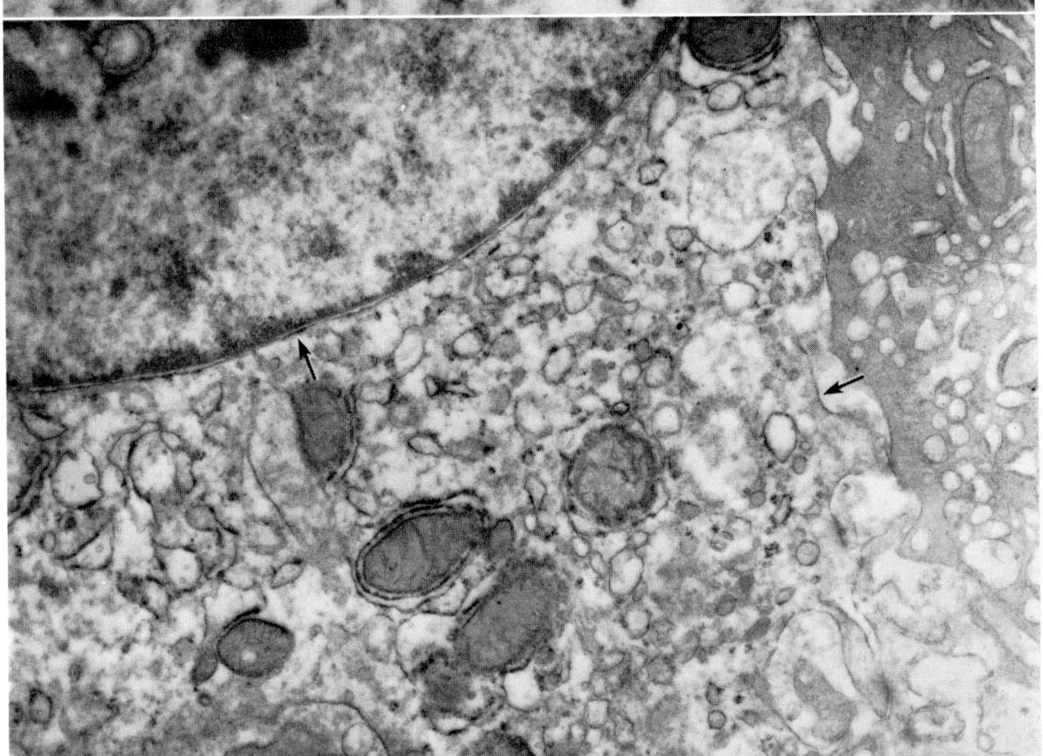
4

PRODUCTION OF α-FETOPROTEIN BY TRANSPLANTABLE RAT HEPATOMA

Hiroyuki WATABE and Hidematsu HIRAI
*Department of Biochemistry, School of Medicine, Hokkaido University**

Production of rat α-fetoprotein (AFP) by transplantable ascites hepatoma was studied. α-Fetoprotein was detected in the serum and ascitic fluid of rats transplanted with some ascites tumors. It was found that 26 out of 78 ascites hepatoma cell lines tested were AFP-producing lines. α-Fetoprotein was detected in 1 of 5 Morris hepatomas and in some sublines derived from Yoshida sarcoma which is a typical nonproducing line. α-Fetoprotein was also detected in the extract of AFP-producing tumor cells.

Rats were fed 4-dimethylaminoazobenzene and developed hepatomas. All the rats were AFP-positive. From the developed hepatoma nodules, 5 ascites tumor cell lines were established. Three of 5 continued to produce AFP.

Since Abelev *et al.* (*1*) reported that an α-globulin in the serum of mice bearing chemically induced hepatomas was immunologically identical to mouse α-fetoprotein (AFP), the appearance of AFP in primary or chemically induced hepatomas has been shown in various mammalian species (*4*, *5*, *8*, *13*, *17*, *18*, *20*). Synthesis of AFP was also demonstrated in some transplantable tumors in rats (*17*) and mice (*1*).

The transplantable cell lines of rat ascites hepatoma established and maintained in Japan were mostly derived from hepatomas induced by 4-dimethylaminoazobenzene (DAB) or 3′-methyl-DAB. On the other hand, Yoshida sarcoma is of spontaneous origin. Recently, some sublines of Yoshida sarcoma designated as LY were established by Satoh *et al.* (*21*). The present investigation was undertaken to study in more detail the production of AFP by such established tumors.

Immunological Analysis of AFP

α-Fetoprotein was detected by the double diffusion method of Ouchterlony (*15*). The concentration of AFP was determined by the method of Mancini *et al.* (*10*). Antiserum used in this study was a monospecific antiserum against rat AFP and the preparation procedure has previously been given in detail (*20*).

* Kita-15-jo, Nishi-7-chome, Kita-ku, Sapporo 060, Japan (渡部博之, 平井秀松).

α-Fetoprotein in Rats Bearing Transplantable Tumors

Most of the transplantable ascites hepatomas (AH), Yoshida sarcoma, and its sublines (LY) are maintained in the Sasaki Institute, Tokyo, and were offered by Dr. H. Satoh for the present study. AH-64 series was supplied by Dr. M. Ishidate, Jr. (National Institute of Hygienic Sciences, Tokyo). The life span of rats transplanted with AH tumors (about 10^7 cells) is usually 10 days to 2 weeks.

Blood was collected by decapitation of rats bearing the tumor 1 or 2 days

TABLE I. α-Fetoprotein in the Sera, Ascitic Fluids, and Cell Extracts from Ascites Hepatoma-bearing Rats

Cell line	S	A	E	Cell line	S	A	E	Cell line	S	A	E
AH-13	—	—	—	AH-64C-2	—	—	—	AH-136B	+++	+++	—
13C	—	—	—	64C-3	—	—	—	143A	+	+	—
13M	—	—	—	64C-4	—	—	—	149	—	—	—
13R	—	—	—	64D	—	—	—	150A	++	+++	+
21	—	—	—	65C	+	+	—	173	—	—	—
34	—	—	—	66	+++	+++	++	173F	—	—	—
39	—	—	—	66F	—	—	—	210A	—	—	—
41A	+	+	—	66FI	—	—	—	225A	—	—	—
41B	—	—	—	70B	+++	+++	+	272	—	—	—
41C	—	—	—	84A	—	—	—	310	++	++	+
42B	++	++	+	99	++	++	+	311	+	++	+
44	—	—	—	100B	—	—	—	322	—	—	—
49	—	—	—	107B	—	—	—	371A	++	++	+
49WH	++	++	—	108A	—	—	—	408	++	++	+
57B	+	++	+	108AF	—	—	—	414	—	—	—
60C	++	++	+	109A	—	—	—	601[a]	++	++	—
61B	—	—	—	122A	+	++	—	602[a]	+	+	—
62	—	—	—	122B	++	++	—	602F[a]	++	++	+
62F	—	—	—	127	—	—	—	712	—	—	—
63F	—	—	—	130	—	—	—	782	—	—	—
64A	—	—	—	130FG	—	—	—	3683[b]	—	N	N
64B	—	—	—	130FN	—	—	—	3924A[b]	++	N	N
64B-1	—	—	—	130FNI	++	++	+	7974	+	+	—
64B-2	—	—	—	130F (S_1)	—	—	—	7974F	—	—	—
64C	—	—	—	131A	+	+	—	H35TC-2[b]	++	N	N
64C-1	—	—	—	131B	—	—	—	FCIII-6[c]	—	—	—

— : AFP-negative; + ++ +++ : AFP-positive, weak, medium, and strong; S=serum, A=ascitic fluid, E=saline extract of tumor cells, N=not done.

All of the lines with no mark were established from rat hepatoma developed by feeding DAB or 3′-Me-DAB.

[a] Original hepatomas were produced in rats fed with *o*-aminoazotoluene (AAT).

[b] Produced by N-2-fluorenyldiacetamide (FAA). These strains were provided by courtesy of Dr. Y. Hashimoto, Tokyo Biochemical Research Institute, Tokyo.

[c] Produced by cycasin. This strain was provided by courtesy of Dr. I. Hirono, Department of Pathology, Gifu University School of Medicine.

TABLE II. α-Fetoprotein in the Sera of Morris Hepatoma-bearing Rats

Cell line		AFP
Morris hepatoma	5123TC	−
	7316 B	−
	7793	−
	7794 A	−
	7795	⧺

These lines were provided by courtesy of Dr. T. Ono, Cancer Institute, Tokyo, and Dr. T. Sugimura, National Cancer Center Research Institute, Tokyo.

before death due to tumor growth. Ascitic fluids and tumor cells were taken by peritoneal puncture and separated by centrifugation. The tumor cells were freed from ascitic fluid by washing several times with a sufficient amount of physiological saline, and were suspended in saline with a volume equal to that of the packed tumor cells. The suspension was then sonicated and centrifuged in order to obtain the cell extracts.

The detection of AFP was carried out on the sera, ascitic fluids, and tumor cell extracts. The results are shown in Table I. α-Fetoprotein was detected in 26 (33%) out of the 78 cell lines tested.

Five lines of Morris hepatoma maintained in Japan were also investigated, and as shown in Table II, 1 of the 5 lines was shown to produce AFP.

Table III gives the results of examination of Yoshida sarcoma and its sublines. α-Fetoprotein was detected in 4 of the 7 LY cell lines.

α-Fetoprotein levels in the serum and ascites of rats transplanted with AH-66 ascites hepatoma were quantitatively determined. The results are shown in Figs. 1 and 2. The serum was collected from the tail vein 3, 5, 7, 9, and 12 days after inoculation of the tumor and after 5, 7, 9, and 11 days in the case of the ascites. The rats usually died on the 13th day as a result of tumor growth. All rats showed AFP production and the level increased with time after transplantation. The levels in serum and ascites were almost identical.

TABLE III. α-Fetoprotein in the Sera of Rats Transplanted with Yoshida Sarcoma (YS) and Its Sublines

Cell line	AFP	Cell line	AFP
YS	−	LY-1[b]	−
YS-G[a]	−	LY-5	++
YS-GH	−	LY-7	+
YS-GV	−	LY-52	++
		LY-54	−
		LY-80	+
		LY-336	−

[a] YS-G, GH, GV: YS sublines of low sensitivity to nitrogen mustard.
[b] LY: Sublines of YS.

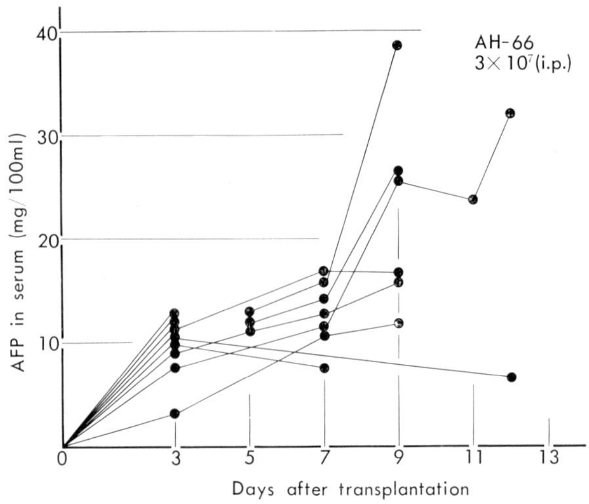

FIG. 1. Change of AFP concentration in the sera of rats transplanted with AH-66 cells

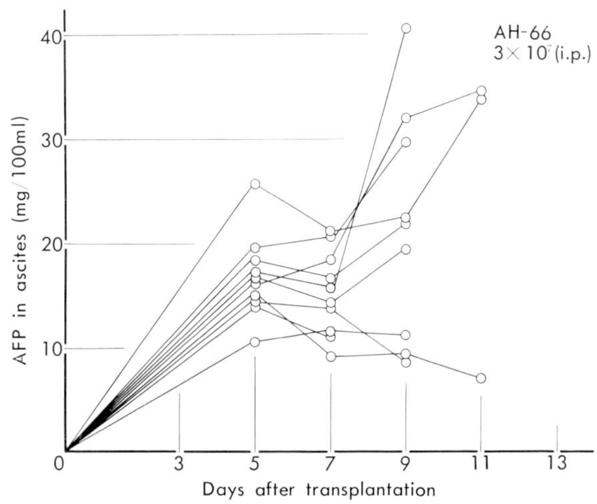

FIG. 2. Change of AFP concentration in ascitic fluids of rats transplanted with AH-66 cells

Production of AFP by Newly Established Ascites Hepatomas

As previously reported by Watabe (*20*) AFP was detected in all the rats having hepatomas induced by DAB. The establishment of new ascites hepatoma cell lines was always undertaken from such " AFP-positive " rat livers.

The hepatic nodules were removed and gently homogenized. The freed tumor cells were inoculated into the peritoneal cavity of healthy rats. By this procedure, 5 cell lines of ascites hepatoma were established. AH-1062M was established from a metastatic nodule in an omentum of No. 1062 rat, AH-1084A was from the tumor cells in the ascitic fluid of No. 1084 rat, and AH-1091 was from No. 1091 rat, A from the tumor cells in the ascitic fluid, B from a large

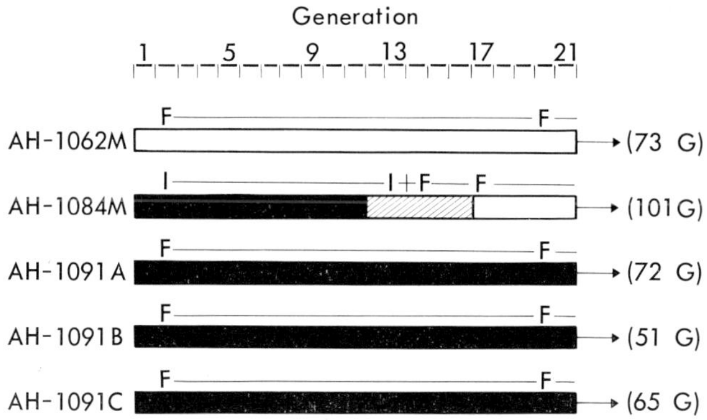

FIG. 3. Production of AFP following serial transplantation
F: free cell; I: island cell. ■ AFP-positive; □ AFP-negative.

hepatoma nodule, and C from a small hepatoma nodule in the liver. The life span of rats transplanted with these ascites tumors was 8 to 10 days.

Three of them (AH-1091A, AH-1091B, AH-1091C) have been AFP-positive for 72, 51 and 65 generations, respectively, to date (Fig. 3). One line (AH-1062M), however, never produced AFP. This line has already passed 73 generations but remains consistently AFP-negative. Another line (AH-1084A) was strongly AFP-positive for 11 generations but after 12 generations AFP became weak, and became entirely undetectable after 17 generations. It has remained negative for 85 generations to date.

DISCUSSION

Abelev *et al.* (*1*) demonstrated that AFP was synthesized by the hepatoma cell itself in mice, and the same result was obtained by Stanislawski-birencwajg *et al.* (*17*) in rats. Since then, many investigators have made similar observations by the immunofluorescence method in man and animals. In the present investigation, synthesis of AFP by the tumor cell was also demonstrated by the extraction of AFP from tumor cells.

Synthesis of AFP by ascites hepatoma was also demonstrated in the tissue culture by Abelev *et al.* (*1*) and Tsukada *et al.* (*19*). The AFP was secreted into the culture medium.

As shown in Table I, AFP was detected similarly in serum, ascitic fluid, and in extract of tumor cells, except in several cases of tumor cell extracts. The negative incidence in these exceptional cases is not significant because of the variable concentration of AFP in the cells and inadequate extraction.

The precipitin reaction in agar gel showed that 33% of transplantable hepatoma cell lines tested synthesized AFP and secreted it into the ascitic fluid and blood stream of the host.

A previous paper by Watabe (*20*) demonstrated that all rats bearing DAB-induced hepatomas in their livers revealed AFP in the sera. Though almost all AH lines were established from hepatoma developed in the liver mostly by

DAB or 3′-Me-DAB, only 33% of them continue to produce AFP. The discontinuance of AFP production may be explained by selection. Most of the cell lines tested have been passaged over 100 generations from rat to rat. During these passages, selection of the tumor cells may occur. The hepatoma nodules formed in the liver of rats by a carcinogen may consist of many types of tumor cells. This mosaic structure was proposed, for example, by Ishidate (*7*) who demonstrated the heterogeneity of the karyotype. Some recent studies (*2*, *3*) indicated, by the immunofluorescence technique, the presence of both AFP-positive and AFP-negative cells in a hepatoma nodule. During serial transplantation the selection of either AFP-positive or AFP-negative hepatoma cells will occur.

As shown in Table I, AH cell lines with the same number, such as 131A and 131B, indicate that these lines originated from the tumor of rat No. 131. However, such cell lines from a rat do not show the same AFP production. The same phenomena are seen in some other cell lines such as AH-66,-130 and-7974. On the other hand, a group of cell lines such as AH-64 established by Ishidate (*7*) all show absence of AFP production, but nevertheless, each line can be clearly distinguished by the difference in cytological properties.

Symbols other than A, B, and C indicate some sublines from a line. 66-F, 66-FI, 130-FNI, 7974-F, *etc.*, proved to be different in AFP production from their original lines. These differences are also explained by selection, as described above.

Most of AH lines were established from hepatomas produced by DAB or 3′-Me-DAB. No difference was observed between the 2 carcinogens. AH-601 and AH-602 were established from hepatomas produced by *o*-aminoazotoluene (AAT). These lines showed positive AFP but the incidence is too small to assume that AAT is responsible for positive AFP. AH-3683, AH-3924A, and AH-35TC-2 were established from hepatomas produced by N-2-fluorenyldiacetamide (FAA), and FCIII-6 by cycasin. No difference between the carcinogens used was observed.

Abelev *et al.* (*1*) reported that rapidly growing transplantable mouse hepatomas appeared to synthesize AFP, but in the present study, such a correlation between AFP production and tumor-cell growth rate was not observed. Some morphological and cytological properties of AH cell lines, such as karyotype, sensitivity to X-irradiation or nitrogen mustard, and rate of malignancy (life span of host animals, or the growth rate of the tumor cells) have been observed and described in detail by Yoshida and his group (*6*, *9*, *11*, *12*, *16*). However, no correlation between these properties and the rate of AFP production was observed, except for the following phenomenon. The AH cells form clusters in ascitic fluid in various grades. Odashima (*14*) summarized data for the grade of cluster formation, which was expressed as free cell percentage; 100% means that all the tumor cells float in ascitic fluid as single cells (free-cell) and 0% means that all the tumor cells form clusters and no single cells are observed. Figure 4 shows a correlation between the intensity of AFP production observed in the present study and the grade of cluster formation cited from the data of Odashima (*14*). It can be seen that AFP-positive lines are always found in the cluster-

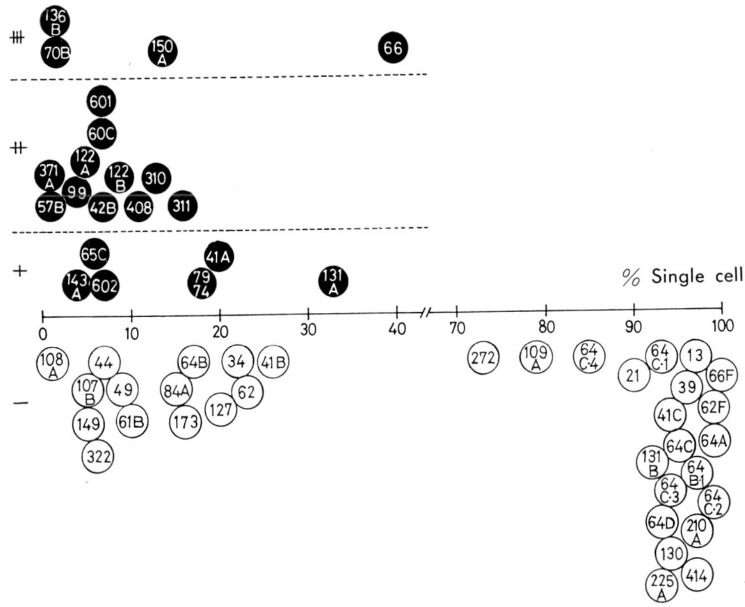

FIG. 4. Production of AFP and degree of hepatoma cell clusters
● AFP-producing; ○ AFP non-producing.

forming lines and not in the free-cell-type lines. It appears that the greater the cluster formation, the higher the AFP production, although this is only qualitative. AH-66 is an exception. This line contains about 40% free cells but AFP production is very high.

Among newly established AH cell lines, on the other hand, 3 lines (AH-1091A, AH-1091B, AH-1091C) consist of about 90% of free cells, but show strong production of AFP. All the lines summarized in Table I and Fig. 4 are quite old strains investigated a long time after their establishment, so that AFP production in our new cell lines should be reinvestigated after the passage of many generations.

Regarding any correlation between cluster formation and AFP production, observations in sublines of Yoshida sarcoma are interesting. Yoshida sarcoma is a typical free-cell-type ascites tumor, but the sublines designated LY, established by Satoh *et al.* (*21*), form large clusters. These sublines showed a decrease in malignancy as indicated by elongation of life span of the host animals. As shown in Table III, 4 out of 7 LY lines were AFP-positive.

The conversion *in vitro* of YS into AFP-producing cells was investigated by Isaka and Tsukada, and the results are reported elsewhere in this issue.

Similar correlation was obtained in the AH-1084A cell line (Fig. 3). This line consisted of large cell clusters for 11 generations and AFP production was strongly positive. However, after 12 generations the number of free cells increased and their content reached about 95% after 17 generations. Simultaneously AFP production became negative.

The formation of clusters is said to be one of the characteristics of epithelial cells such as hepatocytes. The AFP production is a function of normal fetal liver cells and may be an indication of the grade of differentiation of hepatoblastic cells. α-Fetoprotein production, cluster formation, and elongation of life span observed in LY sublines may be correlated to the change in malignancy of Yoshida sarcoma. From these points of view, AFP production in Morris hepatoma, shown in Table II, is quite interesting. These well-differentiated hepatomas having very low malignancy did not show production of AFP, except in one strain.

In clinical observations in Japan, about 80% of primary hepatoma patients show positive AFP but 20% are negative (*4, 13*). This fact has been confirmed by many other investigators. The data presented in this paper may also be significant with regard to the relation between malignancy and AFP production, although a more precise quantitative analysis is necessary.

The sensitivity of the AFP test used in this investigation was 1 mg/100 ml. Further work is in progress with a more sensitive method, *i.e.*, radioimmunoassay, and more detailed information will be obtained.

Acknowledgments

The authors are indebted to Dr. H. Satoh, Sasaki Institute, Tokyo, Dr. T. Ono, Cancer Institute, Tokyo, Dr. T. Sugimura, National Cancer Center Research Institute, Tokyo, Dr. I. Hirono, Department of Pathology, Gifu University School of Medicine, Gifu, and Dr. Y. Hashimoto, Tokyo Biochemical Research Institute, Tokyo, for the gift of the tumors and sera of tumor-bearing rats used in this study. Grateful acknowledgment is made to Dr. Y. Tsukada of this laboratory for establishing the transplantable hepatoma strains.

REFERENCES

1. Abelev, G. I., Perova, S. D., Khramkova, N. I., Postnikova, Z. A., and Irlin, I. S. Production of embryonal α-globulin by transplantable mouse hepatoma. *Transplantation*, **1**, 174–180 (1963).
2. Engelhardt, N. V., Gusev, A. I., Shipova, L. Ja., and Abelev, G. I. Immunofluorescent study of alpha-fetoprotein (αfp) in liver and liver tumors. I. Technique of αfp localization in tissue sections. *Int. J. Cancer*, **7**, 198–206 (1971).
3. Gusev, A. I., Engelhardt, N. V., Masseyeff, R., Camain, R., and Basteris, B. Immunofluorescent study of alpha-fetoprotein (αfp) in liver and liver tumors. II. Localization of αfp in the tissues of patients with primary liver cancer. *Int. J. Cancer*, **7**, 207–217 (1971).
4. Hirai, H., Nishi, S., and Watabe, H. Embryonic α_f-globulin and hepatoma (in Japanese). *Nippon Rinsho* (*Jap. J. Clin. Med.*), **29**, 212–216 (1971).
5. Hull, E. W., Carbone, P. P., Gitlin, D., O'Gara, R. W., and Kelly, M. G. α-Fetoprotein in monkeys with hepatoma. *J. Natl. Cancer Inst.*, **42**, 1035–1044 (1969).
6. Irako, Y. Studies on the effect of X-irradiation upon ascites tumor cells. II. Different sensitivities of various transplant strains of the ascites hepatoma to X-irradiation. *GANN*, **49** (Suppl.), 319–320 (1958).
7. Ishidate, M., Jr. Cytological individuality of hepatoma cell lines derived from a single Donryu rat. *GANN*, **59**, 341–356 (1968).
8. Kahan, B. and Levine, L. The occurrence of a serum fetal α_1 protein in develop-

ing mice and murine hepatomas and teratomas. *Cancer Res.*, **31**, 930–936 (1971).
9. Kajiwara, K., Isaka, H., Nakamura, K., Aruji, R., Kaise, A., Odashima, S., and Satoh, H. Studies on the ascites hepatoma. II. On the transplantation rate of the ascites hepatoma intraperitoneally transplanted. *GANN*, **44**, 307–309 (1953).
10. Mancini, G., Carbonara, A. O., and Heremans, J. F. Immunochemical quantitation of antigens by single radial immunodiffusion. *Int. J. Immunochem.*, **2**, 235–254 (1965).
11. Nakamura, K. Studies on the ascites hepatoma. VIII. Difference of chromosome numbers among tumor cells constituting the same " island " of the ascites hepatoma. *GANN*, **46**, 196–199 (1955).
12. Nakamura, K., Odashima, S., Isaka, H., and Kurata, T. Studies on the ascites hepatoma. X. Further studies on the chromosome number. *GANN*, **47**, 502–504 (1956).
13. Nishi, S. Isolation and characterization of a human fetal α-globulin from the sera of fetuses and a hepatoma patient. *Cancer Res.*, **30**, 2507–2513 (1970).
14. Odashima, S. Establishment of ascites hepatomas in the rat, 1951–1962. *Natl. Cancer Inst. Monograph*, **16**, 51–93 (1964).
15. Ouchterlony, O. Antigen-antibody reaction in gels. IV. Types of reaction in coordinated systems of diffusion. *Acta Pathol. Microbiol. Scand.*, **32**, 231–240 (1953).
16. Satoh, H. Studies on the ascites hepatoma. XI. Different responses by different strains of ascites hepatomas of rats to chemotherapeutic treatment. *GANN*, **47**, 334–337 (1956).
17. Stanislawski-birencwajg, M., Uriel, J., and Grabar, P. Association of embryonic antigens with experimentally induced hepatic lesions in the rat. *Cancer Res.*, **27**, 1990–1997 (1967).
18. Tatarinov, Yu. S. Content of embryo-specific α-globulin in fetal and neonatal sera and from adult humans with primary carcinoma of the liver. *Vopr. Med. Khim.*, **11**, 20 (1965) (*Fed. Proc.*, **25**, 344–346 (1966)).
19. Tsukada, Y., Watabe, H., Kobayashi, K., and Hirai, H. Production of α-fetoprotein by tumor cells in tissue culture. *Proc. Jap. Cancer Assoc., 30th Annu. Meet.*, 226 (1971).
20. Watabe, H. Early appearance of embryonic α-globulin in rat serum during carcinogenesis with 4-dimethylaminoazobenzene. *Cancer Res.*, **31**, 1192–1194 (1971).
21. Yoshida, T., Isaka, H., and Satoh, H. Problem of the origin of Yoshida sarcoma. *Arzneimittelforschung*, **14**, 735–741 (1964).

GANN Monograph on Cancer Research 14, 1973

A COMMENT ON α-FETOPROTEIN-PRODUCING VARIANTS OF YOSHIDA ASCITES SARCOMA, WITH REFERENCE TO THE HYPOTHESIS OF HEPATIC CELL ORIGIN OF THE ASCITES TUMOR*[1]

Hidehiko ISAKA and Yutaka TSUKADA

Sasaki Institute[*2] *and Department of Biochemistry, School of Medicine, Hokkaido University*[*3]

α-Fetoprotein-producing variant tumor cells have been isolated from Yoshida ascites sarcoma. This seems to provide support for Yoshida's hypothesis of a hepatic cell origin for the Yoshida ascites tumor.

The concept seems to be current that the cancer cell has stable characteristics and proliferates to form a clonal population of homogeneous cells with uniform characteristics, as long as it is accepted as a somatic mutant. However, analytical studies on ascites tumors with respect to the chromosome, drug sensitivity, and/or resistance demonstrated that a cancer, even a clonal tumor cell population, was characterized by a considerable degree of variation in the individual cells constituting an apparently uniform tumor cell population (*6*, *7*, *9*). Variant ascites tumor cells with altered characteristics and behavior, some of them being accompanied by chromosomal alterations, were successfully isolated from their parent population both *in vivo* and *in vitro* (*5*, *12–14*, *16*, *18*, *25*, *26*). This means that the cancer cell can undergo further changes which could result in either loss, gain, or alteration of specific cell properties, giving rise to a variant cancer cell population. The exact mechanism underlying such biological changes in cancer cells is not yet clarified. Possible factors for selective and/or competitive growth of variant cells within a tumor should be responsible for the development of variant tumors.

LY-Variants of Yoshida Ascites Sarcoma

An ascites tumor of the rat, which has been referred to as Yoshida ascites sarcoma since 1948, is composed of individually isolated tumor cells proliferating in the ascitic fluid when transplanted intraperitoneally. They invade various peritoneal organs and form multiple tumor nodules in which they have never shown any epithelial growth, histopathologically. The growth morphology of

*1 This work was supported by a Grant-in-Aid for Cancer Research from the Ministry of Education.

*2 Surugadai 2-chome, Kanda, Chiyoda-ku, Tokyo 101, Japan (井坂英彦).

*3 Kita-15-jo, Nishi-7-chome, Kita-ku, Sapporo 060, Japan (塚田　裕).

this ascites tumor was kept stable through animal passage from the beginning of serial transplantation in 1943. However, variant cell lines of the ascites tumor, designated as LY-variants, which had developed in immunologically conditioned Donryu rats, demonstrated the formation of clusters or islands (bound groups of tumor cells) in ascites, presenting an epithelial character (*20*, *32*). This was first recorded by Satoh (*20*) who later established more than 15 different LY-variants. A cluster of LY-variant cells can hardly be distinguished morphologically from the "hepatoma islands" of authentic hepatocarcinoma cells in ascites hepatoma, the ascites form of azo-dye-induced rat hepatoma, as shown in Photo 1. Neighboring cells constituting the same LY cluster showed the development of a terminal bar desmosome at the edge of their free surface under the electron microscope (*23*). They grew in host tissues, showing histopathologically an adenocarcinomatous pattern (Photo 2). Their growth was considerably slower than that of the parent Yoshida sarcoma, as revealed by the longer survival time of their hosts and/or generation time *in vitro* (*15*, *32*). All the LY-variants differed both from each other and from their original tumor line in their karyotypes (*8*). Analogs of such variants have been observed by Ishidate and Isaka (*11*).

The development of LY-variants threw some light on the problem of the origin of Yoshida ascites sarcoma, which had remained unsolved for a long time, although Kupffer's stellate cell, a reticuloendothelial cell of the liver, had been postulated as the mother cell of Yoshida sarcoma (*30*, *33*). Recently, Yoshida (*31*) has dealt with this problem again and stated that the so-called Yoshida ascites sarcoma may not be a sarcomatous tumor, but may be derived from malignant hepatoma cells, based on the following accumulated findings.

(1) The Yoshida ascites sarcoma was discovered by Yoshida in a rat which had been fed *o*-aminoazotoluene (4′-amino-2, 3′-dimethylaminoazobenzene) for 3 months and then painted on the back with KAs_2O_3 solution. Besides the ascites tumor, primary solid hepatoma nodules were noticed in the liver of that rat (*29*).

(2) Azo-dye-induced solid hepatoma is transformed by ascitic conversion into an ascites hepatoma which is characterized by either individually isolated, single hepatoma cells, or both single and clustered hepatoma cells growing in ascites, *i.e.*, "free cell-type" or "island-type" growth of hepatoma cells. It has been frequently noticed that an ascitic growth of hepatoma cells occurs spontaneously in rats with primary hepatomas induced by azo-dye-feeding, presenting a state of primary ascites hepatoma when the cells are vigorously proliferating. Many transplant lines of ascites hepatoma have been established with hepatoma materials regardless of whether the primary material has been solid or ascitic (*18*). The microscopic pictures of both ascitic and invasive growth in free-cell-type ascites hepatomas are practically indistinguishable from those in the Yoshida ascites sarcoma.

(3) It was frequently found that a transformation from the island-type ascites hepatoma into the free-cell-type tumor took place during prolonged animal passage, though the factors responsible for such change were unknown (*21*). In such cases, the free-cell-type variants developed in association with chromosomal alteration of tumor cells. On the other hand, the transformation of ascites

hepatoma from the free-cell-type to the island-type also occurred, though rarely, giving rise to a population of island-type tumor cells with altered chromosomes (*31*). The above LY-variants of Yoshida ascites sarcoma, island-type tumors, are understood to be variant tumors in the latter category, transformed from the free-cell-type ascites tumor. An explanation for the mechanism of LY-transformation was presented by Yoshida (*31*) who suggested that the epithelial cell nature of Yoshida ascites tumor, which had been " masked " for a long time, was " unmasked " by unknown factors and the original island or epithelial nature became apparent. These findings do not suggest the possibility of a nonepithelial cell origin of Yoshida ascites tumor, but strongly support a hepatoepithelial cell (hepatic cell) origin for the tumor.

Biochemical studies on the LY-variants and their parent Yoshida ascites tumor were made by some workers. Ono (*19*), among them, demonstrated that two LY-variants including LY-336 possessed almost no differentiated enzyme activities in spite of their lowered growth, with regard to glucose 6-phosphate dehydrogenase, glutamate dehydrogenase, glucose-6-phosphatase, ornithine transcarbamylase, aspartate transcarbamylase, threonine dehydrogenase, and deoxycytidylate deaminase. He suggested that well-differentiated hepatomas should be slow-growing, but the slow growth rate does not necessarily induce differentiation, and that the lowered growth rate of LY-variants results from repression of thymidine kinase and/or DNA synthesis. Sugimura (*24*) and co-workers (*22*) made a comparative study on hexokinase isozyme patterns in rat liver, an ascites hepatoma AH-109A, a slow-growing variant of AH-109A, Yoshida ascites tumor, and LY-5, an LY-variant. According to them, rat liver possesses 4 different types of hexokinase isozyme, I, II, III, and IV, and AH-109A and Yoshida ascites tumor have only types I and II hexokinases, whereas the slow-growing variant of AH-109A and LY-5 have hexokinases of types I, II, and III. Sugimura emphasized that a restoration of type III hexokinase activity took place in such slow-growing variants, including an LY-variant line. This is an interesting phenomenon to the present authors, in considering the ancestry of Yoshida ascites sarcoma.

Production of AFP in Variants of Yoshida Ascites Sarcoma

Since the report of Abelev *et al.* (*2*) much attention has been paid to α-fetoprotein (AFP) production by malignant hepatoma cells. Data accumulated up to now demonstrate that AFP is synthesized and secreted by hepatic cells of fetal, neonatal, or cancerous origin in the rat (*1*). Not a single case of AFP-producing rat tumors, except for malignant hepatomas, has been recognized yet. However, the presence of AFP was detected in most cases of malignant hepatoma examined so far. Hirai (*4*) and his associates (*17*, *27*, *28*) have enthusiastically studied AFP in human and experimental hepatomas, including the ascites hepatoma, Yoshida ascites tumor and their variants in the rat. For example, Watabe *et al.* (*28*) demonstrated the presence of this fetal-type protein in 24 out of 74 transplant lines of the ascites hepatoma, most AFP-positive lines being of

TABLE I. Growth of AFP-producing Variant Tumor Cells of Yoshida Ascites Sarcoma

Variant cell lines	Doubling time *in vitro* (hr)	Survival of host rats (days)
SB-7-2	28.2	12
UP	14.7	11
UO	44.1	14
Yoshida sarcoma, control	20.9	8

the island type morphology and *vice versa*. An interesting finding was obtained, that 4 lines out of 7 different LY-variants produced AFP, while their parent Yoshida ascites tumor did not.

In 1971, Isaka *et al.* (*10*) established 3 further variant cell lines of Yoshida ascites tumor, characterized by AFP production and lowered growth. They cultivated Yoshida ascites tumor cells *in vitro* for almost 12 months. Their culture experiment consisted of subculture groups, in which cloned and noncloned Yoshida tumor cells were treated *in vitro* for a short period with mutagenic chemicals such as 4-nitroquinoline 1-oxide, N-methyl-bis (2-chloroethyl) amine, and N-methyl-N'-nitro-N-nitrosoguanidine, and control subculture groups. The variant cells were isolated from these subcultures of cloned cells by means of intraperitoneal and intrasplenic transplantation in normal Donryu rats. Details of this experiment have been described already (*10*). Table I indicates the growth of 3 variants by doubling time measured *in vitro* and survival time of the host animals. Marked slowdown of growth was noticed in the variant lines, compared to their parent tumor. Cells of all 3 variants grow in ascitic fluid as individually isolated cells when transplanted intraperitoneally and no sign of cell cluster or island formation can be detected, as shown in Photos 3–5. The variant cells have never shown any sign of epithelial nature in histological pictures of their solid tumors (Photo 6). They are cytogenetically altered cells differing from each other and from the parent Yoshida tumor cells (Photo 7). Production of AFP by these variants is indicated in Table II and Photo 8.

It is impossible to determine whether the chromosome alteration observed in the present 3 variants is related to their ability to produce AFP and/or lowered

TABLE II. Concentration of AFP in Rats and Culture Medium of Variant Cells of Yoshida Ascites Sarcoma and Ascites Hepatoma AH-66 Cells

	SB-7-2	UO	UP	AH-66
Serum[a]	0.4	0.1	0.24	10
Ascites[a]	0.2	0.06	0.1	20
Culture Medium[b]	1.2×10^{-9} (0.23)[c]	3.1×10^{-10} (0.058)[c]	6.3×10^{-10} (0.12)[c]	2.3×10^{-8} (3.2)[c]

[a] Collected from the host rats 7 days after transplantation. Inoculum, 10^7 cells/ml. Numbers indicate mg AFP in 100 ml serum or ascites.

[b] Collected 7 days after cultivation of cells in Eagle's minimum essential medium supplemented with 10% calf serum. Inoculum, 5×10^4 cells/ml. Numbers indicate mg AFP produced per cell per day.

[c] Numbers indicate mg AFP in 100 ml culture medium.

growth tempo, and the mechanism for the development of these variants is quite unknown. It is suggested that the AFP production of hepatoma cells could result from a change in the repressor system which may occur in a random way (*3*). Then, one may assume that the ability to produce this fetal-type protein of Yoshida ascites tumor cells which had been " masked " was " unmasked " *in vitro* by unknown effects in association with possible changes in the gene expression mechanism and altered chromosomes, and an original and functional property of the cells was revealed, in spite of their unchanged pathomorphology. It should be emphasized that the finding of AFP-producing variants of Yoshida ascites sarcoma seems to provide further support for Yoshida's hypothesis on the hepatic cell origin of Yoshida ascites tumor.

REFERENCES

1. Abelev, G. I. Production of embryonal serum α-globulin by hepatomas: Review of experimental and clinical data. *Cancer Res.*, **28**, 1344–1350 (1968).
2. Abelev, G. I., Perova, S. D., Khramkova, N. I., Postnikova, Z. A., and Irlin, I. S. Production of embryonal α-globulin by transplantable mouse hepatomas. *Transplantation*, **1**, 174–180 (1963).
3. Grabar, P., Stanislawski-birencwajg, M., Oisgold, S., and Uriel, J. Immunochemical and enzymatic studies on chemically induced rat liver tumors. *UICC Monograph*, **2**, 20–31 (1967).
4. Hirai, H. α_f-Globulin and hepatomas (in Japanese). *Tohoku Igaku Zasshi*, **82**, 236–245 (1971).
5. Hirono, I., Kojima, K., Kachi, H., Ohashi, A., and Sasaoka, I. Development of free-cell sublines of the ascites hepatoma AH-130 and their biological properties. *GANN*, **55**, 363–372 (1964).
6. Isaka, H. Natural drug resistance of the ascites hepatoma in the rat. *Natl. Cancer Inst. Monograph*, **16**, 131–147 (1964).
7. Isaka, H. Variable drug sensitivity and chromosomal features of a cancer clone. *GANN*, **56**, 443–460 (1965).
8. Isaka, H. Chromosomal features and DNA content of Yoshida ascites sarcoma and its slow-growing variants characterized by island formation in ascites. *GANN*, **59**, 327–339 (1968).
9. Isaka, H., Izumitani, M., Moriwaki, A., and Sakurai, Y. Isolation and characterization of nitrogen mustard-sensitive cells from a nitrogen mustard-resistant subline of Yoshida sarcoma. *GANN*, **57**, 353–366 (1966).
10. Isaka, H., Umehara, S., Hirai, H., and Tsukada, Y. Development of variant tumor cells of Yoshida ascites sarcoma producing α-fetoprotein. *GANN*, **63**, 63–71 (1972).
11. Ishidate, M., Jr. and Isaka, H. Studies on two variant strains of Yoshida sarcoma characterized by island formation in ascites. *GANN*, **57**, 413–426 (1966).
12. Kuroki, T. Studies on *in vitro* growth of Yoshida sarcoma cells. III. Virulence of the long-term cultured cells. *GANN*, **57**, 379–389 (1966).
13. Kuroki, T., Goto, M., and Satoh, H. Studies on tissue culture of tumor. IV. Establishment and characteristics of cultured cell lines from mouse ascites hepatoma MH-129P and MH-129F. *GANN*, **57**, 391–401 (1966).
14. Kuroki, T., Isaka, H., and Satoh, H. Studies on *in vitro* growth of Yoshida

sarcoma cells. II. Cellular alteration of the cultured cells during long-term cultivation. *GANN*, **57**, 367–377 (1966).
15. Kuroki, T., Sato, M., and Satoh, H. The growth of LY-variants of Yoshida sarcoma (in Japanese). *Nippon Rinsho (Jap. J. Clin. Med.)*, **24** 19–21 (1966).
16. Miyata, M., Takaoka, T., and Katsuta, H. Ascites mammary carcinoma-MM2 cells of the mouse in tissue culture. *Jap. J. Exp. Med.*, **39**, 153–166 (1969).
17. Nishi, S., Watabe, H., and Hirai, H. Antigenicity of α-fetoproteins in several mammalian species (in Japanese). *Seibutsu-Butsuri-Kagaku (Physicochem. Biol.)*, **16**, 79–82 (1971).
18. Odashima, S. Establishment of ascites hepatomas in the rat, 1951–1962. *Natl. Cancer Inst. Monograph*, **16**, 51–93 (1964).
19. Ono, T. Enzyme patterns and malignancy of experimental hepatomas. *GANN Monograph*, **1**, 189–205 (1966).
20. Satoh, H. Induction of resistance in animals to tumor transplantation (in Japanese). *Kenkyu Hokoku Shuroku, Gan-hen (Annu. Rep. Co-oper. Res. Min. Educ. Cancer)*, 84–94 (1964).
21. Satoh, H. and Ichimura, H. Variant sublines of ascites hepatomas developed by prolonged animal passage or cold storage at −80° (in Japanese). *Nippon Rinsho (Jap. J. Clin. Med.)*, **24**, 10–12 (1966).
22. Sato, S., Matsushima, T., and Sugimura, T. Hexokinase isozyme patterns of experimental hepatomas of rats. *Cancer Res.*, **29**, 1437–1466 (1969).
23. Sugano, H., Ikawa, Y., and Satoh, H. Ultrafine structures of LY-variants of Yoshida sarcoma (in Japanese). *Nippon Rinsho (Jap. J. Clin. Med.)*, **24**, 14–18 (1966).
24. Sugimura, T. Decarcinogenesis, a newer concept arising from our understanding of the cancer phenotype. *In* " Chemical Tumor Problems," ed. by W. Nakahara, Japan Society for Promotion of Science, Tokyo, pp. 267–284 (1970).
25. Takahashi, M. Alteration of virulence of MN ascites sarcoma after continuous culture *in vitro*. *GANN*, **54**, 295–310 (1963).
26. Takaoka, T., Katsuta, H., Ohta, S., and Miyata, M. Two cell strains of tissue culture, JTC-15 and -16, from rat ascites hepatomas, AH-66 and -7974. *Jap. J. Exp. Med.*, **39**, 267–275 (1969).
27. Watabe, H. Early appearance of embryonic α-globulin in rat serum during carcinogenesis with 4-dimethylaminoazobenzene. *Cancer Res.*, **31**, 1192–1194 (1971).
28. Watabe, H., Hirai, H., and Satoh, H. α-Fetoprotein in rats transplanted with ascites hepatoma. *GANN*, **63**, 189–199 (1972).
29. Yoshida, T. Origin of Yoshida sarcoma (in Japanese). *In* " Yoshida Sarcoma," ed. by T. Yoshida, Nara Shobo, Tokyo, pp. 40–50 (1949).
30. Yoshida, T. Studies on an ascites (reticuloendothelial cell?) sarcoma of the rat. *J. Natl. Cancer Inst.*, **12**, 947–969 (1952).
31. Yoshida, T. Comparative studies of ascites hepatomas. *Methods Cancer Res.*, **6**, 97–157 (1971).
32. Yoshida, T., Isaka, H., and Satoh, H. Problems of the origin of Yoshida sarcoma. *Arzneimittelforschung*, **14**, 735–741 (1964).
33. Yoshida, T., Satoh, H., and Aruji, T. Origin of the Yoshida sarcoma. I. Experimental production of " ascites hepatoma " in the rat. *Proc. Japan Acad.*, **27**, 289–301 (1951).

EXPLANATION OF PHOTOS

PHOTO 1. A picture of ascitic island-type variant LY-336. Tumor cell islands vary in size and shape. Phase-contrast.

PHOTO 2. A histological picture of infiltrative growth of LY-336 cells in the omentum. An adenocarcinomatous pattern of tumor cells surrounded by stroma tissue. Hematoxylin and Eosin stain.

PHOTO 3. An ascitic picture of AFP-producing variant SB-7-2. Individually isolated tumor cells. Phase-contrast.

PHOTO 4. AFP-producing variant UP cells in ascitic fluid. Free-cell type. Phase-contrast.

PHOTO 5. An ascitic picture of variant UO cells producing AFP. Phase-contrast.

PHOTO 6. A histopathological picture of a solid tumor developing in the omentum of rat bearing variant SB-7-2 cells. No sign of tumor cell arrangement in epithelial fashion. Hematoxylin and Eosin stain.

PHOTO 7. Typical metaphase chromosomes in clonal Yoshida sarcoma cells at different culture periods; YS-Clone-Control (I) and YS-Clone-Control (II), and their variant descendants producing AFP, SB-7-2, UP and UO. YS-Clone-Control (II) shows changed chromosome pattern after 22 weeks' cultivation of YS-Clone-Control (I). Chromosomes are arranged from left to right in groups of the same type, telocentrics (T), submeta- and subtelocentrics (S), and metacentrics (M), and in order of decreasing length. In each line, the number of chromosomes of the same type is indicated. Numbers in parentheses show total number of chromosomes. Marked dissimilarities are evident.

PHOTO 8. Double immunodiffusion pattern of the sera of rats bearing ascites hepatoma of AH-66 line (AH-66), 3 variants of Yoshida sarcoma (SB-7-2, UP, and UO), Yoshida sarcoma (YS), and normal adult rat serum (Sm). Anti-AFP horse serum is indicated by aαf. The fused precipitation lines represent antigenic identity and absence of reaction between the antiserum and Yoshida sarcoma or normal rat serum.

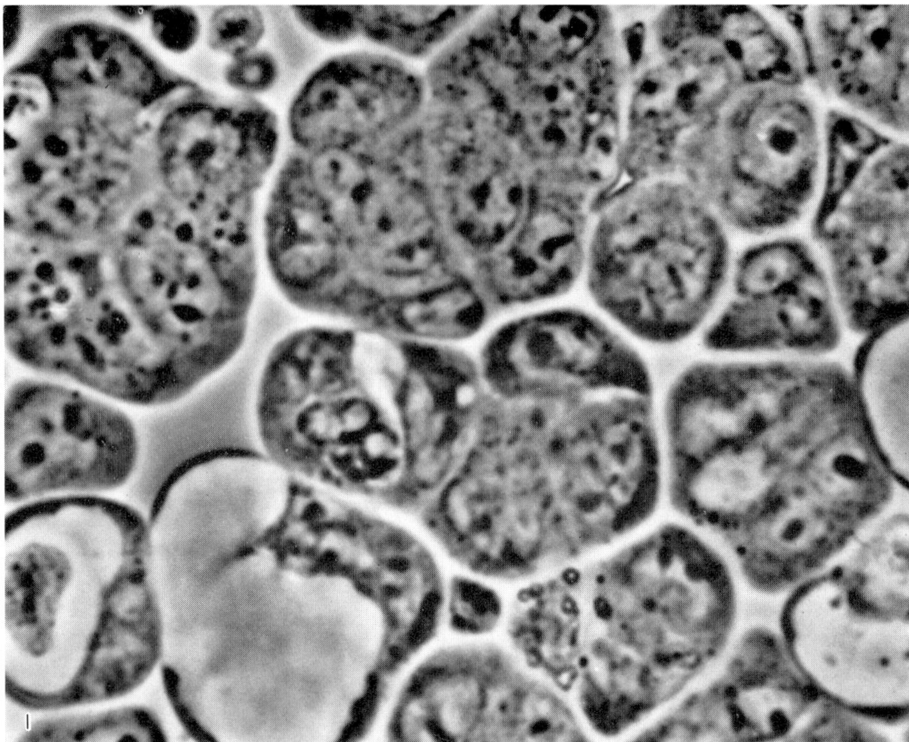

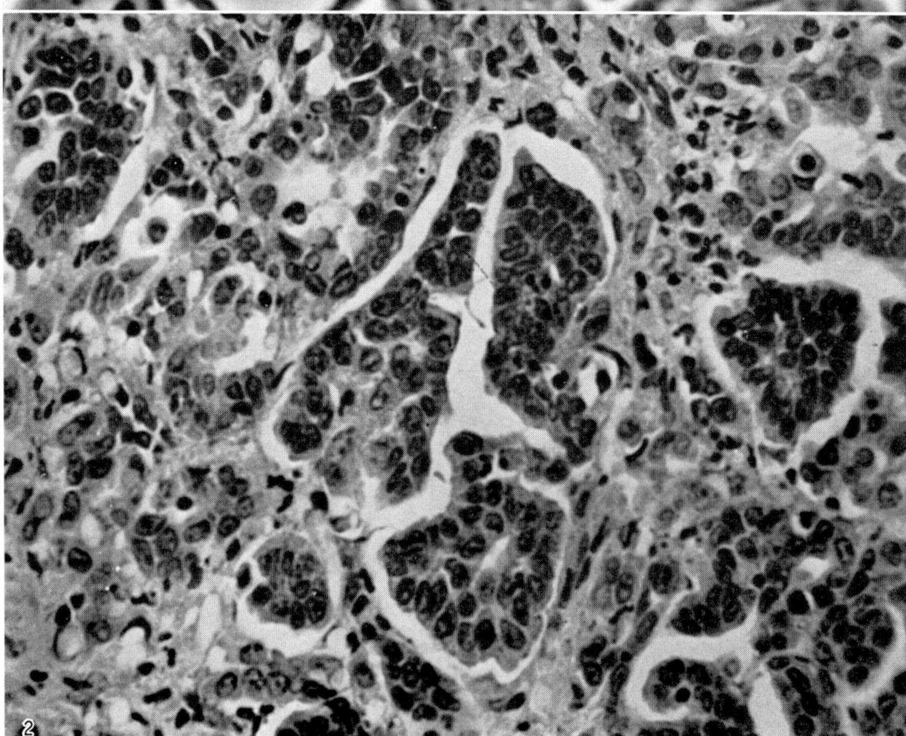

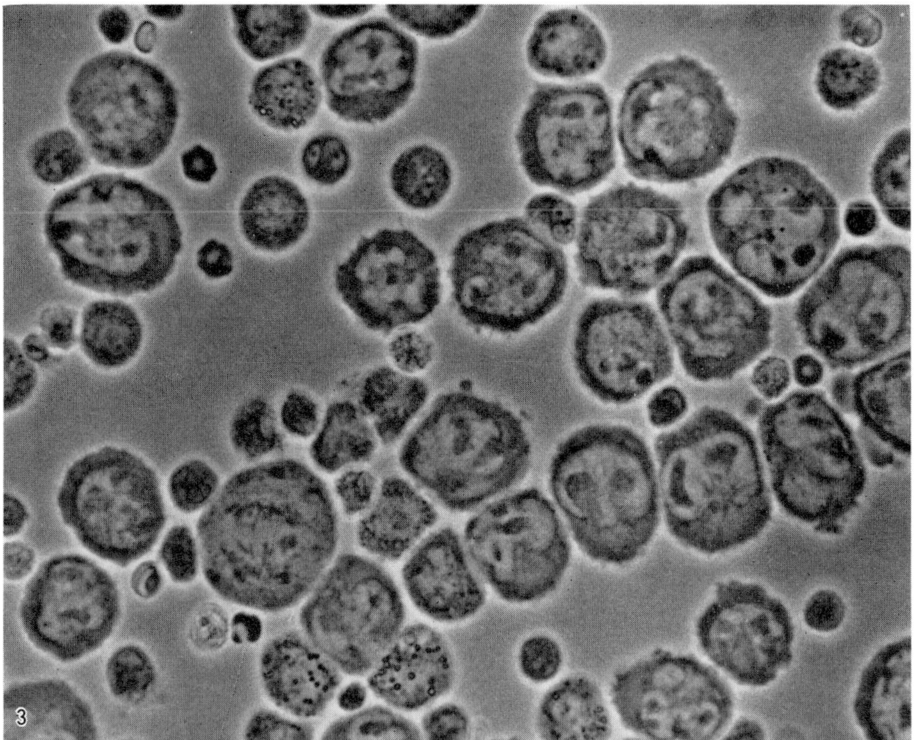
3

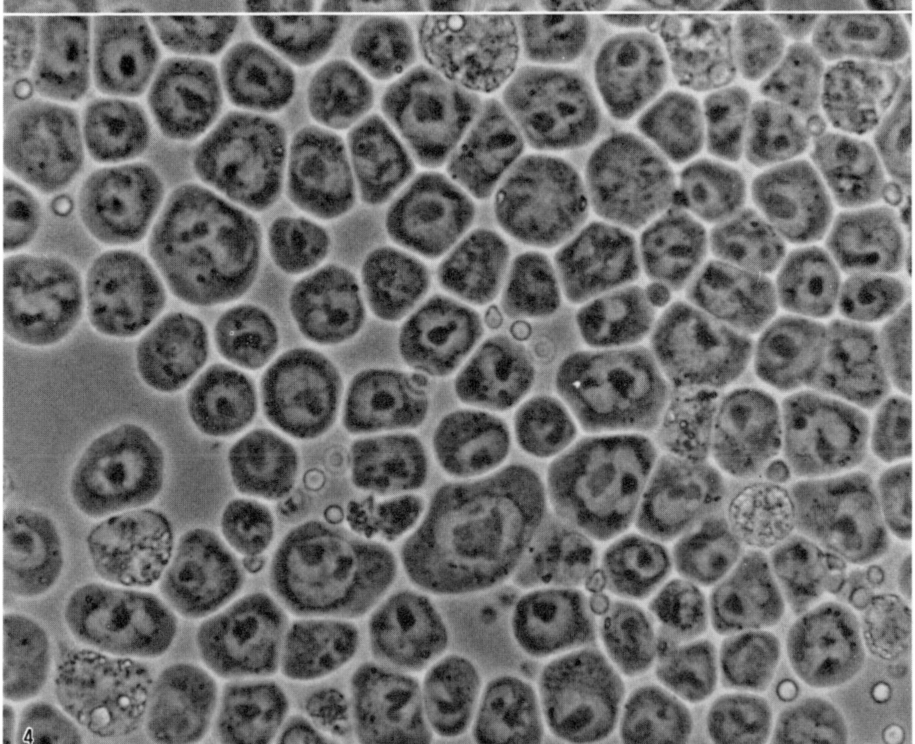
4

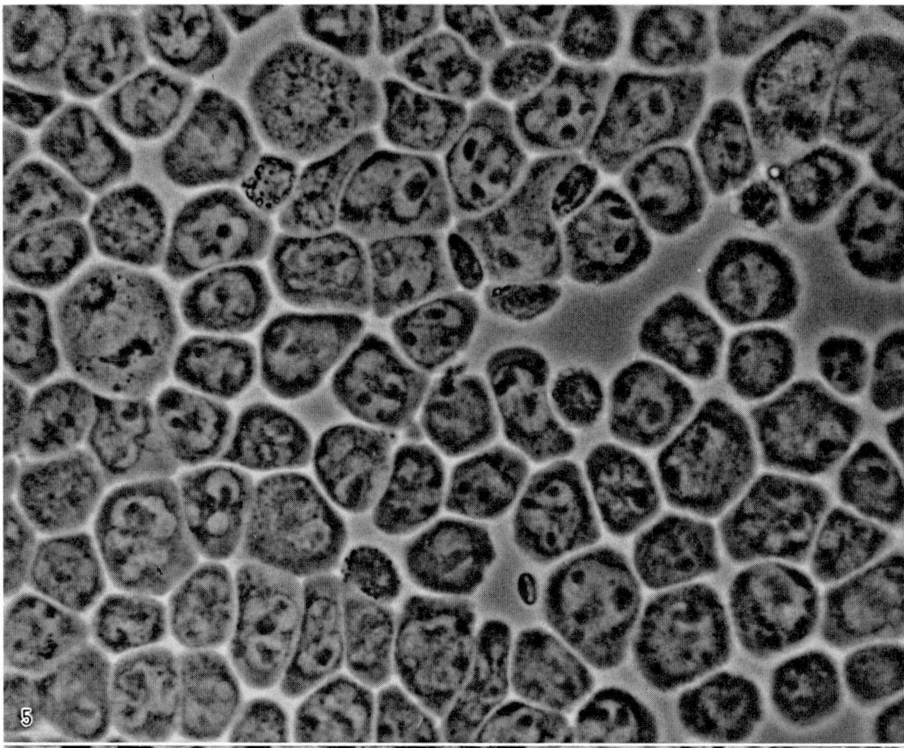
5

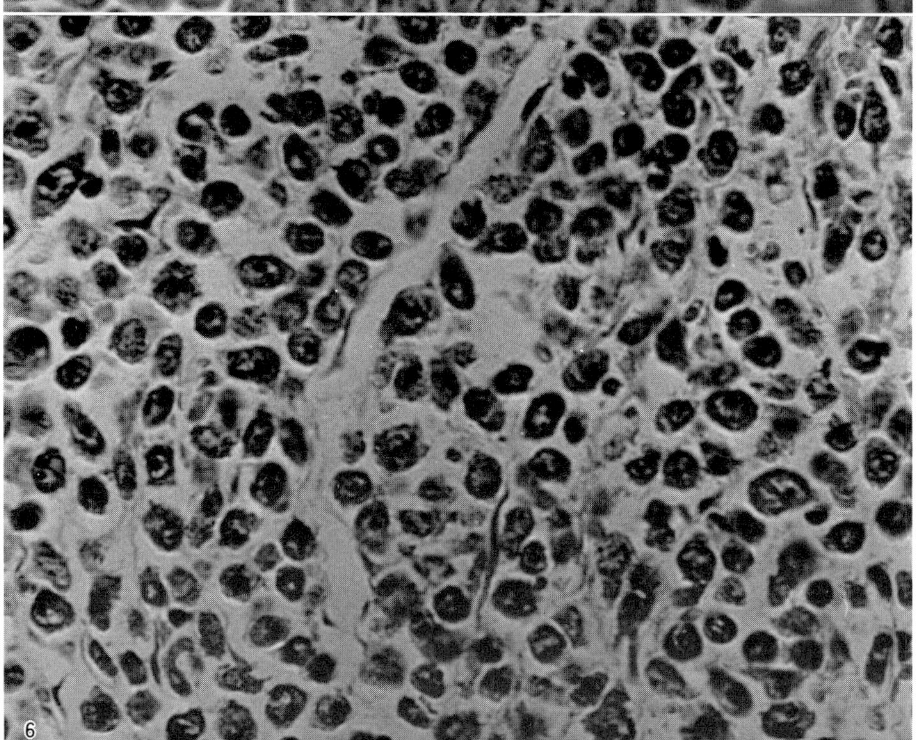
6

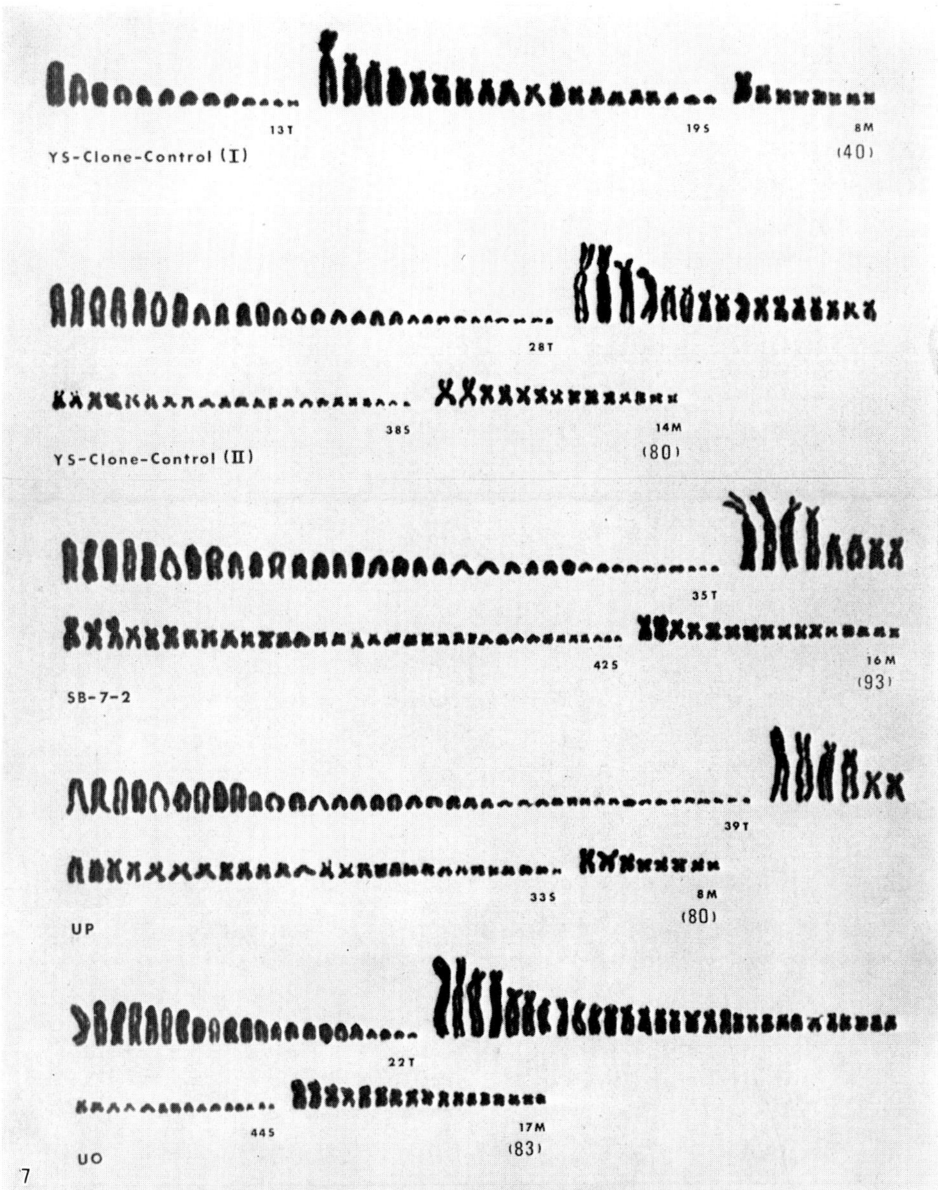
13T
19S
8M
YS-Clone-Control (I)
(40)
28T
38S
14M
YS-Clone-Control (II)
(80)
35T
42S
16M
(93)
SB-7-2
39T
33S
8M
(80)
UP
22T
44S
17M
(83)
UO

7

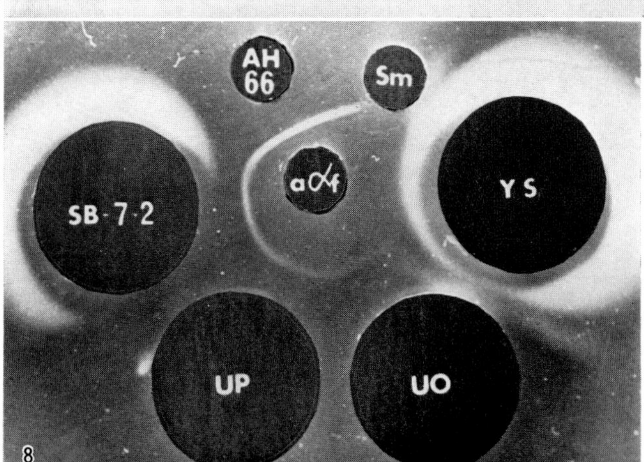
AH
66
Sm
aαf
SB-7-2
YS
UP
UO

8

GANN Monograph on Cancer Research 14, 1973

α-FETOPROTEIN DURING HEPATOCARCINOGENESIS IN DOGS TREATED WITH CHEMICAL CARCINOGENS

Yoichi SHINOMIYA,*[1] Kazuya HIRAO,*[1] Kazutaka MATSUMURA,*[1] Atsushi IMAGAWA,*[1] Yasuhisa ENOMOTO,*[1] Yasutoshi FUKAI,*[1] and Nobuyuki ITO*[2]

The 1st Department of Surgery[1] *and the 1st Department of Pathology,*[2] *Nara Medical University*

In the present work, two chemical carcinogens, N-nitrosodiethylamine and N-nitrosopiperidine, were administered to adult mongrel and beagle dogs. Various changes in α-fetoprotein (AFP) were seen in the sera of most of the mongrel dogs after various periods of carcinogen administration. However, no AFP appeared in the sera of beagle dogs on treatment with either carcinogen.

Among 25 dogs treated with N-nitrosodiethylamine for at least a year, 4 kinds of hepatic tumor were observed: 1 case of hepatocellular carcinoma, 2 of hemangioendothelioma, 1 of leiomyosarcoma, and 1 of fibroma. The present work does not show any clear relationship between the appearance of AFP in the serum and various histological changes of the liver, including hepatocellular carcinoma.

Experimental Hepatocarcinogenesis in Dogs Treated with N-Nitrosodiethylamine or N-Nitrosopiperidine

There are many reports on the carcinogenic effects of various compounds on the livers of small experimental animals (*8*, *12*, *21*, *27*, *38*, *42*). Induction of hepatic cancer in rats by N-nitrosodiethylamine or N-nitrosopiperidine has also been reported from our laboratories (*22*, *28*). For clinical research on the early diagnosis of hepatic cancer, large experimental animals must be used, so that early carcinogenic changes may be detected by clinical, histopathological, and immunological observations. Kelly *et al.* (*23*) produced hepatoma in monkeys by administration of N-nitrosodiethylamine and recently, Hull *et al.* (*20*) reported results on the analysis of α-fetoprotein (AFP) in the sera of monkeys during hepatocarcinogenesis induced by treatment with N-nitrosodiethylamine. In dogs, Rooney reported studies on various spontaneous liver tumors, showing that canine hepatic carcinoma presents both striking differences from and similarities to the comparable disease in man (*35*). Schmähl *et al.* (*39*) reported one case of a large hepatic tumor induced by treating dogs with N-nitrosodiethylamine, and found

*1,*2 840 Shijo-cho, Kashihara, Nara 634, Japan (四宮洋一, 平尾和也, 松村一隆, 今川敦史, 榎本泰久, 深井泰俊, 伊東信行).

that this was a leiomyosarcoma. However, there are no reports of hepatocellular carcinoma in dogs treated with N-nitrosodiethylamine. In the present work on hepatocarcinogenesis in dogs, we used two potent hepatocarcinogens, N-nitrosodiethylamine and N-nitrosopiperidine.

1. Pathological observations on mongrel dogs treated with carcinogens

A total of 25 male mongrel dogs, weighing 10 to 20 kg, were used. These dogs received solutions of 50 to 500 ppm of N-nitrosodiethylamine or 100 to 300 ppm of N-nitrosopiperidine continuously as drinking water for 50 to 90 weeks. In most cases carcinogen administration had to be reduced or stopped for a few weeks during the experiment because of loss of appetite or body weight, or bleeding in the alimentary canal. The effect of N-nitrosodiethylamine was examined in 7 dogs and that of N-nitrosopiperidine in 11 dogs.

Gross findings were that the livers of all dogs treated with the carcinogens had a cirrhotic or irregular surface. Multiple yellow or white nodules, 0.5 cm to 2.0 cm in diameter, were observed in all cirrhotic livers. On treatment with N-nitrosodiethylamine the liver occasionally developed small cystic nodules.

Microscopic examination showed that connective tissue usually proliferated into periportal areas of the liver of dogs treated with either carcinogen, but no fatty changes of parenchymal cells were seen (Photo 1). Occasionally, oval cell infiltration and bile duct proliferation in periportal areas were noticed (Photo 2). Hyperplastic nodules were also frequently seen, but no malignant changes were found in areas of nodular hyperplasia.

Among 7 dogs treated with N-nitrosodiethylamine for at least 1 year, there were 5 cases of hepatic tumors: 1 of hepatocellular carcinoma, 2 of hemangioendothelioma, 1 of leiomyosarcoma, and 1 of fibroma (Photos 3–6). No malignant liver tumor or benign neoplasia of the liver has yet been observed in the 11 dogs treated with N-nitrosopiperidine.

2. Observations on beagle dogs

At present 9 male beagles, weighing an average of 10 kg, have received solutions of 5 mg of N-nitrosodiethylamine or 5 or 10 mg of N-nitrosopiperidine continuously as capsules over a period of 46 weeks, and after 48 weeks the concentrations of carcinogen were doubled. All the beagles are still alive and no remarkable pathological or morphological changes have been observed.

3. Methods of immunological observation of dogs treated with carcinogens

Blood was collected by decapitation from embryos obtained by cesarian section of mongrel dogs after a gestation period of 40 to 50 days. The serum was separated and saturated ammonium sulfate solution was added to a final saturation of 50%. The mixture was allowed to stand for 24 hr at 4°, and was then centrifuged. The supernatant was dialyzed for 4 days against phosphate-buffered saline solution to remove ammonium sulfate. Rabbits were given subcutaneous injections of 0.5 ml of this crude antigen solution emulsified with an equal volume of Freund's complete adjuvant at intervals of 2 weeks for 5 injections. Blood was taken from the femoral artery after the last injection and crude antiserum was obtained. For immunospecific purification of anti-dog AFP serum, we used immunoadsorbents prepared using bromoacetylcellulose. Bromoacetylcellulose was donated by Dr. Miyagawa of the Department of Bacteriology, Nara Medical University. The present investigations were performed by a modification of the bromoacetylcellulose immunoadsorbent technique of Robbins *et al.* (*34*).

Bromoacetylcellulose was allowed to react with normal adult dog serum. The conjugate of bromoacetylcellulose with antigen was dispersed in crude antiserum and stirred for 2 hr at 4°. Then the mixture was centrifuged at 10,000 *g* for 10 min and the supernatant was separated. To elute normal antibodies from the adsorbents, the complex of antibodies and immunoadsorbent was resuspended in 0.1 M acetic acid for 1 hr at 37° and the bromoacetylcellulose-antigen conjugates were redispersed in the supernatant fluid. This procedure was repeated at least 5 times. The antibody solutions were concentrated by ultrafiltration and then dialyzed exhaustively against phosphate-buffered saline, pH 7.0. The purified antibody solutions were stored at −20°. Screening for AFP was done by the double diffusion method and by counter-immunoelectrophoresis (electrosyneresis).

Double diffusion was done by the method of Ouchterlony (*32*) (Photo 7), counter-immunoelectrophoresis (electrosyneresis) by the method of Culliford *et al.* (*7, 17*) (Photo 8), and immunoelectrophoresis as described by Scheidegger (*37*) (Photos 9 and 10). These methods were performed with 1.2% agarose gel in 0.05 M barbital buffer, pH 8.6. Purified anti-dog AFP serum gave only a single precipitation line against dog serum during hepatocarcinogenesis and this line fused completely with that of fetal dog serum, but did not react with normal adult dog serum. Anti-dog AFP serum also reacted with human fetal serum. The 2 precipitation lines fused with spur formation, indicating incomplete antigenecity. Antiserum (anti-human AFP serum) prepared against human AFP and absorbed with normal adult human serum also reacted with fetal dog serum and serum of a dog during hepatocarcinogenesis. On immunoelectrophoresis using anti-human AFP and anti-dog AFP serum, the band of fetal dog serum moved slightly more slowly than that of human serum.

Appearance of AFP in Mongrel Dogs Treated with Carcinogens

The sera of the dogs were examined at intervals of 2 weeks for the presence of AFP. On treatment with N-nitrosodiethylamine, AFP first appeared in the serum after about 20 to 30 weeks and was found in about half of the experimental dogs. Then it disappeared rapidly and reappeared after about 50 weeks. Among the dogs in which AFP temporarily disappeared, only 2 dogs had detectable serum AFP at death. In 2 dogs, no serum AFP was detectable during hepatocarcinogenesis. In 3 other dogs, serum AFP was first detectable only after about 30 to 45 weeks. In general, the appearance of AFP seemed to be related to the period of administration of carcinogen. The changes of AFP in the sera of dogs during hepatocarcinogenesis induced by N-nitrosodiethylamine are shown graphically in Fig. 1.

Serum AFP appeared more rapidly on treatment of mongrel dogs with N-

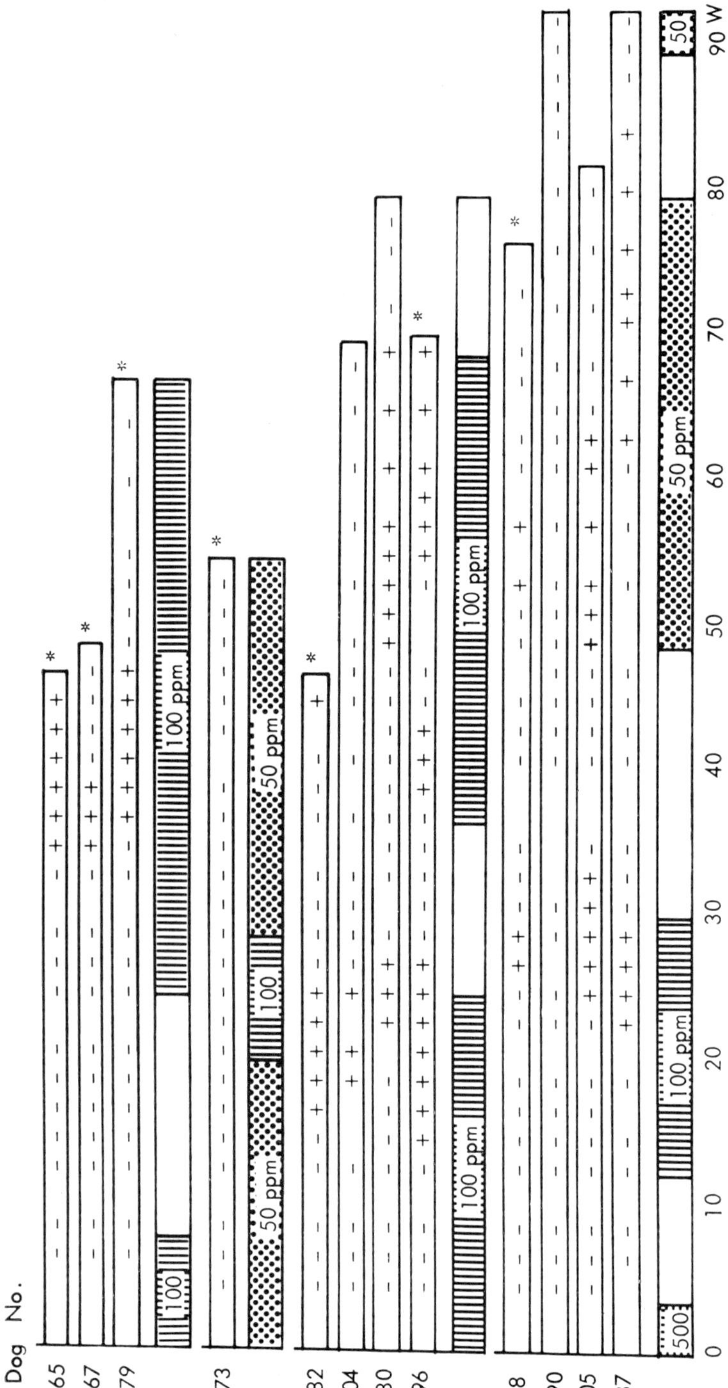

FIG. 1. Changes of AFP in dog sera during hepatocarcinogenesis induced by N-nitrosodiethylamine
▥, ▦ or ⊠ carcinogen treatment; □ without carcinogen treatment.
+, − positive or negative reaction for AFP. * sacrificed for microscopic observations.

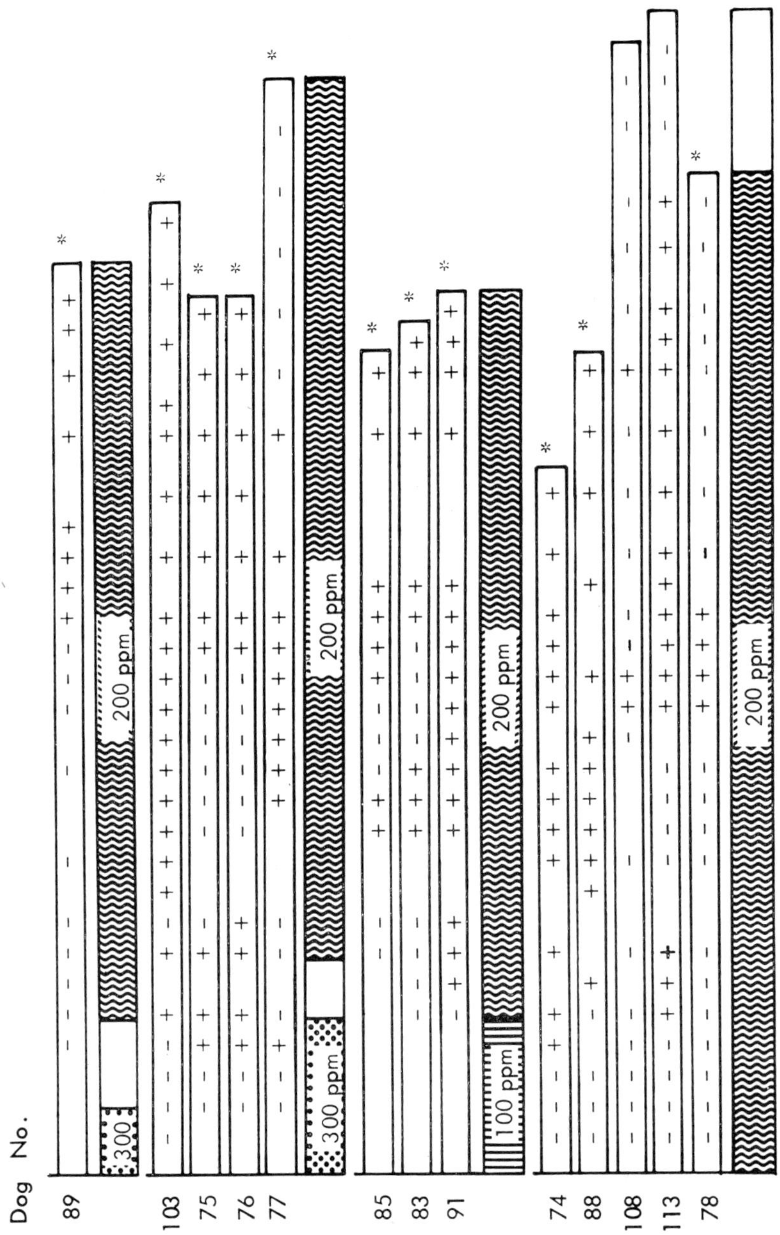

FIG. 2. Changes of AFP in dog sera during hepatocarcinogenesis induced by N-nitrosopiperidine.
⬚, ▨ or ▥ carcinogen treatment; □ without carcinogen treatment.
+, − positive or negative reaction for AFP. * sacrificed for microscopic observations.

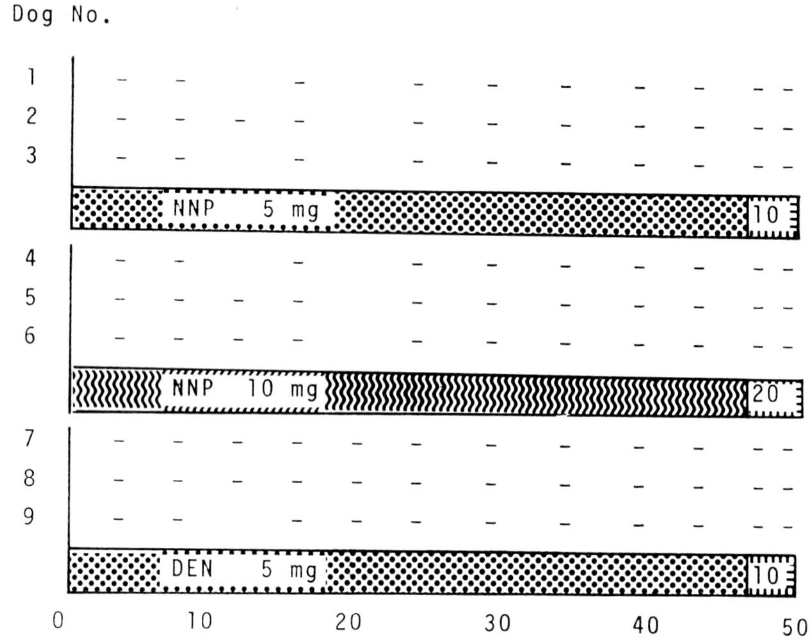

FIG. 3. Absence of AFP in beagle sera during hepatocarcinogenesis induced by N-nitrosodiethylamine (DEN) or N-nitrosopiperidine (NNP)

▦, ▩ or ▣ carcinogen treatment. — negative reaction for AFP.

nitrosopiperidine than on treatment with N-nitrosodiethylamine, and was first seen within 20 weeks. In these dogs, the patterns of change in serum AFP varied, as shown in Fig. 2. No hepatoma or benign neoplasia of the liver has yet been observed in dogs receiving N-nitrosopiperidine but the body weight of all dogs has decreased during the administration.

No AFP was found in 9 beagles on carcinogen administration for 50 weeks, as shown in Fig. 3. The beagles initially received lower concentrations of carcinogens than mongrels and, therefore, after 48 weeks the concentrations were doubled.

DISCUSSION

It has been shown that an embryo-specific AFP may be found in the sera of patients with primary carcinoma of the liver (*2, 4, 5, 29, 31, 33, 43*), and the clinical value of assay of AFP is now well documented. The AFP is specifically present in embryonal and fetal sera of different animal species including primates (*14, 44*). In early ontogenesis, AFP is the main component of the serum, but it cannot be found in normal adults (*6, 15, 25, 40*). The AFP has also been found in the sera of animals with primary or transplantable liver tumors (*1, 3, 20, 41*) and of patients suffering from hepatocellular carcinoma or embryonal carcinoma of the testis and ovary (*4, 14, 44*). The mechanism of regulation of AFP production in ontogenesis and the causes of its synthesis in hepatomas are completely obscure. Nishi *et al.* (*30, 36*) purified AFP and characterized its physicochemical properties. The cellular distributions of AFP in the livers of rat fetuses and human embryos and in human hepatomas have been investigated by the fluorescent antibody technique (*9, 10, 16, 18, 26*).

However, the biological significance of serum AFP is unknown yet and there is little information about the relationship between histological changes of the liver and the presence of AFP in the sera of experimental animals. Chemically induced hepatomas in rats have been studied by many observers and recently, the relationship between the appearance of AFP and pathological changes in the liver of rats induced by 3′-methyl-4-dimethylaminoazobenzene was investigated by Watabe and Hirai (*45*) and Kitagawa *et al.* (*24*). They suggested that the presence of AFP was related to the appearance of oval cells in the liver, induced by the carcinogen. Previously, Farber (*13*) observed that oval cell infiltration was an early histological change induced in rat liver by ethionine, 2-acetylaminofluorene or 3′-methyl-4-dimethylaminoazobenzene. In the livers of dogs treated with N-nitrosodiethylamine, Hirao *et al.*(*19*) and Enomoto *et al.* (*11*) reported that oval cell infiltration, bile duct proliferation, and development of hyperplastic nodules were the most remarkable changes detected in histological, electron microscopic, and histochemical studies. In the present work, the same histological changes were observed in dog liver.

There have been no previous reports of biopsy or histopathological studies on dog liver during hepatocarcinogenesis. In the present studies, no correlation was found between the number of nodular hyperplasia or the grade of oval cell infiltration and the presence or absence of serum AFP in dogs. At autopsy the livers of all dogs examined showed various degrees of oval cell infiltration and only 4 kinds of liver tumors were found. Clues to the relation between epithelial and mesenchymal tumors may be obtained by further experiments through studies on many more tumors in dog liver.

The relationship between histological findings in the liver and the appearance of AFP in dogs treated with carcinogen requires further study.

REFERENCES

1. Abelev, G. I. Production of embryonal serum α-globulin by hepatomas: Review of experimental and clinical data. *Cancer Res.*, **28**, 1344–1350 (1968).
2. Abelev, G. I., Assecritova, I. V., Kraevsky, N. A., Perova, S. D., and Perevodchikova, N. I. Embryonal serum α-globulin in cancer patients: Diagnostic value. *Int. J. Cancer*, **2**, 551–558 (1967).
3. Abelev, G. I., Perova, S. D., Khramkova, N. I., Postnikova, Z. A., and Irlin, I. S. Production of embryonal α-globulin by transplantable mouse hepatomas. *Transplantation*, **1**, 174–180 (1963).
4. Alpert, E., Hershberg, R., Schur, P. H., and Isselbacher, K. J. α-Fetoprotein in human hepatoma: Improved detection in serum, and quantitative studies using a new sensitive technique. *Gastroenterology*, **61**, 137–143 (1971).
5. Alpert, M. E., Uriel, J., and de Nechaud, B. α_1-Fetoglobulin in the diagnosis of human hepatoma. *New Engl. J. Med.*, **278**, 984–986 (1968).
6. Bergstrand, C. G. and Czar, B. Paper electrophoretic study of human fetal

serum proteins with demonstration of a new protein fraction. *Scand. J. Clin. Lab. Invest.*, **9**, 277–286 (1957).

7. Culliford, B. J. Precipitin reactions in forensic problems. *Nature*, **201**, 1092–1094 (1964).
8. Druckrey, H., Steinhoff, D., Preussmann, R., and Ivankovic, S. Erzeugung von Krebs durch eine einmalige Dosis von Methylnitroso-Harnstoff und verschiedenen Dialkynitrosamine an Ratten. *Z. Krebsforsch.*, **66**, 1–10 (1964).
9. Engelhardt, N. V., Shipova, L. Y., Gusev, A. I., Jazova, A. K., and Ter-grigorova, E. N. Detection of α_F-globulin in liver sections from human embryos and newborn mice by means of fluorescent antibodies. *Bull. Exp. Biol. Med. (U.S.S.R.)*, **12**, 62–64 (1969).
10. Engelhardt, N. V., Gusev, A. I., Shipova, L. J., and Abelev, G. I. Immunofluorescent study of α-fetoprotein in liver and liver tumors. I. Technique of AFP localization in the tissue sections. *Int. J. Cancer*, **7**, 198–206 (1971).
11. Enomoto, Y., Hirao, K., Matsumura, K., Imagawa, A., Hayashi, H., Fukai, Y., Kamada, T., Ohishi, H., Sugihara, S., and Ito, N. Clinical, histopathological and electron microscopic observations on dogs treated with N-nitrosodiethylamine. *Acta Hepatol. Japon.*, **13**, 7 (1972).
12. Farber, E. Carcinoma of the liver in rats fed ethionine. *A. M. A. Arch. Pathol.*, **62**, 445–453 (1956).
13. Farber, E. Similarities in the sequence of early histological changes induced in liver of the rat by ethionine, 2-acetylaminofluorene, and 3′-methyl-4-dimethylaminoazobenzene. *Cancer Res.*, **16**, 142–148 (1956).
14. Gitlin, D. and Boesman, M. Fetus-specific serum proteins in several mammals and their relation to human α-fetoprotein. *Comp. Biochem. Physiol.*, **21**, 327–336 (1967).
15. Gitlin, D. and Boesman, M. Sites of serum α-fetoprotein synthesis in the human and in the rat. *J. Clin. Invest.*, **46**, 1010–1016 (1967).
16. Gitlin, D., Kitzes, J., and Boesman, M. Cellular distribution of serum α-fetoprotein in organs of the fetal rat. *Nature*, **215**, 534 (1967).
17. Gocke, D. J. and Howe, C. Rapid detection of Australia antigen by counterimmunoelectrophoresis. *J. Immunol.*, **104**, 1031–1032 (1970).
18. Gusev, A. I., Engelhardt, N. V., Masseyeff, R., Camain, R., and Basteris, B. Immunofluorescent study of α-fetoprotein in liver and liver tumors. II. Localization of AFP in the tissue of patients with primary liver cancer (PLC). *Int. J. Cancer*, **7**, 207–217 (1971).
19. Hirao, K., Matsumura, K., Imagawa, A., Oya, H., Hayashi, Y., Enomoto, Y., Fukai, Y., Hiasa, Y., and Ito, N. Early changes of liver in dogs induced by diethylnitrosamine. *Proc. Jap. Cancer Assoc., 29th Annu. Meet.*, 69 (1970).
20. Hull, E. W., Carbone, P., Gitlin, D., O'Gara, R. W., and Kelly, M. G. α-Fetoprotein in monkeys with hepatoma. *J. Natl. Cancer Inst.*, **42**, 1035–1044 (1969).
21. Ito, N., Fukuoka, Y., Marugami, M., Nakamura, H., and Kitamura, H. Relationship between Congo Red index and quantitative histology in the rat liver during azo-dye carcinogenesis. *GANN*, **52**, 155–164 (1961).
22. Ito, N., Kamamoto, Y., Hiasa, Y., Makiura, S., Marugami, M., Yokota, Y., Sugihara, S., and Hirao, K. Histopathological and ultrastructural studies on esophageal tumors in rats treated with N-nitrosopiperidine. *GANN*, **62**, 445–451 (1971).
23. Kelly, M. G., O'Gara, R. W., Adamson, R. H., Gadekar, K., Botkin, C. C., Reese,

W. H., Jr., and Kerber, W. T. Induction of hepatic cell carcinomas in monkeys with N-nitrosodiethylamine. *J. Natl. Cancer Inst.*, **36**, 323–351 (1966).
24. Kitagawa, T., Yokochi, T., and Sugano, H. 3′-Me-DAB and 2-FAA hepatocarcinogenesis and serum α-fetoprotein in rat. *Proc. Jap. Cancer Assoc., 30th Annu. Meet.*, 5 (1971).
25. Kithier, K. and Prokěs, J. Fetal α_1-globulin of rat serum. *Biochim. Biophys. Acta*, **127**, 390–399 (1966).
26. Linder, E. and Seppälä, M. Localization of α-fetoprotein in the human fetus and placenta. *Acta Pathol. Microbiol. Scand.*, **73**, 565–571 (1968).
27. Magee, P. N. and Barnes, J. M. Carcinogenic nitroso compounds. *Adv. Cancer Res.*, **10**, 163–246 (1967).
28. Makiura, S., Hiasa, Y., Kamamoto, Y., Marugami, M., Konishi, Y., Ito, N., and Kitamura, H. Effects of α-naphthylisothiocyanate and 3-methylcholanthrene on hepatocarcinogenesis in rats treated with N-nitrosodiethylamine. *Proc. Jap. Cancer Assoc., 29th Annu. Meet.*, 57 (1970).
29. Masopust, J., Kithier, K., Rádl, J., Koutecky, J., and Kotál, L. Occurrence of fetoprotein in patients with neoplasms and non-neoplastic disease. *Int. J. Cancer*, **3**, 364–373 (1968).
30. Nishi, S. Isolation and characterization of a human fetal α-globulin from the sera of fetuses and a hepatoma patient. *Cancer Res.*, **30**, 2507–2513 (1970).
31. O'Conor, G. T., Tatarinov, Y. S., Abelev, G. I., and Uriel, J. A collaborative study for the evaluation of a serologic test for primary liver cancer. *Cancer*, **25**, 1091–1098 (1970).
32. Ouchterlony, O. Antigen-antibody reaction in gels. *Acta Pathol. Microbiol. Scand.*, **26**, 507–515 (1949).
33. Purves, L. R., Bersohn, I., and Geddes, E. W. Serum α-fetoprotein and primary cancer of the liver in man. *Cancer*, **25**, 1261–1270 (1970).
34. Robbins, J. B., Haimovich, J., and Sela, M. Purification of antibodies with immunoadsorbents prepared using bromoacetylcellulose. *Immunochemistry*, **4**, 11–22 (1967).
35. Rooney, J. R. Liver carcinoma in the dog. *Acta Pathol.*, **45**, 321–330 (1959).
36. Ruoslahti, E. and Seppälä, M. Studies of carcino-fetal proteins: Physical and chemical properties of human α-fetoprotein. *Int. J. Cancer*, **7**, 218–225 (1971).
37. Scheidegger, J. J. Une micro-méthode de l'immunoélectrophorèse. *Int. Arch. Allerg.*, **7**, 103–110 (1955).
38. Schmähl, D. and Thomas, C. Über die Wirkung von Epiphysenextrakt auf die Epithelkörperchen der Ratte. *Naturwissenschaften*, **52**, 164 (1965).
39. Schmähl, D., Thomas, C., and Scheld, G. Cancergene Wirkung von Diäthylnitrosamine beim Hunb. *Naturwissenschaften*, **51**, 466–467 (1964).
40. Stanislawski-birencwajg, M. Specific antigens of rat embryonic serum. *Cancer Res.*, **27**, 1982–1989 (1967).
41. Stanislawski-birencwajg, M., Uriel, J., and Grabar, P. Association of embryonic antigens with experimentally induced hepatic lesions in the rat. *Cancer Res.*, **27**, 1990–1997 (1967).
42. Takayama, S. and Oota, K. Malignant tumors induced in mice fed with N-nitrosodiethylamine. *GANN*, **54**, 465–472 (1963).
43. Tatarinov, Y. S. Content of embryo-specific α-globulin in fetal and neonatal sera and sera from adult humans with primary carcinoma of the liver. *Vopr. Med. Khim.*, **11**, 20–24 (1965). (*Fed. Proc.*, **25**, 344–346 (1966)).
44. Tatarinov, Y. S. and Afanas'eva, A. V. The development of similar antigenic

determinants in embryo-specific α-globulins of man and certain animals. *Bull. Exp. Biol. Med.* (*U.S.S.R.*), **59**, 65–69 (1965).

45. Watabe, H. and Hirai, H. Early appearance of α-fetoprotein in rat serum during chemical carcinogenesis. *Proc. Jap. Cancer Assoc., 30th Annu. Meet.*, 5 (1971).

EXPLANATION OF PHOTOS

PHOTO 1. Cirrhotic changes in the liver of a dog treated with N-nitrosodiethylamine. H-E: Hematoxylin and Eosin stain. ×84.

PHOTO 2. Marked oval cell infiltration in the periportal area of the liver after N-nitrosodiethylamine treatment. H-E. ×168.

PHOTO 3. Undifferentiated hepatocellular carcinoma in the liver (dog No. 96) induced by N-nitrosodiethylamine. Diffuse growth of tumor cells among hepatic parenchymal cells is seen. H-E. ×84.

PHOTO 4. Hemangioendothelioma in the liver (dog No. 73) induced by N-nitrosodiethylamine. H-E. ×84.

PHOTO 5. Leiomyosarcoma in the liver (dog No. 98) induced by N-nitrosodiethylamine. H-E. ×84.

PHOTO 6. Fibroma in the liver (dog No. 79) induced by N-nitrosodiethylamine. Marked hyalinization is seen in the tumor area. H-E. ×84.

PHOTO 7. Double immunodiffusion pattern of dog fetal (D) and human fetal (H) sera against anti-dog AFP (AD*α*f) and anti-human AFP (AH*α*f) serum.

PHOTO 8. Counter-immunoelectrophoretic pattern of human fetal serum (H), dog fetal serum (D), serum from a dog during hepatocarcinogenesis (DC), and normal and adult dog serum (N) against anti-dog AFP serum (AD*α*f).

PHOTOS 9 and 10. Immunoelectrophoretic pattern of dog fetal (D) and human fetal (H) sera against anti-dog AFP and anti-human AFP serum.

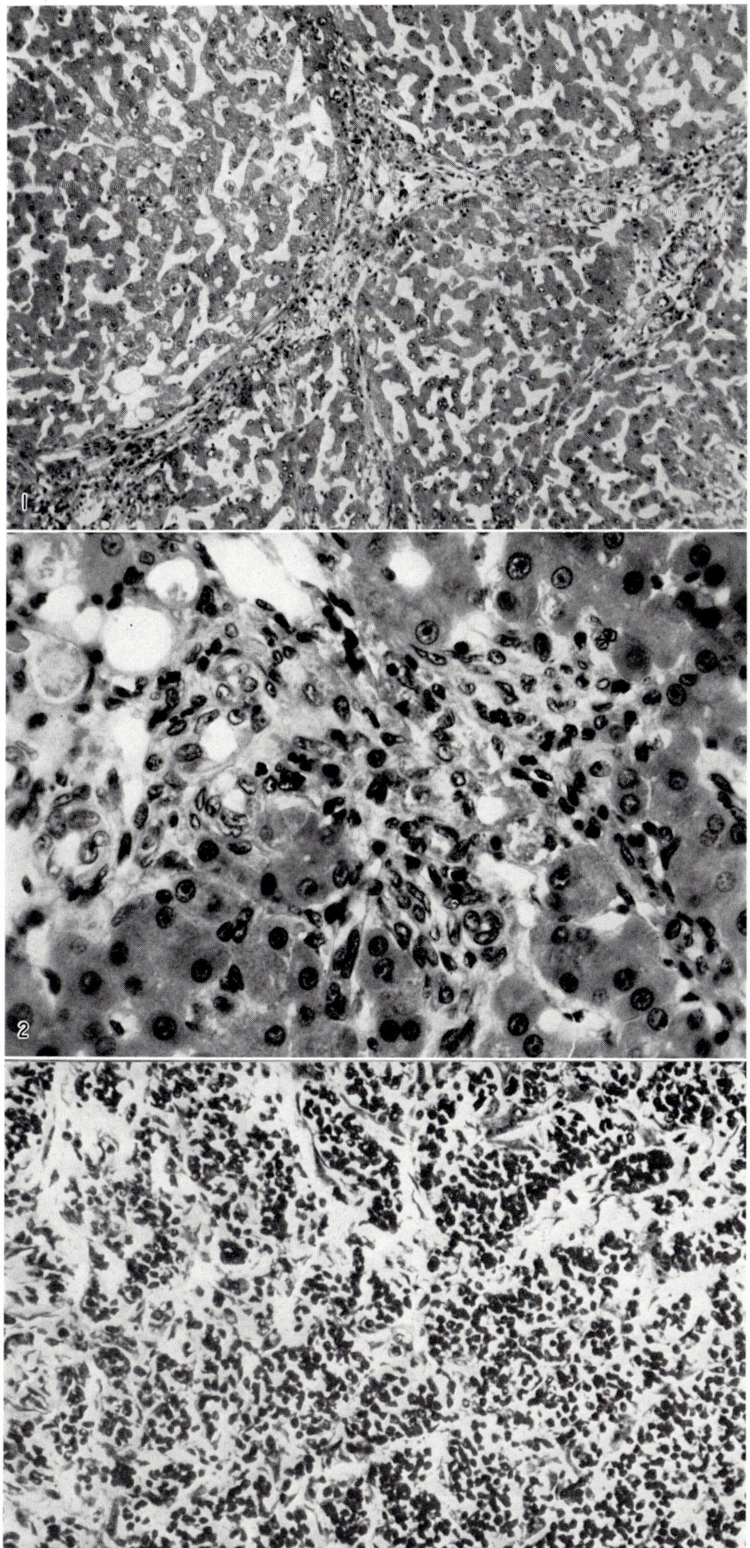
1
2
3

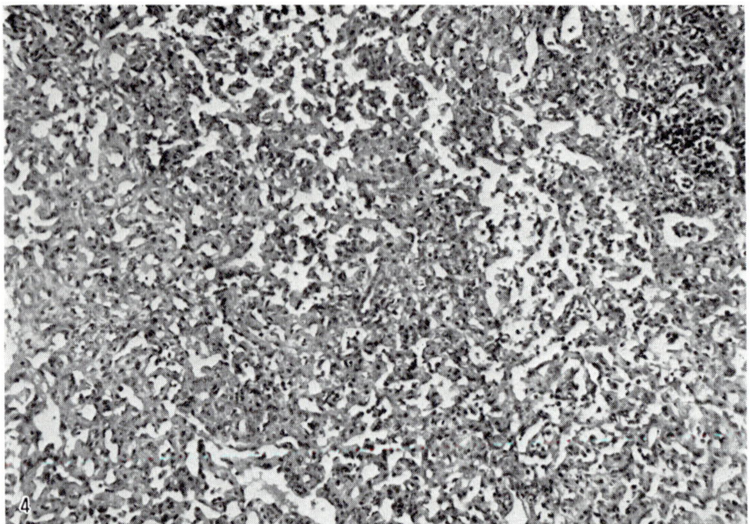
4

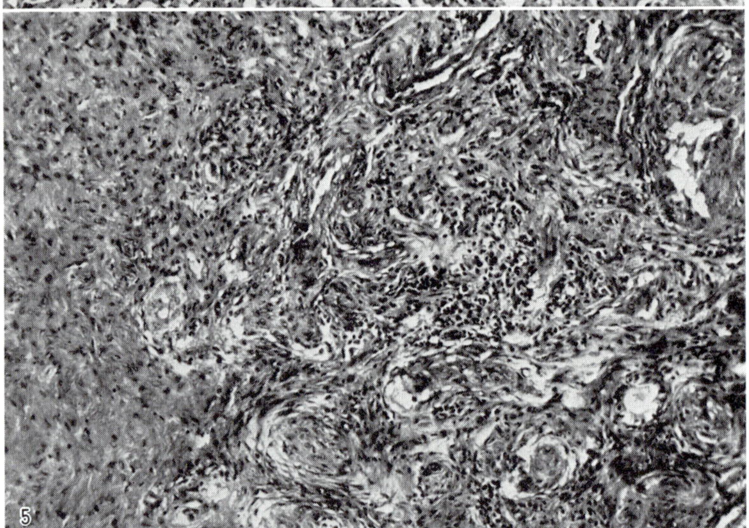
5

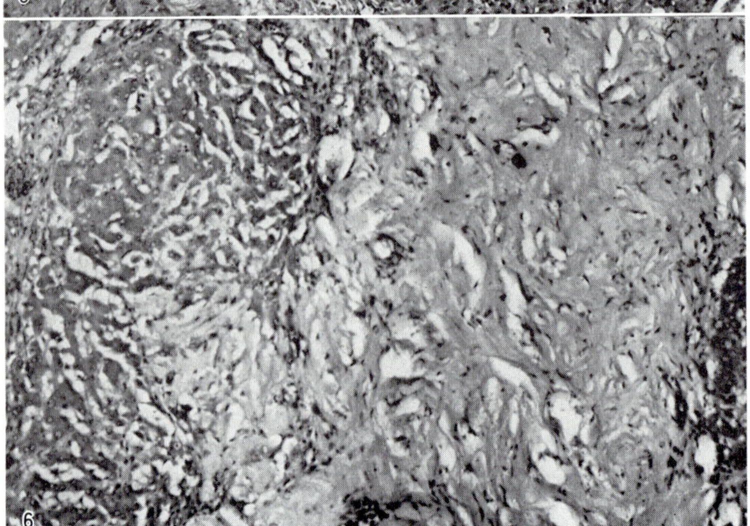
6

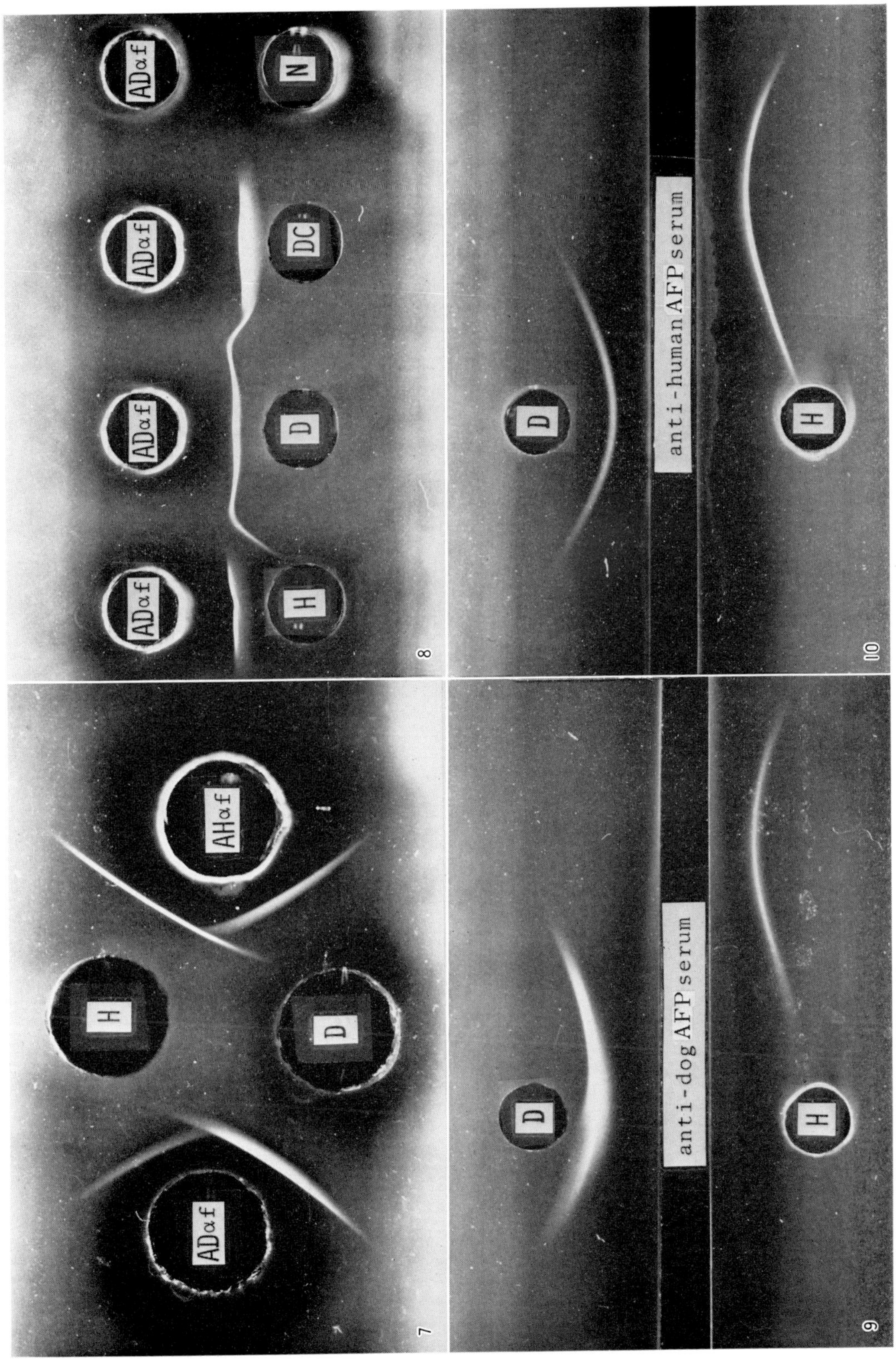
7
ADαf
H
D
AHαf
8
ADαf
ADαf
ADαf
ADαf
H
D
DC
N
9
D
anti-dog AFP serum
H
10
D
anti-human AFP serum
H

INDEX

A

B

C

D

I

J

K

L

M

N

O